W9-ASR-469

OXFORD MEDICAL PUBLICATIONS

Doppler Ultrasound in Perinatal Medicine

Doppler Ultrasound in Perinatal Medicine

Edited by

J. MALCOLM PEARCE

Senior Lecturer,
Department of Obstetrics and Gynaecology,
St George's Hospital, London

OXFORD   NEW YORK   TOKYO
OXFORD UNIVERSITY PRESS
1992

Oxford University Press, Walton Street, Oxford OX2 6DP
Oxford   New York   Toronto
Delhi   Bombay   Calcutta   Madras   Karachi
Petaling Jaya   Singapore   Hong Kong   Tokyo
Nairobi   Dar es Salaam   Cape Town
Melbourne   Auckland
and associated companies in
Berlin   Ibadan

Oxford is a trade mark of Oxford University Press

Published in the United States
by Oxford University Press, New York

A catalogue record for this book is available from the British Library

Library of Congress Cataloging in Publication Data
Doppler ultrasound in perinatal medicine / edited by J. Malcolm
Pearce.
(Oxford medical publications)
Includes index.
1. Ultrasonics in obstetrics.   2. Doppler ultrasonography.
I. Pearce, J. Malcolm (John Malcolm)   II. Series.
[DNLM: 1. Pregnancy Complications–ultrasonography.
2. Ultrasonography, Prenatal.   WQ 210 D692]
RG628.3.U58D67   1992   618.3'207543–dc20   91–39325
ISBN 0–19–262019–3 (h/b)

Typeset by Footnote Graphics, Warminster, Wiltshire
Printed in Hong Kong

To my wife, Marie

Preface

It is fitting that the first textbook on Doppler ultrasound in perinatal medicine should be published exactly 150 years after Doppler's original paper (Doppler, J. C. (1842)).* Just as Doppler-shifted frequencies rise as the source and the observer approach each other so the interest in perinatal medicine has risen as ultrasound technologies have allowed non-invasive access to pregnancies.

The authors in this book come from several disciplines but share a common love of screening for, and managing high-risk pregnancies. The links with medical physicists not only helped obstetricians to understand the tremendous potential of Doppler ultrasound but also began the process of scientific thinking within the art of obstetrics. This has led to serious attempts at proper evaluation of the technique rather than its introduction based upon the feeling that any technology is better than clinical methods. Understanding statistics is difficult for clinicians but I was surprised to learn that statisticians have to work hard to understand it as well. Having struggled, however, explaining it to others often becomes easy. This explains why the chapter in this book is a model of clarity and will allow clinicians the understanding to evaluate the statistics of Doppler studies and to plan future studies properly!

The remaining chapters are excellent reviews of the literature interpreted in the light of the experience of the authors, many of whom are pioneers in this field. I am grateful to them for allowing me to attempt to amalgamate them in a cohesive fashion. The management of fetal cardiac dysrhythmias stands out as having little association with Doppler ultrasound but is included as it complements the role of Doppler ultrasound in high-risk pregnancies.

It is not difficult to envisage a future that includes the ability to map both fetal and maternal blood vessels in detail. I hope those who read this book become as caught up in perinatal medicine as those who contributed to it.

London   J. M. P.
April 1992

* Über das farbige licht der Doppelsterne und einger ander hestirne des Himmels. Abhandlungen d. Königl. Böhmischen Gesellschaft der Wissenschaften V. Folge 102.

Contents

Contributors

Dr S. Lee Adamson Associate Professor, University of Toronto.

Dr Widad Al-Ghazali Research Fellow, Departments of Obstetrics and Gynaecology and Perinatal Cardiology, Guy's Hospital, London.

Lindsey Allan Professor of Fetal Cardiology, Guy's Hospital, London.

Dr Douglas G. Altman Head of the Medical Statistics Laboratory, Imperial Cancer Research Fund, Lincoln's Inn Fields, London.

Dr R. Bryan Beattie Clinical Lecturer, University of Birmingham, Birmingham Maternity Hospital.

Dr Susan Bewley Research Registrar, King's College Hospital, London.

Dr Martin Bland Senior Lecturer in Medical Statistics, Department of Public Health Sciences, St George's Hospital Medical School, London.

Dr Sarah Bowers Research Registrar, King's College Hospital, London.

Dr James C. Dornan Senior Lecturer/Consultant, Department of Obstetrics and Gynaecology, The Queen's University of Belfast and Royal Maternity Hospital, Belfast.

David H. Evans Professor of Medical Physics, University of Leicester.

William Dunlop Professor and Head of the Department of Obstetrics and Gynaecology, University of Newcastle upon Tyne.

Dr Alan Fenton Research Fellow, University Department of Paediatrics, Leicester Royal Infirmary.

Mr Gerald A. Hackett Senior Registrar, Department of Obstetrics and Gynaecology, Addenbrooke's Hospital, Cambridge.

Dr Frank D. Johnstone Department of Obstetrics and Gynaecology, Edinburgh University, Edinburgh.

Dr Petros Kaminopetros Research Fellow, Harris Birthright Research Centre for Fetal Medicine, Department of Obstetrics and Gynaecology, King's College School of Medicine and Dentistry, London.

Malcolm Levene Professor of Paediatrics and Child Health, The General Infirmary, Leeds.

Dr Peter McParland Assistant Manager, National Maternity Hospital, Holles Street, Dublin 2, Ireland.

Karel Marsal Professor, University of Lund, Department of Obstetrics and Gynaecology, Malmo General Hospital, Malmo, Sweden.

Mr Darryl J. Maxwell Director, Fetal Medicine Unit, Consultant Obstetrician and Gynaecologist, Guy's Hospital, London.

Robert J. Morrow Assistant Professor of Obstetrics and Gynaecology, University of Toronto and Mount Sinai Hospital, Toronto, Ontario, Canada.

Dr Alfred Ng Fellow in Maternal-Fetal Medicine, Westmead Hospital, Australia.

Mr Kypros Nicolaides Director, Harris Birthright Research Centre for Fetal Medicine, Department of Obstetrics and Gynaecology, King's College School of Medicine and Dentistry, London

Mr J. Malcolm Pearce Senior Lecturer, The Fetal Welfare Laboratory, Department of Obstetrics and Gynaecology, St George's Hospital, London. UK.

J. W. Knox Ritchie Professor of Obstetrics and Gynaecology, University of Toronto; Obstetrician and Gynaecologist-in-Chief, Mount Sinai Hospital, Toronto, Ontario, Canada.

Mr Stephen C. Robson Training Fellow in Fetal Medicine, Department of Obstetrics and Gynaecology, University College and Middlesex School of Medicine, London. UK.

Dr Judith M. Steel Associate Specialist, Department of Diabetes, Royal Infirmary, Edinburgh.

Dr Patricia A. Stewart Department of Obstetrics and Gynaecology, Division of Prenatal Diagnosis, Academic Hospital Dijkzigt Rotterdam, Dr Molewaterplein 40, 3015 GD Rotterdam, The Netherlands.

Brian Trudinger Associate Professor of Obstetrics and Gynaecology, The University of Sydney at Westmead Hospital, Australia.

Mr Simon N. Tyrrell Consultant in Obstetrics and Gynaecology, Hull Maternity Hospital.

Juriy W. Wladimiroff Professor of Obstetrics and Gynaecology, Division of Prenatal Diagnosis, Academic Hospital Dijkzigt Rotterdam, Dr Molewaterplein 40, 3015 GD Rotterdam, The Netherlands.

Mr Sanjay Vyas Registrar, Department of Obstetrics and Gynaecology, King's College Hospital, London

I BASIC CONSIDERATIONS

1. The physics of Doppler ultrasound

David Evans

INTRODUCTION

The Doppler principle, stated in its simplest form, is that the frequency of oscillation an observer measures is affected by relative movement between the observer and the source of the oscillation. If the source and the observer are moving towards each other then the observer crosses more wavefronts every second than the source is emitting, and therefore measures a higher frequency (see Observer 1, Fig. 1.1). If, however, the source and the observer are moving away from each other, the measured frequency falls (see Observer 2, Fig. 1.1). This principle is widely used to measure velocities in astronomy, in radar systems and within the human body.

Doppler ultrasound in medical use is a slight modification in that the source and the receiver of the ultrasound (the transducer) are stationary and the ultrasound is bounced off moving structures. Such structures may be solid objects such as heart walls or valves but by far the most important use of Doppler ultrasound is for detecting, measuring or imaging moving blood.

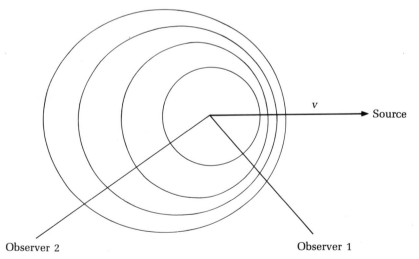

Fig. 1.1 An illustration of the Doppler principle. See text for explanation.

THE DOPPLER PRINCIPLE

When a single transducer is used both to transmit and receive ultrasound (Fig. 1.2) it may be shown that the Doppler-shifted frequency is given by

$$f_d = f_t - f_r$$
$$= 2.v.f_t.\cos \theta /c$$

where f_d is the Doppler-shifted frequency; f_t is the transmitted frequency; f_r is the received frequency; v is the velocity of the target; θ is the angle between the ultrasound beam and the direction of the velocity vector; and c is the velocity of ultrasound in blood.

This equation is completely valid only under unattainable ideal conditions, but for practical purposes holds for most obstetric applications. The most important aspect of this equation is that the Doppler-shifted frequency (f_d) is directly proportional to the velocity (v) of the target but is affected by the angle of the ultrasound beam to the blood vessel. It follows that the maximum Doppler-shifted frequency will occur at angles of 0° (maximum positive Doppler-shifted frequency) and at 180° (maximum negative Doppler-shifted frequency). At an angle of 90° no Doppler-shifted frequencies will be recorded as cosine 90° is zero. Doppler-shifted frequencies obtained from moving blood in the uteroplacental and fetal circulations fortunately lie in the audible range (up to 12 KHz) and can therefore be monitored by loudspeakers and stored on magnetic audio-tape.

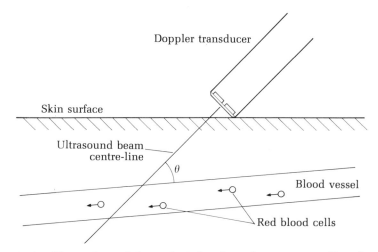

Fig. 1.2 An illustration of the principle of continuous wave Doppler ultrasound equipment. The single transducer contains separate transmitting and receiving crystals that measure the velocity of moving blood.

The Doppler spectrum

It is probable that single red blood cells do not produce Doppler-shifted signals as their diameter is only a fraction of the wavelength of the ultrasound beam. Scattering of the ultrasound beam therefore probably occurs from random changes in density of groups of red blood cells in the plasma. The Doppler equation applies only to a single target so that interrogation of a vessel at a single moment in time produces many Doppler-shifted frequencies, known as the Doppler spectrum.

There are a number of ways of processing such complex signals, but the most useful is to separate the Doppler-shifted signal into its individual frequency components which, by reference to the Doppler equation, may then be related to individual velocities. This is most commonly achieved by performing a Fourier transform on samples of the Doppler-shifted signal to produce a series of Doppler spectra (Fig. 1.3). Since the Doppler-shifted frequency is proportional to velocity, and the power in any frequency band is proportional to the number of targets moving with velocities that correspond to that frequency band, in ideal circumstances the shape of the Doppler power spectrum will be the same as a velocity distribution histogram for the targets within the ultrasound beam. From this it follows that a considerable amount of information about blood flow can be extracted from the power spectrum.

The maximum velocity can be found by substituting the maximum Doppler-shifted frequency into the Doppler equation. At any one moment in time the mean velocity (instantaneous mean velocity) may be found by calculating the intensity-weighted mean Doppler-shifted frequency (IWMF) and substituting it into the Doppler equation.

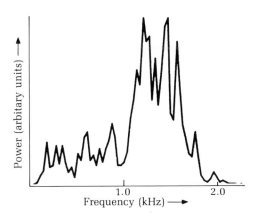

Fig. 1.3 Power spectrum of a 12.5-ms segment of the Doppler signal taken from a human carotid artery at peak systole.

The IWMF is usually calculated by the software on Doppler equipment and involves consideration of the grey scale of the Doppler sonogram. At any one moment in time the grey scale represents the number of targets that are producing a particular Doppler-shifted frequency; the nearer to white the signal the greater the number of targets (see also Fig. 1.6). Finally, the shape of the Doppler spectrum may be used to infer the type of flow in the vessel. For example, a relatively flat spectrum (Fig. 1.4(a)) implies that the instantaneous velocity profile in the blood vessel is parabolic whilst a spectrum with most of the power close to maximum frequency suggests plug flow (Fig. 1.4(b)).

Flow velocity profiles   The distribution of velocities of a fluid flowing in a long, smooth-sided, non-branching tube is radially symmetrical about the centre of that tube and is known as laminar blood flow. Close to the heart and at the time of maximum ventricular contraction (peak systole) blood flow in the aorta demonstrates a plug flow velocity profile (Fig. 1.5). As the

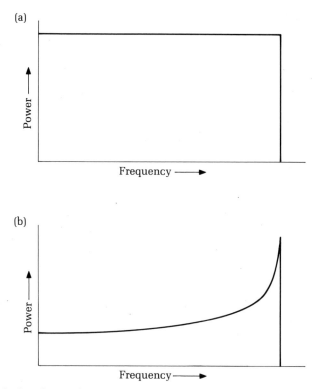

Fig. 1.4 Idealized Doppler power spectra resulting from (a) a parabolic velocity profile and (b) a plug velocity profile.

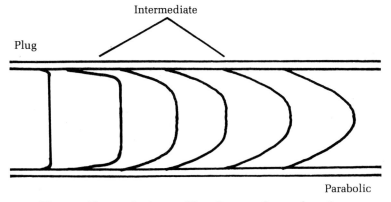

Fig. 1.5 Flow velocity profiles. See text for explanation.

force of the ventricular contraction reduces, the blood vessel walls slow the blood in contact with them by friction and hence the flow velocity profile gradually becomes parabolic.

Arterial blood flow is also pulsatile and examination of the spectral characteristics of the Doppler-shifted signal at a single instant in time gives little information. It is therefore necessary to calculate new spectra at frequent intervals, usually 80–200 times a second. This makes it impossible to examine each spectrum in detail so the data have to be presented in a different form to allow interpretation. The most usual method of displaying the spectral data is in the form of a sonogram (Fig. 1.6).

The Doppler sonogram
In this type of data display the Doppler-shifted frequency is plotted along the vertical axis and time is plotted along the horizontal axis (Fig. 1.6). The

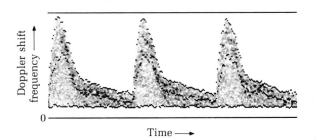

Fig. 1.6 Sonogram from the fetal aorta. The grey-scale level of each pixel relates to the number of targets giving rise to the particular Doppler-shifted frequency envelope. The maximum envelope and the intensity-weighted mean envelope are picked out by the upper and lower dotted lines respectively.

power of the Doppler-shifted signal at a given time is represented by the grey scale at a position corresponding to that frequency band and time. The Doppler information may be further summarized, for example by extracting either the maximum frequency envelope or the IWMF envelope (Fig. 1.6) from the full spectral information. This has merit when calculations are to be performed on the Doppler information but it is imperative that before this is done the operator observes the sonogram to ensure that the signal is of high quality and is not influenced by spurious factors such as inappropriate filtering or signals from other vessels.

DOPPLER ULTRASOUND EQUIPMENT

Doppler equipment ranges in complexity and cost from simple continuous wave (CW) devices up to real-time, colour flow imaging systems which are capable of portraying complex flow patterns. All, however, are based on detecting changes in frequency that occur when an ultrasound beam strikes a moving target.

Continuous wave equipment

Continuous wave equipment continually transmits a beam of ultrasound into the tissue and, at the same time, continuously detects the echoes. In general such devices use separate crystal for transmitting and receiving. The disadvantage of CW equipment is that because transmission is continuous the devices have little or no range resolution, being sensitive to any movement within the ultrasound beam. The lack of range sensitivity is balanced in obstetric practice by the following advantages of CW systems:

1. It is easier to find signals from small vessels with CW because of the inability of the pulsed equipment to image small vessels. Although this may be overcome by using colour flow Doppler combined with pulsed wave the latter is much more expensive.

2. Power levels from CW equipment are much lower than those from both pulsed Doppler and colour flow Doppler systems.

Whilst simple CW devices are acceptable in much of obstetric practice it is vital that they should be truly directional in that they should be able to process forward and reverse flow signals simultaneously; this is best achieved by a spectrum analyser. Continuous wave devices may also be used in conjunction with real-time imaging systems to allow easier location of the area of interest. Such Doppler transducers may be an integral part of the imaging transducer or may be attached to one end. Whatever the case, the path of the Doppler ultrasound beam in the tissue is indicated by a bright line superimposed on the real-time image. The operator can then manipulate the entire probe or simply the direction of the Doppler beam to interrogate the area of interest.

Pulsed wave equipment

These systems have the advantage over CW in that the operator may not only choose the direction of the Doppler beam but may also determine the depth from which the signals are gathered. Pulsed wave (PW) devices emit short pulses of ultrasound several thousand times a second, switching to receive mode between uses. By allowing the receiver to gather signals only from a particular time-window, the operator is able to control the depth from which the signals are gathered; the length of the sample volume is thus either a single vessel or, in the case of larger vessels, a particular region within the vessel.

The disadvantages of a PW system are as follows

1. They cannot be used without a coexistent real-time image system (duplex system) or colour flow Doppler system to guide placement of the sample volume.

2. They suffer from velocity limitations. The maximum frequency shift that can be detected by a PW system is limited by the Nyquist theory. This states that the maximum Doppler-shifted frequency that can be detected is one-half of the pulse repetition frequency. Because the resulting waveform is reconstructed from a series of samples of the original waveform if the samples do not occur often enough, then the phenomenon known as aliasing occurs (Figs 1.7 and 1.8).

3. They have range limitations. This occurs because it is necessary to wait for the returning echo from the most distant target before a further pulse of ultrasound is transmitted.

Major fetal vessels are generally located at a distance of up to 15 cm from the surface of the maternal abdomen, and peak systolic velocities from the descending fetal aorta may approach 1.5 m/s. With insonating angles of 45–55°, and using transmitting frequencies of 2–3 MHz, a pulse repetition frequency (PRF) of 5–7.5 kHz is required. For pulse repetition frequencies of up to 2.5 kHz it is technically possible to interlace the Doppler and real-time ultrasound equipment such that a simultaneous real-time image may be displayed. At higher PRF values the real-time image has to be frozen, but is usually updated about once a second.

Real-time colour flow imaging systems

These are the most sophisticated and expensive Doppler devices available. They overlay a colour-coded map of the Doppler-shifted frequencies on

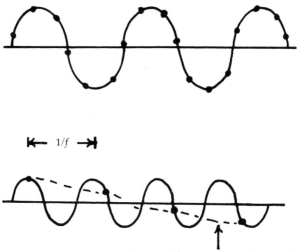

Incorrectly reconstructed waveform

Fig. 1.7 An illustration of how aliasing occurs. If the waveform is sampled at more than half of its frequency then it will be accurately reconstructed as illustrated in the top diagram. If the pulsed repetition frequency (sampling points) is less than half of the frequency of the waveform, then the waveform will be incorrectly reconstructed (lower diagram).

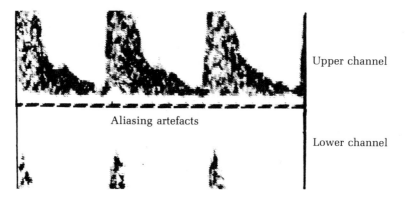

Fig. 1.8 Screen output from a spectrum analyser, demonstrating aliasing artefacts.

part or all of a grey-scale, real-time image of a slice of tissue (Fig. 1.9). The Doppler information is derived by interrogating each line through the tissue with 8 to 10 pulses (as opposed to the single pulse used for pulsed echo information), and therefore either the frame rate or the scan area, or

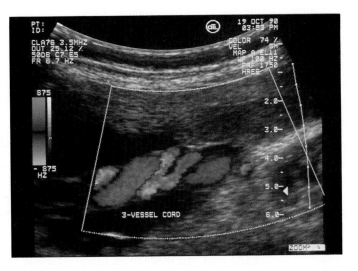

Fig. 1.9 Colour flow Doppler image which clearly delineates the three vessels in the umbilical cord. (Courtesy of ATL Ltd.)

both, are relatively reduced. It is important to note that Doppler informa-tion displayed on colour flow images is subject to the same restrictions as PW Doppler information. That is to say colour flow images are susceptible to aliasing and, more importantly in relation to obstetric scanning, the measured Doppler shift is angle dependent; therefore, great care must be exercised in the quantitative interpretation of such scans.

FACTORS AFFECTING DOPPLER POWER SPECTRA

Under ideal circumstances the Doppler power spectrum is the same as the velocity distribution histogram for the targets within the ultrasound beam. This simple relationship is upset by a number of factors (for details see Evans *et al.* 1989, pp. 115–93). The most important of these are: non-uniform vessel insonation and high-pass filtering.

Non-uniform insonation   The Doppler power spectrum only reflects the velocities of targets that are actually in the ultrasound beam; therefore, if the beam does not uniformly insonate the vessel a distorted picture of the velocities may be obtained. In general, unless the ultrasound beam is very badly placed, the centre of the vessel will be properly insonated but parts of the periphery may well be missed. This is less important if subsequent analysis of the Doppler information relies only on the maximum frequency envelope, but intensity-weighted mean velocity and volumetric flow calculations may be markedly altered by non-uniform insonation. Failure of uniform insonation leads to an under-representation of slow velocities with subsequent overestimates of both mean velocity and mean volume flow. In order to ensure uniform insonation it is usual practice to set the width of the range gate to a value that exceeds the diameter of the vessel that is interrogated.

High-pass filtering   Doppler-shifted signals contain not only the required signal from the moving blood but also high-amplitude, low-frequency signals from slow-moving, strong reflectors of ultrasound such as the vessel walls or other solid boundaries. When processing Doppler-shifted signals it is therefore necessary to apply very sharp filtering in order to reject such low-frequency signals (high-pass filtering). Unfortunately the filter cannot distinguish between low-frequency signals from slow blood flow and signals from unwanted sources. At best this leads to an incorrect estimate of flow velocity when an intensity-weighted mean follower is used to calculate velocity, but more seriously it can completely remove velocities in end-diastole. This completely changes the shape of both the maximum and the mean frequency envelope and may produce a serious misdiagnosis.

In order to keep this effect to a minimum the high-pass filter (also called the thump filter or the vessel wall filter) should be kept as low as possible consistent with obtaining a noise-free sonogram. The finding of absent end-diastolic frequencies should cause the operator to review the machine settings and to reduce the filter to its lowest level (usually 50 Hz). If the sonogram is interpreted solely from the maximum frequency envelope there is a strong argument for switching off the filter completely as vessel wall movements rarely influence maximum frequency. The velocity cut-off point for a given high-pass filter setting is influenced by the transmitting frequency, the angle between the Doppler beam and the vessel, the gain, and the vessel depth, so the numerical value of the filter should not be treated as absolute.

BLOOD FLOW MEASUREMENTS IN OBSTETRICS

Most duplex scanners are equipped with facilities and the software necessary to make volumetric flow measurements. These, however, are currently little used in obstetrics because of: (1) errors associated with calculating the time-averaged, intensity-weighted mean velocity; (2) the difficulties in measuring the angle between the Doppler beam and the blood vessel; and (3) the difficulties of measuring the diameter of small vessels. The fetal aorta averages 2–10 mm, and other vessels are much smaller.

Volumetric flow is calculated as the product of time-averaged, intensity-weighted mean velocity and the cross-sectional area of the vessel. Some of the problems of calculating the intensity-weighted mean volume are detailed above, but in obstetrics the biggest source of error in volumetric flow is associated with errors in measuring the cross-sectional area of the blood vessel.

Errors in measurement of cross-sectional area may be grouped as: (1) those due to vessel movement; (2) those inherent in making a reliable diameter measurement; and (3) those due to deviation of the vessel's cross-sectional shape from circular.

Leaving aside all these factors, the accuracy of making a single diameter measurement cannot be any better than approximately one wavelength of the ultrasound beam. This means that for vessels of 3 mm in diameter interrogated with a 5 MHz ultrasound beam, a minimum error of 10 per cent will occur in calculations of velocity. Because cross-sectional area depends upon the square of the radius, errors in calculating volume flow are therefore much greater. Fig. 1.10 summarizes the magnitude of error in volume flow calculations that can be expected under ideal conditions for vessels of varying sizes.

WAVEFORM ANALYSIS

Even if measurements of volumetric flow are accurate, they are unlikely to

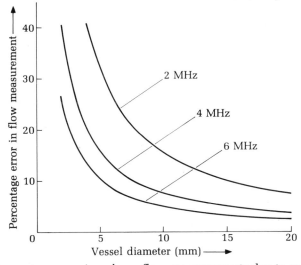

Fig. 1.10 Percentage error in volume flow measurements due to an error of one wavelength in the vessel diameter measurement, for various interrogating frequencies.

provide the investigator with as much information as can be obtained from waveform analysis, for two reasons:

1.   In many cases small changes in the circulation have a marked effect on the pulsatile components of blood flow before mean flow rates are affected: therefore, waveform shape is more sensitive to these changes than volume flow.

2.   Waveform analysis may give a clue to the site of the circulatory change.

To date, waveform analysis in obstetrics has been fairly crude and depends largely upon indices that are derived from the maximum frequency envelope (see Fig. 3.4). These techniques, however, are extremely easy to apply and have been widely used, with justifiable claims of success (see Section II). It should be remembered, however, that although the maximum frequency envelope is immune from many sources of error it is still dependent upon the equipment and techniques used to record it. Each of the indices that describes the envelope (see Fig. 3.8, p. 71) is strongly dependent upon the presence and the amount of diastolic flow. Signals from end-diastole may be lost artefactually for the following reasons: (i) a high-pass filter with too high a setting; (ii) a high angle of vessel insonation; and (iii) fetal breathing movements.

   As absence of end-diastolic frequencies is so significant in obstetric practice care, the above should be carefully sought in each case. This problem is dealt with in the clinical setting in Chapter 3.

   Several more complex indices have been described (for example, see Thompson *et al.* 1985) and there is still scope for these to be thoroughly investigated in obstetric practice (Evans 1984).

SAFETY

When an ultrasound wave is transmitted into the body the vast majority of its energy is dissipated within the tissues, with only a tiny fraction of 1 per cent escaping. The dissipated energy must cause physical change, and such change has the potential to cause damage.

   Ultrasonic energy is propagated as a pressure wave, and the energy crossing a unit pre second is called the intensity; it is generally expressed in watts/cm^2. The highest intensities are generated along the beam axis, and as the beam spreads out beneath the skin the intensity is reduced. The intensity across the beam may be spatially averaged (SA) whilst the intensity at the beam axis is usually measured as a spatial peak (SP) intensity. Pulsed echo systems may also have the intensity described in the following terms:

(1) temporal average (TA), the intensity of ultrasound averaged from one pulse to the next;

(2) pulse average, the average intensity of the pulse (not including the listening period to the next pulse);

(3) temporal peak (TP), the intensity of the maximum amplitude reached within a pulse.

In practice, diagnostic ultrasound intensity levels are usually quoted as spatial peak, temporal average (SPTA), and levels of less than 100 mW/cm^2 are usually considered safe. However, all ultrasound users—but particularly those practising obstetric ultrasonography—should be aware of the potential hazards, for two reasons:

1. While it is often possible to demonstrate that a technique is unsafe, it is never possible to demonstrate complete safety.

2. Manufacturers are tending to introduce machines with higher and higher powers. For example, all currently available pulsed Doppler equipment is capable of SPTA intensities in excess of 100 mW/cm^2. This is particularly important in obstetrical practice, where machines designed for cardiology or peripheral vascular investigations may be used. Such equipment often operates at high intensities.

A number of potential hazards of ultrasound have been described (for example, see Wells 1987) but to date there have been no confirmed reports of deleterious effects in patients who have been exposed to diagnostic levels of ultrasound. Potential hazards may result from heating of the tissue that has absorbed the ultrasound wave or to the possible disruptive effect of large swings in pressure. These two effects are independent in the sense that a pulsed ultrasound regimen that may cause large pressure swings may result in only very small temperature changes and vice versa. This is the reason why there are so many methods of quantifying ultrasonic output.

As far as temperature changes are concerned, the time-averaged intensity appears to be most important, and the most widely reported intensity is SPTA. Pressure changes are usually reported in terms of peak-positive (p^+) and peak-negative (p^-) pressures. SPTA intensities are highly dependent on both pressure swings within the ultrasound pulse and on pulse length and pulse repetition frequency. More recently, research has turned away from abstract measurements to easily comprehended and biologically meaningful qualities such as the maximum *in vivo* temperature rise that an ultrasound field produces.

Simple codes of good practice should be carried out by all ultrasound operators as these can easily reduce the total amount of ultrasonic energy that the patient receives by a factor of 1000 (Evans *et al.* 1989, pp. 229–30):

1. Use the lowest transmitted power that will give a result.
2. Use the minimum duration of examination.
3. Use the lowest pulse repetition frequency of a pulsed Doppler unit that will allow the highest velocity to be recorded.
4. Use CW rather than PW Doppler if possible.
5. Do not leave the Doppler beam insonating the region for any longer than necessary. With a duplex system, switch back to imaging mode as soon as the Doppler recording is complete.

REFERENCES

Evans, D. H. (1984). The interpretation of continuous wave ultrasonic Doppler blood velocity signals viewed as a problem in pattern recognition. *Journal of Biomedical Engineering*, **6,** 272–80.

Evans, D. H., McDicken, W. N., Skidmore, R., and Woodcock, J. P. (1989). *Doppler ultrasound: physics, instrumentation, and clinical applications.* John Wiley, Chichester.

Thompson, R. S., Trudinger, B. J., and Cook, C. M. (1985). Doppler ultrasound waveforms in the fetal umbilical artery: quantitative analysis techniques. *Ultrasound in Medicine and Biology*, **11,** 707–18.

Wells, P. N. T. (1987). The safety of diagnostic ultrasound. *British Journal of Radiology*, Supplement 20.

2. Statistics as applied to Doppler ultrasound studies

Martin Bland and Douglas Altman

INTRODUCTION

In this chapter several aspects of the statistical design and analysis of studies of Doppler blood flow measurements are considered. These include the evaluation of blood flow measuring devices, including the repeatability of measurements using a particular device and the agreement between two different devices, the construction of gestational age-related reference ranges, and the evaluation of diagnostic tests, including sensitivity, specificity, allied indices and receiver operating characteristic curves.

Apart from the specific references given in the chapter, further details of the statistical methods discussed can be found in Altman (1991), Armitage and Berry (1987), and Bland (1987).

SOURCES OF VARIATION IN DOPPLER FLOW MEASUREMENTS

In this section the sources of measurement error in Doppler blood flow indices are considered. The term 'error' is used in the statistical sense, to mean the variation in measurements that occurs due to the lack of precision in instruments, the limitations of reading numbers from scales, the natural variability of blood flow from heartbeat, and so on. It does not mean mistakes.

Repeated measurements

When an index of blood flow is measured, the number obtained is one of many possible measurements on that subject. Table 2.1 shows six repeated measurements of umbilical resistance index (RI) on each of 10 patients (Pearce 1988). Inspection of the table suggests that there is variation in RI from measurement to measurement, and also variation from subject to subject. Here, time and subject are different sources of variation. Data such as these can be used to estimate the repeatability of blood flow measurements.

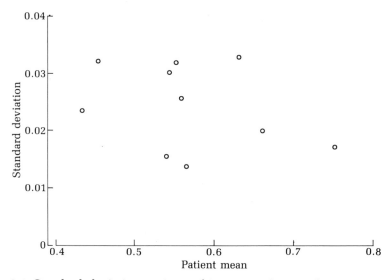

Fig. 2.1 Standard deviation against subject mean for simulaneous measurements of umbilical resistance index on the same subject (for data of Table 2.1).

The basic measure of repeatability is the standard deviation of repeated blood flow measurements on the same subject. To calculate a general value for this, the rather strong assumption must be made that this variability is the same for everybody, in particular that it is not related to the level of blood flow. This assumption is often not true for blood flow indices, and that case is dealt with below.

The general method for the estimation of the measurement error is analysis of variance, using subjects as a factor and estimating the standard deviation of the repeated measurements from the residual sum of squares. Table 2.2 shows the analysis of variance for the data of Table 2.1. The within-subjects standard deviation is the square root of the residual mean square. For the example, this is $\sqrt{0.000636} = 0.025$. The highly significant F ratio indicates that the differences between subjects are much greater than those that can be explained by the variation in RI from measurement to measurement (the measurement error).

The standard deviation can be estimated for each subject individually to see how it varies, in particular, across the range of the index. The standard deviation of repeated measurements can be plotted against the mean for that subject, to see whether there is any evidence of a relationship. Figure 2.1 shows that there is little evidence of such a relationship for the umbilical RI data. This could be tested formally using correlation, here $r = -0.31, p = 0.4$. If there is a relationship, this is likely to be positive and the method described below under 'Coefficient of variation' can be used.

Table 2.1 Umbilical resistance index measurements on 10 patients (Pearce 1988)

				Patient no.					
1	2	3	4	5	6	7	8	9	10
0.52	0.48	0.67	0.55	0.43	0.67	0.76	0.55	0.57	0.58
0.55	0.42	0.64	0.56	0.43	0.63	0.74	0.53	0.58	0.57
0.51	0.46	0.63	0.57	0.46	0.60	0.73	0.52	0.52	0.55
0.56	0.41	0.67	0.58	0.42	0.60	0.74	0.53	0.50	0.59
0.59	0.46	0.67	0.58	0.40	0.67	0.77	0.56	0.54	0.53
0.58	0.49	0.68	0.55	0.46	0.61	0.77	0.55	0.55	0.53

Table 2.2 One-way analysis of variance for repeated measurements of umbilical resistance index in 10 patients illustrated in Table 2.1

Source of variation	Degrees of freedom	Sums of squares	Mean square	F ratio	Probability
Total	59	0.5063			
Between patients	9	0.4745	0.05272	82.9	$p < 0.0001$
Within patients	50	0.0318	0.000636		

When there are only two observations per subject, a simple formula based on the differences between the pairs of observations can be used (see Bland 1987, para. 15.1):

$$s = \sqrt{\frac{1}{2n} \Sigma (x_i - y_i)^2}$$

where x_i and y_i are the pair of measurements on the ith subject.

The measurement error can be presented and used in several ways:

1. The within-subjects standard deviation, s, can be reported as it stands.

2. The largest difference that is likely to occur between the observation and the true mean blood flow index for the subject, which is $1.96s$. For the umbilical RI this is $1.96s = 1.96 \times 0.025 = 0.049$. For 95 per cent of measurements, the subject's true mean umbilical RI will be within 0.049 of that observed. This calculation implies the assumption that observation on the same subject will follow a normal distribution. This is usually reasonable in this context.

3. The repeatability coefficient, as defined by the British Standards Institution (1979), which is the maximum difference likely to occur between two successive measurements. This is defined as $r = 2\sqrt{2}s = 2.83s$. To correspond to a probability of 95 per cent, $1.96\sqrt{2}s = 2.77s$ would be better, but the difference is unimportant. For the umbilical RI data, the estimated repeatability is $r = 2.83s = 2.83 \times 0.025 = 0.071$. This tells us that two measurements on the same subject are unlikely to be more than 0.071 apart, when there has been no change in the true value.

4. The coefficient of variation, defined as $s/\bar{x}$ and usually quoted as a percentage. This is not appropriate when the error is independent of the mean, although it is often given. It would be reasonable if the error, s, were proportional to the mean, but in that case calculation of s, assuming a constant error, as described above, is incorrect. The appropriate circumstances for the use of the coefficient of variation and its calculation are discussed below.

Coefficient of variation

Indices of blood flow typically have positively skew distribution between subjects. For example, Fig. 2.2 shows the distribution of RI in a group of women (Steel *et al.* 1988). Under these circumstances, the variability

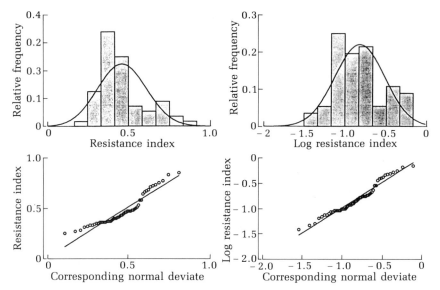

Fig. 2.2 Distribution of resistance index (RI) and log RI, with normal quantile plots.

between repeated measurements is likely to depend on the level of blood flow, higher flows being associated with greater variability. When standard deviation varies with the subject mean, a single estimate of standard deviation cannot be provided. In the common situation where the standard deviation is proportional to the subject mean, it can be expressed as a percentage of the subject mean, the coefficient of variation.

When the standard deviation is proportional to the mean, the logarithmic transformation will make the standard deviation independent of the mean on the transformed scale. Because this is the only transformation that allows a simple interpretation related to the untransformed scale, it is the one recommended for this application. Although there is no reason to apply the log transformation to the data of Table 2.1, it will be done for illustration. The prior analysis is now carried out on the log scale and s is determined (Table 2.3). On the log $_{10}$ scale this gives $s = \sqrt{0.000419} = 0.020$.

Table 2.3 One-way analysis of variance for the data of Table 2.1 after log transformation

Source of variation	Degrees of freedom	Sums of squares	Mean square	F ratio	Probability
Total	59	0.2943			
Between patients	9	0.2734	0.030375	72.49	$p < 0.0001$
Within patients	50	0.0210	0.000419		

The interpretation of the within-subject standard deviation calculated in this way is different from the previous result. This s does not have the same units as the original data. If s is back-transformed by taking the antilog ($10,^x$ or exp as appropriate) to give antilog$_{10}$ (s) = 1.04826, the result is not a standard deviation on the RI scale. This is because to obtain s, the mean on the log scale was subtracted from the observations on the log scale. The difference between the logs of two numbers is the log of their ratio. By subtracting the mean on the log scale, in effect the individual RI measurements were divided by the mean to get a dimensionless ratio. The antilog or exponent of s is a ratio, the ratio of the subject means plus one within-subject standard deviation to the subject mean. If one is subtracted from this ratio, the result is the ratio of the within-subject standard deviation to the subject mean. Because the within-subject standard deviation is proportional to the subject mean, this ratio is a constant, the coefficient of variation. For the umbilical RI example, the coefficient of variation is $1.048 - 1 = 0.048$, or 4.8 per cent. The coefficient of variation will give a true picture of repeatability only when the within-subject standard deviation is proportional to the subject mean. In other circumstances it may be quite misleading. From the coefficient of variation, the standard deviation of repeated measurements can be estimated at any point within the range of measurement.

The $1.96s$ limit and the repeatability can be calculated on the logarithmic scale. $\text{Antilog}_{10}(1.96s) = \text{antilog } 1.96 \times 0.020 = 1.095$ for the umbilical RI data, so about 95 per cent of the observations will be between the subject's mean value divided by 1.095 and the true value times 1.095, or within about 10 per cent of the subject's mean value. For the repeatability, $\text{antilog}_{10}(2.83s) = \text{antilog } 0.0566 = 1.139$, so for any two random measurements of a single patient, the ratio of one to the other will be at most 1.139, with probability 95 per cent. The $1.96s$ and repeatability could also be estimated directly from the coefficient of variation.

The effect of averaging multiple measurements

When measuring flow using Doppler ultrasound it is customary to take the average value of the index calculated from each of a series of waveforms. A better (i.e. more precise) estimate of the individual's flow is obtained in this way. The gain in precision which this brings can be calculated. The standard error of the mean of several measurements is given by the usual formula, $s/\sqrt{n}$. About 95 per cent of means will lie within two standard errors of the mean of all possible measurements, i.e. the true or mean index for the subject. Table 2.4, taken from Erskine and Ritchie (1985), shows the effect of taking different numbers of measurements, presented in terms of coefficients of variation, the ratio of standard deviation to mean.

This gain in precision applies only to the measurement of instantaneous flow. The longer-term, say diurnal, variation may be much greater than this. There will be two components to the variation, the very short term,

Table 2.4 Percentage error (coefficient of variation) for each averaged index of impedance as sampling number increases (Erskine and Ritchie 1985)

Sampling number	Pulsatility index	A/B ratio	Resistance index	Impedance index
1	8.3	7.5	5.5	18.2
3	4.8	4.3	3.2	10.5
5	3.7	3.3	2.5	8.1
10	2.7	2.4	1.8	5.8
20	1.9	1.7	1.2	4.1

waveform-to-waveform variation, and the longer-term variation over time. The total variation will be given by:

$$\sigma_L^2 + \frac{\sigma_S^2}{n}$$

where σ_S^2 is the short-term variance between individual wave measurements, σ_L^2 is the long-term variance, and n is the number of waves. Once there are sufficient waves to make σ_S^2/n small compared with σ_L^2 taking more waves will not help. For example, Table 2.1. shows umbilical RI measurements which are each the average of five waves. The average standard deviation of these groups of five umbilical RI measurements in Table 2.1 was 0.025, which is an estimate of σ_S. From Table 2.2, the variance within subjects, which includes both short-term variability and longer-term variability and longer-term variability over a day, was 0.000636. Thus σ_L^2 can be estimated by putting:

$$0.000636 = \sigma_L^2 + \frac{\sigma_S^2}{n} = \sigma_L^2 + \frac{0.025^2}{5}$$

This gives:

$$\sigma_L^2 = 0.000636 - \frac{0.025^2}{5} = 0.000511$$

Thus the long-range component of the variation is estimated as $\sigma_L^2 = 0.00051$, $\sigma_L = 0.023$, which is most of the variability. There would be little advantage to taking more measurements.

Observer variation

Table 2.5 shows repeated measurements of umbilical artery A/B ratio made by three observers for 10 subjects. The variability from observer to observer and from patient to patient can be separated, to see what effect these different sources of variability have. An analysis of variance could be performed, just as for repeated measurements. However, the observers are the same three throughout, and there may be systematic differences between them. The appropriate analysis is two-way analysis of variance, with observers and patients as factors. The results of this analysis for the umbilical A/B ratio (Table 2.5) is shown in Table 2.6.

The sum of squares between observers looks at systematic effects, the tendency for one observer to measure consistently higher or lower than another. In Table 2.6 this is small, indicating little systematic bias relative to the other source of variation. The other variations in observation are measured in the residual sum of squares. The variance of measurements by

Table 2.5 Measurements of umbilical A/B by three observers on 10 patients (Pearce 1988)

Patient no.	Observer no. 1	2	3
1	5.15	4.80	5.80
2	4.24	2.35	3.33
3	3.27	3.09	3.94
4	2.60	3.70	2.60
5	2.69	5.28	4.98
6	2.65	5.48	3.86
7	4.95	4.44	3.77
8	4.66	3.69	4.76
9	5.64	2.66	4.59
10	3.65	2.91	3.55

Table 2.6 Two-way analysis of variance for measurements by three observers on 10 patients, for data of Table 2.5

Source of variation	Degrees of freedom	Sums of squares	Mean square	F ratio	p
Total	29	30.7300	1.0597		
Between patients	9	12.8829	1.4314	1.48	0.2
Between observers	2	0.3920	0.1960	0.20	0.8
Residual	18	17.4550	0.9697		

different observers on the same subject can be calculated from the residual variance.

Comparing Doppler blood flow measuring devices

Sometimes blood velocity waveform indices obtained from two different measurement instruments must be compared. For example, van Vugt *et al.* (1988) compared indices obtained by pulsed Doppler and continuous wave Doppler. The analysis of studies comparing methods of measurements seems to cause much difficulty, and incorrect methods of analysis have often been used (see Bland and Altman 1986). In this section a simple technique is described for comparing two methods of measurement.

Asking the right question

The questions to be asked in method comparison studies fall into two categories:

1. Properties of each method: How repeatable are the measurements, i.e. how variable are measurements obtained on the same subject by the same method?
2. Comparison of methods: Do the methods measure the same thing on average? That is, is there any relative bias?

These ideas are often called accuracy and precision respectively. This is a question of estimation, both of variability and bias, not of testing. What is needed is a design and analysis that provide estimates of both. No single statistic can do this.

It is difficult to produce a method that will be appropriate for all circumstances, and therefore a relatively simple pragmatic approach is preferable to more complex analyses. What follows is a brief description of the basic strategy; clearly the various possible complexities that could arise might require a modified approach, involving additional or even alternative analyses.

The analysis will be illustrated using the data in Table 2.7 (van Vugt *et al.* 1988), which shows A/B ratio in the umbilical artery measured by pulsed Doppler and by continuous wave Doppler.

Table 2.7 Measurements of A/B ratio for the umbilical artery by pulsed Doppler (PD) and continuous wave Doppler (CW) for 14 patients (van Vugt *et al.* 1988)

Patient no.	PD	CW	(PD + CW)/2	PD − CW
1	3.63	3.57	3.600	0.06
2	4.13	4.17	4.150	−0.04
3	2.84	2.65	2.745	0.19
4	2.90	3.33	3.115	−0.43
5	3.11	3.47	3.290	−0.36
6	2.64	2.79	2.715	−0.15
7	3.19	2.55	2.870	0.64
8	2.46	2.41	2.435	0.05
9	2.95	3.33	3.140	−0.38
10	2.81	2.71	2.760	0.10
11	2.13	2.32	2.225	−0.19
12	2.59	3.20	2.895	−0.61
13	2.12	1.93	2.025	0.19
14	1.95	2.34	2.145	−0.39

Comparison of methods

The main emphasis in method comparison studies clearly rests on a direct comparison of the results obtained by the alternative methods. The question to be answered is whether the methods are comparable to the extent that one might replace the other with sufficient accuracy for the intended purpose of measurement.

The obvious first step, one which should be mandatory, is to plot the data. Figure 2.3 shows A/B by pulsed Doppler (PD) against A/B by continuous wave Doppler (CW). Plots of this type are very common and often have a regression line drawn through the data. The data will always cluster around a regression line by definition, whatever the agreement. For purposes of *comparing* the methods, the line of equality or identity (PD = CW) is much more informative, and is essential to obtain a correct visual assessment of the relationship. Although this type of plot is very familiar and in frequent use, it is not the best way of looking at this type of data, mainly because much of the plot will often be empty space. Also, the greater the range of measurements the better the agreement will appear.

It is preferable to plot the difference between the methods (PD − CW) against (PD + CW)/2, the average. This plot shows explicitly the differences in A/B ratio, and also indicates whether the magnitude of the differences varies according to the level of A/B ratio. Figure 2.4 shows the

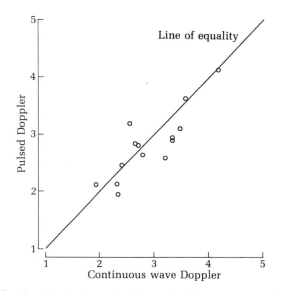

Fig. 2.3 Umbilical A/B ratio by pulsed Doppler (PD) against A/B by continuous wave Doppler (CW), with line of equality (van Vugt *et al.* 1988).

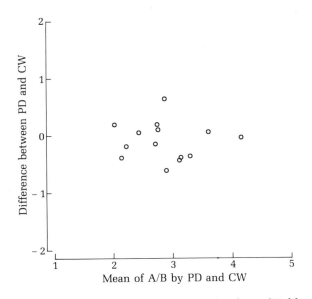

Fig. 2.4 Difference against subject mean for data of Table 2.7.

data from Fig. 2.3 replotted in this way. From this type of plot it is much easier to assess the magnitude of disagreement (both error and bias), spot outliers, and see whether there is any trend, for example an increase in PD − CW for high values. This way of plotting the data is a very powerful way of displaying the results of a method comparison study. It is closely related to the usual plot of residuals after model-fitting, and the patterns observed may be similarly varied.

The quantification of agreement is based on both the average difference between the methods of measurement and the variability in the differences. The average agreement between the two sets of A/B ratio measurements is the mean of the differences from each subject (and is equal to the difference between the overall means). There are several approaches to the assessment of the variability component of agreement.

The best method is to calculate the standard deviation of the within-subject differences. Using the assumption that the differences will have a normal distribution, which is usually reasonable for blood flow data, the range of values that would encompass the large majority of within-subject differences can be calculated. For example, about 95 per cent of differences would be expected to lie between mean − 2SD and mean + 2SD. These two values are called the 95 per cent limits of agreement (Bland and Altman, 1986). These values can also be superimposed on the scatter diagram. For the data of Table 2.7, the mean difference = − 0.094 and the standard deviation of the difference = 0.330. Thus the 95 per cent limits of agreement are − 0.75 and 0.57. Figure 2.5 shows 95 per cent limits of agreement superimposed on the data from Fig. 2.4. This type of figure gives a splendid summary of the comparison of the two methods.

If there is to be a single estimate of the standard deviation of the differences, the standard deviation must be unrelated to the magnitude of the measurement. In other words, the differences between the two methods should not be related to the mean. This can be checked visually from Fig. 2.5, and by correlation between the mean of the two methods and the difference. For the data of Table 2.7 this is $r = − 0.07$, $p = 0.8$, showing that there is no evidence for a relationship. The relationship between the absolute difference (ignoring sign) and the mean should also be examined; here $r = − 0.10$, $p = 0.7$. If there is a relationship, a log transformation can be used (Bland and Altman 1986). The correlation between PD and CW themselves is not of much interest. This would merely tell us that the methods are related, and it would be very surprising indeed if they were not.

This method does not require an assumption that the differences follow a normal distribution, but it may be misleading if the distribution of the differences is highly skewed or if there are one or more outliers (extreme discrepancies between methods). If the distribution of the differences is skewed (an uncommon occurrence) or has two long tails, a log or other

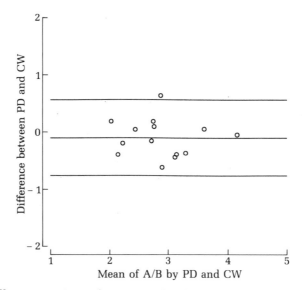

Fig. 2.5 Difference against subject mean for data of Table 2.7, with 95 per cent limits of agreement.

suitable transformation on the original data should make the data more suitable for the analysis. If occasional extreme outlying values are present, an empirical approach may be preferable. One approach is to calculate the proportion of differences that are more than some reference value, say 0.2 for A/B ratio. The reference values can be superimposed on the scatter diagram like the 95 per cent limits of agreement. Alternatively, the values outside which a certain proportion, say 5 per cent, of the observations fell can be calculated directly. This is done simply by ordering the differences and taking the range of values left after removing a percentage of the sample from each end. These values can also be superimposed on the scatter diagram.

Neither of these methods requires any assumptions about the distribution of the differences, but they are generally less reliable than those obtained using normal distribution theory, especially in small samples. To estimate the 2.5 per cent point for the differences directly, values must be found such that 2.5 per cent of differences lie below it. Several hundred observations are necessary to obtain a reasonable number of differences in the 2.5 per cent tail.

Properties of each method: repeatability

The assessment of repeatability is an important aspect of studying alternative methods of measurement. Replicated measurements are, of course, essential for an assessment of repeatability, but to judge from the medical literature the collection of replicated data is rare.

Repeatability is assessed for each measurement method separately using replicated measurements on a sample of subjects. A measure of repeatability can be obtained from the within-subject standard deviation of the replicated, as described above. Replicated data can be used to calculate 95 per cent of agreement. Bland and Altman (1986) give details.

REFERENCE RANGES

Rationale and interpretation

In many clinical areas it is valuable to be able to describe the usual range of values of some measurement in healthy people. Almost always this is done by considering the range in which a high proportion of healthy people fall, most often 90 per cent or 95 per cent. Such a range is called *normal range* or, preferably, a *reference range*.

There are two rather different clinical applications of a reference range. First, it can be used to determine where an individual is placed in relation to the distribution of measurements in the population of healthy individuals. Here an unusual value may be considered potentially abnormal, even though no specific abnormality is detected. Interpretation is by no means straightforward, as it must be remembered that 10 per cent of normal subjects will have values outside the 90 per cent reference range. Second, the range can be used to suggest whether or not a specific abnormality might be present or be likely to occur, i.e. as a diagnostic test. Such an assessment requires information about the measurement in subjects with the abnormality as well as in healthy subjects. Whatever the purpose, it is preferable to use the reference range to determine how far a value is from the average (by quoting a specific centile), and not just whether it lies within or outside the range.

In clinical practice it is unwise to put too much reliance on a single measurement. Other aspects to take into account include the accuracy of the measurement, the accuracy of the dating of the pregnancy, and the centiles of other measurements. The interpretation of a series of two or more measurements of the same subject poses further difficulties. Dramatic changes in centile may arise through measurement error on either occasion or through a genuine change. To this end it is useful to be aware of the likely difference between two measurements when no real change has occurred.

Interpretational difficulties have tended to obscure some fundamental issues relating to the statistical design and analysis of studies that aim to construct reference ranges. Further, when the measurement changes over time, such as during pregnancy, the reference range needs to be *age related*, which poses several additional problems of design and analysis. In particular, there is the possibility of taking measurements from the same women at different times. This section considers all of these problems in relation to gestational age-related references ranges for Doppler measurements. Particular emphasis is placed on design issues because these are rarely considered.

The sample

The sample used to construct a reference range should be representative of the whole relevant population. Thus, for example, for Doppler measurements the sample should represent all pregnant women. In theory, a random sample could be taken of all pregnant women in the country in a given time interval, but in practice such a scheme is unworkable. Most often the sample is taken as an unselected sequence of women seen in the antenatal clinic in a single hospital during a certain time period. This procedure may lead to some small degree of unrepresentativeness, because booking patterns are related to social class and other factors, but such a sample would be representative of women seen in that antenatal clinic. When using the ranges elsewhere, any geographical variation, e.g. in altitude or racial mix, may need to be taken into account. For Doppler measurements such effects may be minimal.

There will usually be some pre-specified reasons for excluding some subjects from the sample. As already noted, a reference range is obtained using data from healthy people. Defining 'healthy' is not always straightforward, but in this context it may be taken to mean without complicating factors such as diabetes or kidney disease. It may also be decided in advance to exclude women with multiple pregnancies. All of these examples relate to information known early in the pregnancy. Apart from such exceptions, all subjects should be included. In particular, it is desirable to have a general rule that one does not exclude individuals on the basis of information not available at the time of the measurement, such a low birthweight, pre-term delivery, and so on. There is perhaps a case for excluding neonatal deaths, but these will be so uncommon as to have a negligible effect on the overall data. The recommendation to make minimal exclusions is based on the fact that when using published standards to evaluate a set of measurements from a pregnant woman at, say, 26 weeks, birthweight and gestational age at delivery are unknown. It is thus inappropriate for reference ranges to take such information into account.

In other specialties it is usual to take an unselected sample, but in obstetrics it is common for pre-term pregnancies to be excluded, and also measurements relating to babies weighing less than the 10th centile for gestational age. Such pregnancies are not neccessarily clinically abnormal, and indeed their Doppler measurements may not be any different. Apart from the disadvantage of throwing away data, such exclusions lead to a supernormal group of patients of uncertain relevance. It is better to keep all pregnancies in the study, and use the opportunity to examine whether there is a relation between mid-pregnancy measurements and outcome.

The sample selection may be seen to relate to the aim of the reference range. The use of an unselected series is more appropriate in the case where there is no specific abnormality that is being screened for, and for tracking pregnancies over time. However, if the aim is to use the measurements to predict some existing or future abnormal condition, then it may be possible to create a diagnostic test (see below). For example, Vyas *et al.* (1990) created reference ranges using data from babies who were of appropriate weight for gestational age (AGA) (i.e. greater than the 10th centile) and showed that a high proportion of small-for-gestational age babies had flow velocity waveform values below the reference range (see Chapter 14), although they did not consider how well a Doppler index outside the reference range would predict which babies would be SGA. Their reference ranges calculated for AGA babies only are of unclear value in routine clinical use.

The issue of sample selection for reference ranges in obstetrics should receive more attention, in relation to the uses to which these ranges are put. It seems illogical routinely to make exclusions related to length of gestation and birth-weight in Doppler studies when such exclusions are not usually made in studies of fetal growth.

Design

Two types of study can be distinguished—cross-sectional and longitudinal. A cross-sectional study collects data about the distribution of the size of the measurement at each of several times (such as at each week of gestation) using subjects at different stages of pregnancy, each woman being measured once. In a longitudinal study, several measurements are taken on each subject at different times and these are used to obtain information about the within-subject changes over time in the measurement. These different ideas are well understood in studies of child growth, where they lead respectively to standards (reference ranges) for distance (size) and velocity (rate of growth). In fetal growth and Doppler studies, however, some confusion has arisen as a result of a different use of these terms. In particular, longitudinal is used to describe a data-set in which several measurements are taken from each subject, even though in virtually all cases such data are used to create reference ranges for size and not for change (i.e. they are analysed as if they were cross-sectional data). For example, Pearce *et al.* (1988) collected longitudinal data from 40 women with the intention of looking at changes (see Chapter 4). In the event, however, the data were used to derive reference ranges for size, not change. There do not seem to have been any analyses of within-subject changes in Doppler ultrasound measurements.

To avoid confusion the terms cross-sectional and longitudinal will be used to refer to the nature of the *data*, as is common in this field. A further complexity arises because the distinction between cross-sectional and longitudinal data can itself be blurred. In some studies there is no deliberate intention to measure the same people at regular intervals throughout pregnancy, but nevertheless some subjects are measured more than once. Such data are likely to arise through the use of whatever data are collected in routine clinical practice. Here the repeat measurements (and thus those later in pregnancy) are likely to be made when there is some clinical concern. This type of data must raise serious worries about representativeness. The women about whom there is concern will tend to be those with the greatest number of measurements. For this reason, routinely collected clinical data ideally ought not to be used to create reference ranges.

An often-stated advantage of longitudinal data is that, in principle, reference ranges derived from them should be more valid for the evaluation of a series of measurements than reference ranges derived from cross-sectional data. However, because of pre-term deliveries and other reasons, data will be incomplete for some subjects. If these are excluded the sample is not really representative, but if they are included the ranges for the later weeks will be less reliable and the overall shape of the reference range might be misleading. In addition, there is the serious statistical problem of dealing with non-independent data. In other words, the data represent a mixture of between-subject within-subject variation. As described below, the analysis of such data is by no means straightforward, and so the collection of longitudinal data is inadvisable unless the express purpose is to study the pattern of a series of measurements over time for individual women.

When designing a study to produce an age-related reference range the question arises about *when* and *how often* to measure each person. These aspects will be seen to relate particularly to cross-sectional and longitudinal data respectively. The essential requirement is that measurements are taken at pre-specified times and not for clinical reasons, especially concern about fetal or maternal well-being. Cross-sectional data should comprise a single measurement from each subject. In order to obtain an adequate spread through the gestational range of interest, some form of balanced randomization can be used to determine when each women will be measured. Other measurements taken for ordinary clinical reasons should not be included in the study. If certain weeks of gestation are of particular interest, then it might be advisable to include extra women at these times.

Longitudinal data should ideally comprise a sequence of measurements on each woman throughout the gestational range of interest. In general these would be equally spaced, although they need not be, and the frequency would relate to practical considerations. One obvious possibility is to take readings every 4 weeks. In order to obtain good coverage of gestational age, the starting point can be chosen at random from the first 4 weeks of the period of interest. The important point is that the times of measurement are pre-determined and unrelated to clinical progress.

The above discussion presumes that the pregnancy has already been reliably dated. This may be by any definable method, but it is vital that dates are reliable. Errors will have serious consequences for the quality of the data and will increase the width of the reference range. A reference range should relate to exact age of gestation. Thus, if length of gestation is recorded as completed weeks, half a week should be added to each gestational age before analysing the data.

A final point is that the data used to construct the reference range should reflect the measurements that are used in clinical practice. Thus, if the standard clinical procedure is to take the largest of a series of three readings, then equivalent data should be used for the reference range. If it is usual to take only a single reading, then this is what should be used for constructing a reference range.

Sample size

For simple (non-age-related) reference ranges the desirable sample size can be calculated in relation to the (im)precision of the limits of the reference range. Assuming that the data have, or can be transformed to have, a normal distribution (see below), the width of the 95 per cent confidence interval for the limits of the reference range calculated using the parametric approach is about $4s\sqrt{3/N}$, where N is the sample size and s is the standard deviation. A graph of this quantity against N (Altman 1991, p. 422) suggests that 100 is a bare minimum sample size, and 200 or more is desirable. However, because the precision is related to the square root of N, beyond 200 the sample size has to increase considerably to gain much further precision. Note the distinction here between the reference range, which describes between-subject variation in a measurement, and the confidence interval, which indicates the range of uncertainty of some statistical estimate. It is important not to confuse these ideas (although such confusion is common in published papers). In practice most published studies presenting reference ranges for Doppler measurements have been rather small. Because of the uncertainty associated with estimates from small samples, differences between the reference ranges obtained in different studies should be expected. With small samples there is also the possibility of failing to detect a curved relation with gestational age.

For a non-parametric reference range (see below), a much larger sample is needed to have equivalent precision. Clinical data-sets are often too small for non-parametric analysis to be a realistic option. Also, as explained below, there are some important advantages to the parametric approach.

For age-related reference ranges the analysis is more complex, and the appropriate samples size is less clear. A similar minimum sample size of at least 200 measurements is desirable. However, because of the need to detect curvature and possibly also changes in variability with gestational age, even larger sample sizes are desirable. An incidental advantage of larger samples is that they allow for the exploration of possible effects of other variables, such as parity and race. With longitudinal data analysed cross-sectionally it seems likely that the total number of observations is what matters most, so that many fewer subjects are needed in longitudinal data-sets. Practical considerations will mean that, for example, 200 observations would require at least 40 or so subjects, and probably rather more.

Constructing a non-age-related reference range

For non-age-related observations there are two basic approaches to the calculation of a reference range. The parametric method requires the data to have a nearly normal distribution, or to be able to be transformed to a normal distribution. For skewed data, a logarithmic transformation is often effective in producing near normality, but this needs to be verified in each case. It should not be assumed that the raw data or log data are normally distributed. Although a simple histogram can give a good idea of whether the data have a suitable distributional shape, a Normal plot is far better, and formal hypothesis tests are available. As in any statistical analysis, extreme values (outliers) should not usually be excluded unless they are clinically impossible or known to be suspect in some way, but it may be · useful to examine the sensitivity of the answers to the inclusion of such measurements.

Having achieved normality, the reference range is obtained simply from the mean and standard deviation (SD) of the data as mean $\pm$ k SD, where k is obtained from a table of the normal distribution. For a 95 per cent reference range, $k = 1.96$, for a 90 per cent range $k = 1.645$, and so on. If the data had to be transformed to obtain normality, then the transformation needs to be inverted to convert the range back to the original units. Thus, if the data were log transformed then the calculated values should be antilogged to give the reference range in the original units. Any new value x can be expressed as a number of standard deviations above or below the mean, by calculating $z = (x - \text{mean})/\text{SD}$, again after transforming x if necessary, where z is known as a standard deviation score (SDS).

The non-parametric approach makes no assumptions about the distribution of the data values, and involves finding the appropriate centiles of the empirical distribution of the sample data. Thus the observations are ranked and, for example, the 90 per cent reference range is obtained by taking the estimated 5th and 95th centiles, i.e. the values below and above which 5 per cent of the sample lies. This method makes no assumptions about the shape of the distribution, but it is much less precise in those situations when the data have a reasonably normal distribution.

Gestational age-related reference ranges

There are several important requirements of a gestational age-related reference range. It should: (a) change smoothly with gestational age; (b) be a good fit to the data at all ages: and (c) be as simple (mathematically) as possible. In addition it is desirable if an individual's value can be placed at a precise centile of the distribution rather than just as either inside or outside the reference range. This last feature is really only practicable with a parametric approach.

A common feature of age-related data is that both the mean and standard deviation change with age. Methods that assume a constant standard deviation are thus inappropriate for general use, although they may work well in some situations. Cross-sectional and longitudinal data will be considered in turn. A worked example is given later.

The methods proposed are not specific to the analysis of Doppler data. However, Doppler measurements raise one particular problem. Two of the common measurements are the A/B ratio and the resistance index (RI), which is $(A - B)/A$ (see p. 71). The RI can be rewritten as $1 - 1/(A/B)$, and is thus a simple transformation of the A/B ratio. Separate reference ranges constructed for each of these indices will not agree exactly, so that it may be possible for someone to be within one reference range and outside the other. To avoid this logical inconsistency it is probably best to choose whichever data-set can best be modelled and then to transform the range for that variable to obtain a range for the other. Thus, a range for RI can be found from one for the A/B ratio using the relation $RI = 1 - 1/(A/B)$, and conversely $A/B = 1/(1 - RI)$.

Cross-sectional data

A common simple approach is to calculate the mean and standard deviation (SD) at each gestational age and produce a graph showing lines connecting the values of the mean, mean $-$ 2SD and mean $+$ 2SD at each gestational age. These outer lines represent a 95 per cent reference range. (The value of 2 should strictly be 1.96, but the difference is minimal.) A 90 per cent range is obtained as mean $\pm$ 1.645SD. If the data are sparse, it may be necessary to group them into intervals of 2 or 3 weeks. This approach is based on some sound ideas but it fails to meet the criteria stated above, especially that of smoothness. It is based on the implicit assumption that the data have a close to normal distribution at each gestational age, one that is not usually examined formally or even informally. Unless a published reference range is presented superimposed upon a scatter diagram of the raw data, then its appropriateness cannot be judged.

Many approaches to the derivation of smooth age-related reference ranges have been suggested. A common simple method is to describe the mean level by a polynomial regression line (nearly always linear or quadratic). The usual way of deriving the reference range is then to take the fitted curve plus or minus twice the residual SD. This is reasonable in principle, but it assumes not only normality but also a constant between-subject variation (SD) over the range of gestation. Royston (1991) has explained the method in detail, and also offers a simple method for dealing with non-constant SD. A slightly more general approach described below works well in many situations. It will be seen that it is a relatively obvious extention of the simple parametric method outlined above.

The basic idea is to consider separately the mean and SD of the variable at each gestational age. Either the mean or the SD may effectively be constant over gestation, but more often the trend will need to be described by a straight line or a curve. If necessary, each is described by a separate regression model with gestational age as the independent variable. Having obtained satisfactory models for the mean and SD, the predicted values at w weeks of gestation can be denoted mean (w) and SD(w). Then, for example, a 90 per cent reference range is estimated as mean $(w) \pm 1.645$SD(w) and a 95 per cent reference range as mean$(w) = 1.96$SD(w). By definition, this approach will yield centiles that change smoothly with gestational age. Further details of the method are given in the next section.

It is assumed that the data have a normal distribution at each gestational age, and this may require that the data are transformed before analysis, most often by taking logarithms. A more detailed explanation is given below, under goodness of fit. As noted above, the need for a transformation must be verified, as should the success of a transformation in achieving near normality. The validity of the method does not depend upon achieving exact normality, but clearly the nearer to normal the data are the better the reference range will fit the data.

A simpler approach to modelling the SD is to separate the data into three equal-sized groups according to gestational age, and to compare the SDs of the residuals from the model fitted to the mean in the first and last groups (see Royston 1991). If these are significantly different then a linear regression of these SDs on the mean gestational age in the three groups should give a reasonable description of the variation in SD. This approach will work best when the SD changes roughly linearly with gestation, in which case it will give a similar result to the more general method.

Other approaches are considered by Cole (1988), Bland *et al.* (1990), and Thompson and Theron (1990). Non-parametric approaches to age-related reference ranges are not common—a considerable amount of data is required.

Details of method for constructing a reference range

This section gives a more technical explanation of the method just proposed for constructing an age-related reference range. A similar approach is described in detail by Royston (1991). The method presumes that the data have a normal distribution at each gestational age, or can be transformed so that this is so. The appropriateness of this assumption is examined in the next section.

The mean can be modelled by applying standard techniques of polynomial regression to the raw data, as described below. Where there is a curved relation between the measurement and gestational age, a better fit is sometimes achieved by first calculating the mean of the data in small age groups (e.g. for each week of gestation) and fitting a regression model to these means. For such grouped data it is usually appropriate to use weighted regression, in which the number of observations in each (gestational age) group is used as a weight in the analysis, so that the weeks with more observations have greater influence.

It is customary for the degree of polynomial curve that is appropriate to be decided using significance testing. The first model is a linear regression of the observations on gestational age. If the slope of this line is significantly greater than zero, then one odds a quadratic term; this is done by adding to the model a variable equal to age squared. Again, if the coefficient for this variable is significant, a cubic term is added, and so on. Extra terms are added until no significant improvement is achieved. In practice, linear or quadratic curves are usually adequate, and a curve beyond a cubic is unlikely to be needed. The rigid adherence to the use of significance tests to decide which model is best is not really satisfactory. Visual inspection of alternative models superimposed on a scatter diagram of the data may override *p* values.

To describe the relation between the SD and length of gestation, the data have to be grouped, most obviously by single weeks of gestation. The correct approach is to use the SD of the residuals from the model fitted to the mean. However, for small intervals of gestational age the actual SDs of the raw (or transformed) data can be used, especially if the mean is not changing quickly with gestational age. Again, polynomial regression analysis is used to determine the nature of the relation between the SD and gestation. A better fit may be achieved by considering the relation between log(SD) and gestation. It is unusual to require a model more complex than a quadratic curve.

The two regression models are then combined to derive the required reference range. The models fitted to the mean and SD provide estimated values at w weeks of gestation of mean(w) and SD(w). Any centile at each gestational age can then be estimated as mean(w) + kSD(w), where k is the appropriate centile of the standard normal distribution. For example, for a 90 per cent reference range the estimated 5th and 95th centiles are obtained using $k = \pm 1.96$.

Goodness of fit

It is essential to check the fit of the reference range to the data. The first step is to plot the raw data with the estimated mean and reference range superimposed. Usually there will not be enough data at each gestational age to make it easy to assess normality at each age. Grouping gestational age is possible when the measurement changes only slowly with gestational age, but is unwise for a rapidly changing measurement because mixing the ages can create non-normality where none exists. In any case, because the models are fitted to all the data at once, it makes sense to assess the fit of the model all at once. Two useful procedures are as follows. First, the difference between the observed and fitted values can be calculated for each subject in the reference data-set. The difference is expressed as a standard deviation score (SDS), z_i, by:

$$z_i = \frac{x_i - \text{mean}(w)}{\text{SD}(w)}$$

where x_i is the observed value for subject i. A graph of the z_i against gestational age should show: (a) the appropriate proportion of observations outside the range $\pm k$; (b) an even spread across gestational age of positive and negative values and values that are outside $\pm k$; and (c) no obvious patterns such as curvature or changing spread with gestation. In addition the z_i can be assessed for normality by constructing a normal plot and calculating the Shapiro–Wilk W test or the Shapiro–Francia W' test of non-normality. Again p values should not be the sole criterion. In particular, in large samples even minor deviations from normality can be statistically significant while having negligible effect on the reference range. In any case, the percentage of individuals included within the reference range is not highly dependent on having an exactly normal distribution (Healy 1974).

An unsatisfactory fit is most likely to be due to the assumption of normality being unreasonable. Some transformation of the original data needs to be made and the complete modelling process repeated. If, as is most common, the data have a positive skewness and thus an excess of high values, the obvious first step is to try the logarithmic (log) transformation. While this is often successful, sometimes a better fit is obtained by using $\log(x + c)$, where c is some constant (not necessarily positive). Here, of course, there is the further step of needing to identify the best value of c. Considerable trial and error is sometimes needed before arriving at a final reference range.

If a transformation is necessary, the models will predict mean(w) and SD(w) on the transformed scale. The reference range will then have to be back-transformed. For example, if the log transformation is used, the 90 per cent reference range is given by antilog(mean(w) $\pm$ 1.645SD(w)). The back-transformation of the mean, calculated as antilog(mean(w)), is most appropriately thought of as the estimated median (50th centile).

Having fixed the reference range the models can be used to calculate for any new subject the centile on which they are located. For example, for an observed value of x at a gestational age of 31 weeks the SDS is calculated as $(x - \text{mean}(31))/\text{SD}(31)$. This value can itself be used in subsequent analyses, for example to see whether some particular group of new subjects tends to have values that are consistently higher (or lower) than those in the reference population. It can be converted into a centile by use of a table of the standard normal distribution. For example, a value of −0.8 means that that subject is on the 21st centile. Similarly, the residuals for subsets of the original sample can be compared. For example, Thompson *et al.* (1988) compared the Pourcelot ratio for nulliparous and multiparous women at each week of gestation using *t* tests. As they acknowledged, this is not a powerful procedure because of the small numbers at each week. By contrast, using the approach just outlined, the data for all gestational ages could be compared in a single analysis.

Longitudinal data

For longitudinal data there are several options. One obvious possibility is to ignore the fact that the data comprise several sets of measurements on one individual and to proceed as for cross-sectional data: this is commonly done. While not a good idea in principle, it is impossible to say in what way this approach might produce misleading answers, and indeed it may well be that in many cases it is not too serious a problem. As noted earlier, the main worry is that there might be a relation between the number of measurements per individual and the actual level of those measurements or some other clinical information. Some insight into this possibility could come from an analysis relating the number of measurements to their mean SDS. Another possibility is to use just one measurement from each person, perhaps chosen at random, and to see whether the reference range using these values is similar to that for the whole set of data.

There are methods of analysis that take account of the linked nature of the data for each individual, but none is both simple and generally applicable. If all the curves for each person can be considered parallel, then it is possible to use analysis of covariance (see Pearce *et al.* 1988), in which parallel curves are fitted to each person's data. However, as noted above, the between-person variability often changes with gestation so that individual curves are not parallel. Although Goldstein (1986) has proposed a complex statistical analysis for such data, and other methods are available, it is advisable to seek expert statistical advice for the analysis of longitudinal data. It is clearly simpler to avoid the problem by collecting cross-sectional data.

Lastly, if longitudinal data are used to derive a reference range for changes over time, this can be done by using pairs of values on the same individual to calculate the expected change (and range) during each part of gestation. This approach is probably feasible only when there is quite a rapid change over time, or when each person's data lie on a reasonably smooth line, neither of which is generally the case for Doppler measurements.

Presentation

The sample source and inclusion/exclusion criteria should be stated. The omission of any subjects should be explained. The exact method used to calculate the measurements should be described, e.g. the mean of three readings. Statistical methods used to derive the reference range should be clearly described, including the possible transformation of the data and any attempts to assess goodness of fit. The regression equations should be presented, with the coefficients all given to the same number of significant figures (usually three or four), rather than the same number of decimal places.

A graph of the raw data with the fitted median and reference range is essential. It is desirable also to include a table of the mean and SD of the raw data for each week of gestation. If space permits, it may also be useful to include a table giving the median and reference range for each week of gestation.

Worked example

The methods outlined above will be illustrated using 201 measurements of the uterine artery A/B ratio (UAB) obtained from 33 women. These data were originally analysed by analysis of covariance (Pearce *et al.* 1988). Here, the fact that the data come from only 33 women will be ignored and they will be treated as 201 independent observations.

Figure 2.6 shows the raw data. It can be seen that there is a general tendency for the A/B ratio to drop with increasing gestation, and a suggestion that the variability also decreases. These are two rather high values at early gestations which might be thought suspect; the effect of these is considered later.

Preliminary analyses including histograms of the data within 4 week spans of gestation showed that the data are positively skewed, so an obvious first step was to try log transformation. The equations relating the mean and SD of log UAB to gestation were:

$$\text{mean}(w) = 1.5905 - 0.02096w$$

$$\text{SD}(w) = 0.4255 - 0.007700w$$

The fit of these straight lines was not appreciably improved by adding a quadratic term. The limits of the 90 per cent reference range for UAB calculated from these data is thus $\exp[\text{mean}(w) - 1.645\text{SD}(w)]$ and $\exp[\text{mean}(w) + 1.645\text{SD}(w)]$. Figure 2.7 shows these curves and the estimated median, given by $\exp[\text{mean}(w)]$. Although the fit appears reasonably good, the standard deviation scores are significantly non-normal using the Shapiro–Francia test ($p = 0.0002$).

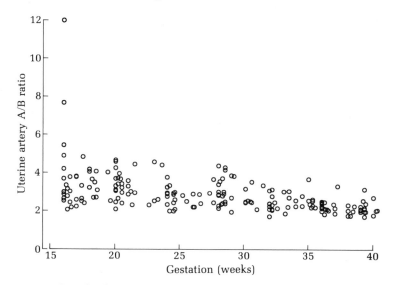

Fig. 2.6 Two hundred and one values of uterine artery A/B ratio (from Pearce *et al.* 1988).

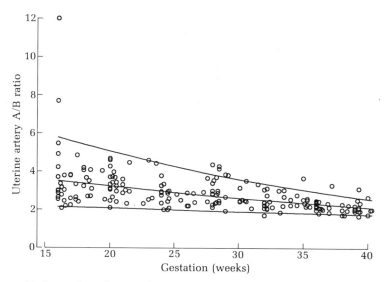

Fig. 2.7 Estimated median and 95 per cent reference range using log transformation.

The most likely reason for the lack of fit is that the log transformation is not quite right, and that the more general transformation log(UAB-constant) should be tried. Inspection of the distribution of UAB in 4 week segments for different values of the constant suggested that the transformation log(UAB-1) would be more appropriate. Accordingly, the whole analysis was repeated after making this transformation.

Figure 2.8 shows the mean and SD of log(UAB-1) for each week of gestation, together with the fitted curves, which were:

$$\text{mean}(w) = 1.432 - 0.03310w$$

$$\text{SD}(w) = 0.5402 - 0.007725w$$

Again, a straight line was found to give an excellent fit. (Note that there was only one observation at 22 weeks, so that the SD was undefined (but plotted as zero). This point was omitted in fitting regression models.)

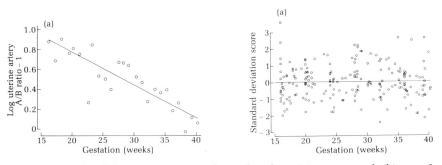

Fig. 2.8 Weighted linear regression lines fitted to (a) mean and (b) SD of log(UAB−1) by gestation.

Figure 2.9 shows the fitted reference range, and Fig. 2.10 shows the raw data with the back-transformed reference range, calculated as exp[mean(w) − 1.645SD(w)] + 1 and exp[mean(w) = 1.645SD(w)] + 1. Figure 2.11 shows the standard deviation scores plotted against gestational age and a normal plot. Although the normal plot is slightly curved, the test of non-normality gives $p = 0.07$, indicating a better fit than for the simple log transformation. Further, there are 13 points both above and below the reference range compared with the 10 expected. Thus, the range shown in Fig. 2.9 is an acceptable fit to the data.

As noted above, there were two very high values of UAB at early gestations. While log transformation reduces their deviation from the main body of the data, they will still exert some influence on the modelling process. The whole analysis was repeated excluding these two values to

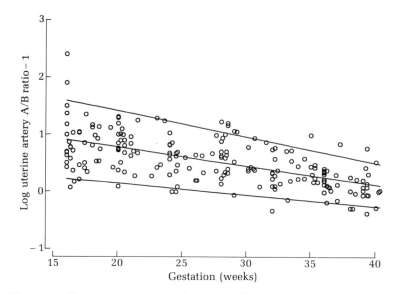

Fig. 2.9 Reference range derived from log(UAB−1) shown on log scale.

assess their influence, using both log UAB and log (UAB − 1). In neither case was there an appreciable improvement in the goodness of fit, and the resulting reference range was not greatly different from that using all the data. Figure 2.12 shows that there was little difference between the reference range from Fig. 2.10 and that obtained if those two outliers were excluded.

DIAGNOSTIC AND SCREENING TESTS

Test results and the true diagnosis

In this section diagnostic tests and their relationship to true diagnosis are considered. These may be tests used in the clinical situation to identify one of several possible diagnoses in a patient or, in screening, to find people with a particular disease in an apparently healthy population. In either case, there is a test that may be compared later with a true diagnosis. The situation is similar to that of comparing two different methods of measurement, where the true diagnosis forms one of the methods. Here, however, the two measures have very different weight: one is regarded as true and the other as an attempt to predict that true measure. The situation is not symmetrical in another way, too. The consequences of misdiagnosis may not be the same for false positives and false negatives, and these cases

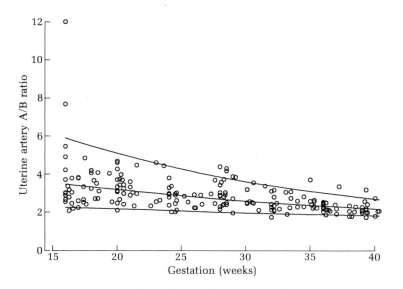

Fig. 2.10 Reference range derived from log(UAB−1) shown on natural scale.

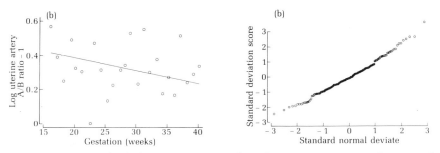

Fig. 2.11 (a) Standard deviation scores plotted against gestation; (b) normal plot of standard deviation scores.

should be considered separately. The test will be called positive if it indicates the disease and negative if not, and the diagnosis positive if the disease is later confirmed, negative if not.

For Doppler ultrasound indices, the test is based on a continuous variable and the disease indicated if it is above or below a given level. The effect of varying the cut-off point on diagnosis must be considered.

How can the effectiveness of a test be measured? It is tempting to take as an index of test effectiveness the proportion for whom the test gives the correct diagnosis. Unfortunately, this is a poor indicator of the value of a

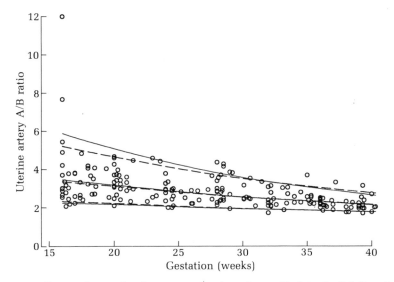

Fig. 2.12 Comparison of reference range based on all data (solid lines) and omitting two extreme values at 16 weeks of gestation (dashed lines).

test, as the following example shows. Table 2.8 shows three artificial sets of test and diagnosis data. For test 1, the proportion of subjects for whom the test is correct is 94 per cent. Now consider test 2, which always gives a negative result. Test 2 will never detect any cases of the disease. It is correct whenever the true diagnosis is negative. Test 2 is correct for 95 per cent of the subjects, better than test 1! However, the first test is useful, in that it detects some cases of the disease, and the second is not because it never detects any cases of the disease. Test 2 is clearly a poor test, yet it has a high proportion of agreement, because most subjects are true negatives. Proportion of agreement is a poor index of the usefulness of a diagnostic test.

A coefficient of agreement could be used, for example Cohen's kappa (κ). This is an index of the agreement over and above that expected by chance, and is 1.0 for perfect agreement and 0.0 if agreement is only that expected by chance. For test 1, this is $\kappa = 0.54$; for test 2 it is $\kappa = 0.00$, indicating much better agreement for test 1 than for test 2. Kappa is better than the proportion agreeing, but still not good enough. Compare test 3, which has almost the same value of κ as test 1, $\kappa = 0.56$. However, test 3 is not as good as test 1 in one respect: it detects only two of the five true positives, compared with four. On the other hand, it is a better test in another way: it does not diagnose as positive any true negatives. As with method comparison studies, a single statistic cannot provide sufficient information.

Sensitivity and specificity

There is no one simple index that enables us to compare different tests in all the ways that are needed. This is because there are several things that need to be measured. One is how good the test is at finding true positives, i.e. those with the condition. Another is how good the test is at excluding true negatives, i.e. those who do not have the condition. The indices conventionally employed to do this are:

$$\text{Sensitivity} = \frac{\text{number who are both true positive and test positive}}{\text{number who are true positive}}$$

$$\text{Specificity} = \frac{\text{number who are both true negative and test negative}}{\text{number who are true negative}}$$

In other words, the sensitivity is the proportion of true positives who are also test positive, and the specificity is the proportion of true negatives who are also test negatives. Sensitivity and specificity are often multiplied by 100 to give percentages.

For the three tests in Table 2.8, the sensitivity and specificity are shown in Table 2.9. Test 2, of course, misses all the true positives and finds all the true negatives, by saying all are negative. The difference between tests 1 and 3 is brought out by the greater sensitivity of test 1 and the greater specificity of test 3. Tests are compared in two dimensions. Test 3 is better than test 2, because its sensitivity is higher and its specificity is the same. However, it is more difficult to see whether test 3 is better than test 1. A judgement must be based on the relative importance of sensitivity and specificity in the particular case.

For example, Table 2.10 shows a comparison of three tests for predicting intra-uterine growth retardation (IUGR). Both low umbilical vein (UV) flow and low oestriol (E_3) or human placental lactogen (HPL) are better than serial biparietal diameter measurements (BPD), as low UV flow has higher sensitivity and equal specificity, and low E_3 or HPL has equal sensitivity and higher specificity. However, it is difficult to say which will be the better test, as low UV flow is better at detecting IUGR than is low E_3 or HPL, and low E_3 or HPL is better at eliminating IUGR in normal fetuses than is low UV flow.

Sensitivity and specificity are estimated by collecting test results on subjects with a positive diagnosis to obtain the sensitivity, and on subjects with a negative diagnosis to obtain the specificity. What is actually observed are sensitivity and specificity relative to the diagnosis, when what is required are sensitivity and specificity relative to the true disease. Provided the diagnosis is always correct, these two pairs of indices are the same and are properties of the test only. They can thus be applied to any

Table 2.8 Some artificial test and diagnosis data

	True diagnosis		
	Positive	Negative	Total
Test 1			
Positive	4	5	9
Negative	1	90	91
Total	5	95	100
Test 2			
Positive	0	0	0
Negative	5	95	100
Total	5	95	100
Test 3			
Positive	2	0	2
Negative	3	95	98
Total	5	95	100

Table 2.9 Sensitivity, specificity and kappa (κ) for artificial test data.

	Sensitivity	Specificity	κ
Test 1	0.80	0.95	0.54
Test 2	0.00	1.00	0.00
Test 3	0.40	1.00	0.56

population. However, when the diagnosis itself is subject to error, the sensitivity and specificity relative to diagnosis depend on the prevalence of the disease in the population, are not a property of the test alone, and cannot be generalized to other populations.

The effect of uncertainty in the diagnosis is to reduce the estimates of both sensitivity and specificity with respect to the true disease. The sensitivity and specificity are always underestimated for a valid test, that is, a test in which test positives have a greater probability of being true positives than do test negatives. The underestimate is greatest for the sensitivity when the prevalence is small, i.e. when the number of incorrect diagnoses

Table 2.10 Three tests for predicting intra-uterine growth retardation (Gill. *et al.* 1984)

	Serial BPD	Low UV flow	Low E$_3$ or HPL
Number of subjects	81	81	34
Sensitivity	0.64	0.91	0.64
Specificity	0.79	0.79	0.91
κ	0.76	0.80	0.86
Positive predictive value	0.32	0.40	0.78

BPD, biparietal diameter; UV, umbilical vein; E$_3$, oestriol; HPL, human placental lactogen; κ, kappa.

is relatively large, and it is greatest for the specificity when the prevalence is high. That is what would be expected, for when the prevalence is high most diagnosed cases will be true cases of the disease. As the prevalence of true disease falls, an increasing number of diagnosed cases will not in fact have the disease and so will be less likely to be test positive. On the other hand, when the prevalence is low, most subjects for whom the diagnosis is negative will not have the disease, whereas as the prevalence rises more of those with a negative diagnosis will be undiagnosed true cases. Pearce (1988) notes, for example, that the sensitivity of the maternal serum α-fetoprotein test for neural tube defect increases with prevalence, suggesting that, as prevalence in the UK is falling, the value of the test may be reduced.

Kraemer (1988) criticizes the practice of using a high-prevalence clinic population to estimate sensitivity and a low-prevalence community population to estimate specificity, on the grounds that these populations will have quite different specificity and sensitivity relative to the diagnosis. This is true, but if the sample sensitivity and specificity are regarded as estimates of the sensitivity and specificity relative to the true disease state, this technique will reduce the bias and is to be recommended.

Standard errors for estimated sensitivity and specificity
Sensitivity and specificity are both binomial proportions, so their standard errors and confidence intervals are found using the binomial distribution. Unless numbers are small, the normal approximation can be used. If there are n_P true positives, of whom a proportion P_{sens} are test positive (i.e. P_{sens} is the sensitivity), then the standard error of P_{sens} is estimated by:

$$\sqrt{\frac{P_{sens}(1 - P_{sens})}{n_P}}$$

Provided the normal approximation is reasonable, i.e. if $n_P P_{sens} > 5$ and $n_P(1 - P_{sens}) > 5$, the 95 per cent confidence interval is estimated by:

$$P_{sens} - 1.96\sqrt{\frac{P_{sens}(1 - P_{sens})}{n_P}} \text{ to } P_{sens} + 1.96\sqrt{\frac{P_{sens}(1 - P_{sens})}{n_P}}$$

The standard error and 95 per cent confidence interval for the specificity are found in the same way. If there are n_N true negatives of whom P_{spec} are negatives, than the estimated standard error of P_{spec} is:

$$\sqrt{\frac{P_{spec}(1 - P_{spec})}{n_N}}$$

and the 95 per cent confidence interval is estimated by:

$$P_{spec} - 1.96\sqrt{\frac{P_{spec}(1 - P_{spec})}{n_N}} \text{ to } P_{spec} + 1.96\sqrt{\frac{P_{spec}(1 - P_{spec})}{n_N}}$$

For example, Table 2.11 shows the umbilical A/B ratio used as a test to predict low birth-weight. The test is sensitive, with sensitivity = 90.2 per cent, but not specific, specificity = 28.1 per cent. The standard error of the sensitivity is:

$$\sqrt{\frac{P_{sens}(1 - P_{sens})}{n_P}} = \sqrt{\frac{0.0902 \times (1 - 0.902)}{51}} = 0.0416$$

and the 95 per cent confidence interval is estimated by:

$$0.902 - 1.96 \times 0.0416 \text{ to } 0.902 + 1.96 \times 0.0416 = 0.82 \text{ to } 0.98$$

The standard error of the specificity is estimated by:

$$\sqrt{\frac{P_{spec}(1 - P_{spec})}{n_P}} = \sqrt{\frac{0.281 \times (1 - 0.281)}{114}} = 0.0421$$

and the 95 per cent confidence interval is estimated by:

$$0.281 - 1.96 \times 0.0362 \text{ to } 0.281 + 1.96 \times 0.0362 = 0.20 \text{ to } 0.36$$

The sensitivity is close enough to one to make the normal approximation a bit suspect, the number of normal A/B ratios, $n_P(1 - P_{sens})$, being equal to 5. There is an exact method, using the individual probabilities of the binomial distribution, which may be preferable (Pearson and Hartley 1970). The confidence interval by this method is 0.78–0.97, compared with 0.82–0.98 by the normal approximation.

Comparison of the sensitivity or specificity of two diagnostic tests can be done using confidence intervals or significance for the difference between two proportions. If the data are collected on the same subjects, as is often the case when comparing different Doppler indices, a matched analysis

Table 2.11 Umbilical A/B ratio as a test to predict low birth-weight
(Pearce 1988)

Umbilical A/B ratio	Birth-weight	
	Below 5th centile	Above 5th centile
Abnormal	46 (90.2%)	82 (71.9%)
Normal	5 (9.8%)	32 (28.1%)
Total	51 (100%)	114 (100%)

(McNemar's method) should be used. This can give either a test of significance or a confidence interval.

When considering a group of tests, one of them will appear to be the best in the sample, due to random variation, even if they are all identical in the whole population. This may lead to an over-optimistic view of the sensitivity and specificity of the test. The test picked out as having the best sensitivity and specificity may be one which by chance had sample sensitivity and specificity at the high end of the sampling distribution, i.e. rather larger than the population values. The actual sensitivity and specificity of the test may be less than those indicated by the data.

Sampling and sample size for estimating sensitivity and specificity

To estimate the sensitivity and specificity of a test, samples of subjects are needed both with the disease and without the disease. There may be a few difficulties in ensuring that subjects in the true negative group are free from the disease, especially if the definitive diagnostic tests are invasive. In the case of Doppler ultrasound, this is not usually a major problem, as the outcome will be observed later in the pregnancy or after birth. As with reference ranges, it is important that samples be collected for the purpose of evaluating the test, not because of concern about the pregnancy.

The sample size is determined as for any binomial proportion. The accuracy of an estimate is measured by its confidence interval, which for a large sample will be 1.96 standard errors on either side of the estimate. Thus, to estimate a proportion to any given accuracy 1.96 standard errors is set equal to the maximum difference that would be accepted between estimate and population value. As always with the binomial distribution, the size of the proportion to be estimated must be guessed. Guesses might be the minimum values of sensitivity and specificity required for our application, or the values expected from published data or from a pilot study. A reasonable level of precision can be chosen, and hence a rough estimate of the required sample size arrived at.

For example, suppose the test is expected to have a sensitivity of about 90 per cent, specificity of about 80 per cent, and it is required to estimate these to within five percentage points (0.05). For the sensitivity sample, the number of subjects needed is given by:

$$0.05 = 1.96\sqrt{\frac{P_{sens}(1 - P_{sens})}{n}} = 1.96\sqrt{\frac{0.90 \times 0.10}{n}}$$

$$n = \frac{1.96^2 \times 0.90 \times 0.10}{0.05^2} = 138$$

For the specificity sample:

$$0.05 = 1.96\sqrt{\frac{P_{spec}(1 - P_{spec})}{n}} = 1.96\sqrt{\frac{0.80 \times 0.20}{n}}$$

$$n = \frac{1.96^2 \times 0.80 \times 0.20}{0.05^2} = 246$$

As with most sample size calculations, these are only approximate but will serve as a guide to what is necessary.

Because indices are continuous measurements, an estimate of the cut-off point to give a particular sensitivity or specificity may be needed. Provided the index has a normal distribution, using a log transformation if necessary, this can be calculated from the mean and standard deviation (SD). The required number of SDs from the mean can be found from a table of the normal distribution. For example, suppose low values of the index are test positive and a sensitivity of 90 per cent is required. For the standard normal distribution, the probability of being below 1.28 is 90 per cent. Thus, a cut-off point of the mean + 1.28 SDs (obtained from the true-positive subjects) would give sensitivity 90 per cent. The standard error of this estimate is approximately:

$$\sqrt{s^2\left(\frac{1}{n} + \frac{z^2}{2(n - 1)}\right)}$$

where z is the number of SDs from the mean, $z = 1.28$ in the example. This standard error can be used for confidence-interval and sample-size calculations as above. If the cut-off point is estimated directly from the frequency distribution, there is a direct, non-parametric confidence interval for a centile which can be used. For Doppler indices, the normal distribution method is usually appropriate.

False positives, false negatives, and positive predictive value

The interpretation of different values for sensitivity and specificity depends on the prevalence of the disease in the population in which the test is to be used. It may be very different in the differential diagnostic situation, where patients present with a problem, and the screening situation, where apparently healthy, symptom-free individuals are offered the test. Two indices that help to quantify the effects of a test in a given population are the false-positive rate and the false-negative rate. A false positive is a subject who is test positive but who is true negative, i.e. someone who the test indicates to have the disease but in reality does not do so. A false negative is a subject who is test negative but who is true positive, i.e. has the disease. False-positive and false-negative rates are defined by:

$$\text{False-positive rate} = \frac{\text{patients who are both true negative and test positive}}{\text{all patients who are test positive}}$$

$$\text{False-negative rate} = \frac{\text{patients who are both true positive and test negative}}{\text{all patients who are test negative}}$$

The complements of these rates, known as the positive and negative predictive value, are often used. The positive predictive value is one minus the false-positive rate, the proportion of test-positive subjects who will be true positive. The negative predictive value is one minus the false-negative rate, the proportion of test-negative subjects who will be true negative.

These rates depend on the prevalence in the population. Denote the sensitivity by P_{sens}, the specificity by P_{spec}, and the prevalence of the disease by P_{prev}. The proportion of all subjects who will be false positive, i.e. will both be positive on the test and not have the disease, will be $(1 - P_{spec}) \times (1 - P_{prev})$, because $1 - P_{prev}$ do not have the disease and the proportion of these who will be test positive is one minus the specificity $1 - P_{spec}$. The proportion of all subjects who will be true positives, i.e. both positive on the test and have the disease will be $P_{sens} \times P_{prev}$. The total number of positives is thus $P_{sens} \times P_{prev} + (1 - P_{spec}) \times (1 = P_{prev})$. The false-positive rate (FPR) and false-negative rate (FNR) are given by:

$$\text{FPR} = \frac{(1 - P_{spec}) \times (1 - P_{prev})}{(1 - P_{spec}) \times (1 - P_{prev}) + P_{sens} \times P_{prev}}$$

$$\text{FNR} = \frac{(1 - P_{sens}) \times P_{prev}}{(1 - P_{sens}) \times P_{prev} + P_{spec} \times (1 - P_{prev})}$$

As the prevalence decreases, the false-positive rate increases and the false-negative rate decreases. The false-positive rate is important, as it is the positives on whom action is taken. Thus, a high false-positive rate means that most of those on whom an intervention is carried out, either treatment or further testing, are true negatives. The false-negative rate is not so important, as it is not usual to do anything to negatives. The proportion of true cases missed, given by $1 - P_{sens}$, is of more interest.

First, an idealized example will be considered. Suppose there is a very good test, with both sensitivity and specificity of 0.95 or 95 per cent. This test will be positive for the large majority of people with the disease and negative for the large majority of those without it. Table 2.12 shows the false-positive rate for several different prevalences. When the prevalence is 50 per cent, as it might be for patients requiring differential diagnosis, the false-positive rate is small and most test positives will have the disease. However, when the prevalence is 1 per cent, quite high for a screening situation, the false-positive rate is 84 per cent; the majority of positives are false positives. Table 2.12 also shows what would happen with a test that has a very high specificity of 99 per cent. When the prevalence is 1 per cent, half of the positives are expected to be false positives, and when it is 1 per 1000, 90 per cent of positives are expected to be false positive. Thus, for any screening test that is not totally specific, most positives would be expected to be false positives.

The lower the prevalence, the greater the disparity between the numbers of false positives and false negatives. The relative importance of sensitivity and specificity depends on the prevalence of the condition as well as on the particular test.

For the prediction of low birth-weight (Table 2.11), the prevalence is by definition 5 per cent. Hence the positive and negative predictive values can be calculated by:

$$\mathrm{FPR} = \frac{(1 - P_{\mathrm{spec}}) \times (1 - P_{\mathrm{prev}})}{(1 - P_{\mathrm{spec}}) \times (1 - P_{\mathrm{prev}}) + P_{\mathrm{sens}} \times P_{\mathrm{prev}}}$$

$$= \frac{(1 - 0.281) \times (1 - 0.05)}{(1 - 0.281) \times (1 - 0.05) + 0.902 \times 0.05} = 0.94$$

$$\mathrm{FNR} = \frac{(1 - P_{\mathrm{sens}}) \times P_{\mathrm{prev}}}{(1 - P_{\mathrm{sens}}) \times P_{\mathrm{prev}} + P_{\mathrm{spec}} \times (1 - P_{\mathrm{pre}})}$$

$$= \frac{(1 - 0.902) \times 0.05}{(1 - 0.902) \times 0.05 + 0.281 \times (1 - 0.05)} = 0.02$$

Alternatively, the positive predictive value is $1 - 0.94 = 0.06$, and the negative predictive value is $1 - 0.02 = 0.98$. A fetus that is positive on this test (abnormal A/B) has only a 6 per cent chance of being of low birth-weight (compared with 5 per cent for all births), whereas a fetus that is negative on the test (normal A/B) has a 98 per cent chance of being of normal or high birth-weight (compared with 95 per cent for all births). This is because, although the test is sensitive, it is not specific.

Table 2.12 False-positive rates expected with tests of sensitivity and specificity of 95 per cent, or sensitivity and specificity of 99 per cent

	False-positive rate (%)	
Prevalence (%)	$P_{spec} = P_{sens} = 95\%$	$P_{spec} = P_{sens} = 99\%$
50	5	1
10	32	8
1	84	50
0.1	98	91

Youden's index

Deciding on the best test involves consideration of both sensitivity and specificity. If a test does best on both dimensions there is no problem, but the test with higher sensitivity often has lower specificity. In Table 2.10, for example, low umbilical vein (UV) flow was more sensitive than low oestriol (E_3) or human placental lactogen (HPL) as a predictor of IUGR, but was less specific. It is often the case that there must be a compromise between higher sensitivity and higher specificity. It then becomes a matter of judgement as to the likely effects of low sensitivity compared with those of low specificity. This will depend on the use to which the test is to be put and the frequency of the condition being diagnosed.

One proposed method of getting round the two-dimensional nature of the problem is Youden's index:

$$J = \text{sensitivity} + \text{specificity} - 1$$

This has the property that $J = 1$ if the test is invariably correct, $J = -1$ if the test is invariably wrong, and $J = 0$ if there is no relationship between test and true diagnosis. The test with the maximum J is chosen. For our example, the criterion of low UV flow gives $J = 0.91 + 0.79 - 1 = 0.70$, and the criterion of low E_3 or HPL gives $J = 0.64 = 0.91 - 1 = 0.55$. Thus, by this index the criterion of low UV flow is better. However, Youden's index implies the arbitrary decision that sensitivity and specificity should have equal weight. This is not necessarily a good idea. As seen in the previous section, their relative importance depends both on the context and on the prevalence of the condition to be detected.

Continuous test measurement and ROC curves

When the test is based on a continuous variable, such as a Doppler index, a cut-off point to define a positive test must be chosen. Changing the cut-off point alters the sensitivity and specificity. If high values of the test index indicate the disease, raising the cut-off point means fewer cases are detected and so the sensitivity is decreased. However, there are fewer false positives and the specificity is increased. The opposite effect is obtained if the cut-off point is lowered. A cut-off value is needed which gives the best compromise between sensitivity and specificity.

For example, Vyas *et al.* (1990) reported a 95 per cent reference range by gestational age for fetal middle cerebral artery pulsatility index, constructed from a cross-sectional study of 162 appropriate-for-gestational age (AGA) fetuses (see Chapter 12). They presented the pulsatility index for a sample of small-for-gestational age (SGA) fetuses plotted on the same graph (Fig. 2.13). (For the purposes of illustration, the data of Vyas *et al.* have been recreated from a published graph, and are only approximate.) The pulsatility index for the SGA fetuses is less than that for AGA fetuses of corresponding age, only one SGA fetus being above the AGA mean. This could be used as a test for SGA. One possibility would be to take the lower boundary of the 95 per cent reference range. This would have a high specificity, since by definition 97.5 per cent of AGA fetuses are above this level, giving a specificity of 0.975. The sensitivity would not be very good, as only 40 of the 81 SGA fetuses are below this boundary, giving a sensitivity of 40/81 = 0.494. Raising the boundary would increase the sensitivity, but reduce the specificity.

The sensitivity and specificity can be calculated for any boundary parallel to those in Figure 2.13. Sensitivity can be estimated by counting the

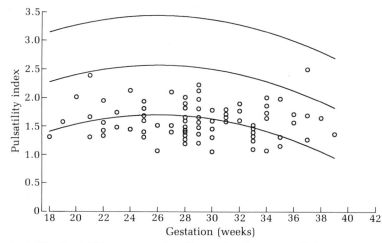

Fig. 2.13 Fetal middle artery pulsatility index for 81 small-for-gestational-age (SGA) fetuses with 95 per cent reference range (from Vyas *et al.* 1990).

number of SGA observations below the boundary. Specificity can be estimated by converting the vertical distance from the mean curve into a standard deviation score and finding from tables what proportion of the standard normal distribution is expected to be above this value.

It is often convenient to examine graphically the way sensitivity and specificity vary. This is usually done by plotting the sensitivity against the specificity (Fig. 2.14). This is called the receiver operating characteristic (ROC) curve. ROC is a term that comes from the study of the subjective assessment of an objective external stimulus, where it is the plot of subjective assessment against objective stimulus (e.g. perceived loudness against sound level in decibels). Why the name should be used in medical applications is unclear. Also shown on the graph is a line from specificity = 0, sensitivity = 1, to specificity = 1, sensitivity = 0, which would be the curve if the test did not discriminate between true positives and true negatives at all. Sometimes the sensitivity is plotted against one minus the specificity, to give a rising graph which can be compared to the line of equality, as in Fig. 2.15. It does not matter which version is used.

The ROC curve plots the proportion of SGA cases who would be correctly identified (i.e. positive) against the proportion of AGA normals who would be correctly identified (i.e. negative). The straight line represents a set of tests which would record positive with equal probability on AGA and SGA fetuses, and would therefore be useless, the position along the line being determined by the probability with which positive is recorded.

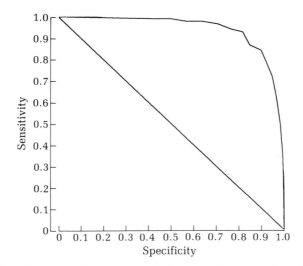

Fig. 2.14 Receiver operating characteristic curve for a test based on cerebral artery pulsatility index.

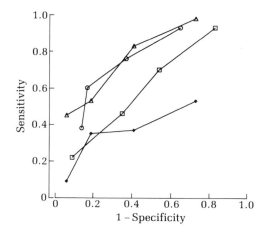

Fig. 2.15 Receiver operating characteristic curves for four Doppler indices, used as tests to predict perinatal death (Pearce 1988). ○, Placental resistance index (RI); □, nonplacental RI; △, umbilical A/B; ◆, aorta A/B.

The height of the curve above the line of equality is Youden's index, but as noted above this index is not really very useful. The relative importance of sensitivity and specificity depends on the consequences of incorrect diagnosis in either direction and on the prevalence of the disease. However, the curve shows us very easily what the trade-off between sensitivity and specificity is for any cut-off point. For example, lowering the specificity of the test from 0.975 to 0.090 would increase the sensitivity from 0.49 to 0.82. Lowering sensitivity further to 0.80 would increase sensitivity only to 0.88.

The ROC technique can be used to compare several different tests. Figure 2.15 shows ROC curves for four different tests, as predictors of perinatal death. From this it can be seen that placental RI and umbilical A/B are similar tests, and are clearly superior to non-placental RI or aorta A/B.

The major defect of ROC curves is that they ignore the prevalence of the condition. This is reflected in their relationship to Youden's index. Kraemer (1988) proposes prevalence-corrected ROC curves.

REFERENCES

Altman, D. G. (1991). *Practical statistics for medical research*. Chapman and Hall, London.

Armitage, P. and Berry, G. (1987). *Statistical methods in medical research*. Blackwell, Oxford.

Bland, M. (1987). *An introduction to medical statistics*. Oxford University Press, Oxford.

Bland, J. M. and Altman, D. G. (1986). Statistical methods for assessing agreement between two methods of clinical mesurement. *Lancet*, **i**, 307–10.

Bland, J. M., Peacock, J. L., Anderson, H. R., Brooke, O. G., and de Curtis, M. (1990) The adjustment of birthweight for very early gestational ages: two related problems in statistical analysis. *Applied Statistics*, **39**, 229–39.

British Standards Institution (1979). *Precision of test methods 1: guide for the determination and reproducibility of a standard test method*. BSI, London.

Cole, T. J. (1988). Fitting smoothed centile curves to reference data (with discussion). *Journal of the Royal Statistical Society A*, **151**, 385–418.

Erskine, R. L. A. and Ritchie, J. W. K. (1985). Umbilical artery blood flow characteristics in normal and growth retarded fetuses. *British Journal of Obstetrics and Gynaecology*, **92**, 605–10.

Gill, R. W., Kossoff, G., Warren P. S., and Garrett W. J. 1984). Umbilical venous flow in normal complicated pregnancy. *Ultrasound in Medicine and Biology*, **10**, 349–64.

Goldstein, H. (1986). Efficient statistical modelling of longitudinal data. *Annals of Human Biology* **13**, 129–41.

Healy, M. J. R. (1974). Notes on the statistics of growth standards. *Annals of Human Biology*, **1**, 41–6.

Kraemer. H. C. (1988). Assessment of 2 × 2 associations: generalizations of signal-detection methodology. *The American Statistician*, **42**, 37–49.

Pearce, J. M. (1988). An evaluation of Doppler waveforms in the assessment of complicated pregnancies. MD thesis, University of Sheffield.

Pearce, J. M., Campbell, S., Cohen-Overbeek, T., Hackett, G., Hernandez, J., and Royston, J. P. (1988). Reference ranges and sources of variation for indices of pulsed Doppler flow velocity waveforms from the uteroplacental and fetal circulation. *British Journal of Obstetrics and Gynaecology*, **95**, 248–56.

Pearson, E. S. and Hartley, H. O. (1970). *Biometrika tables for statisticians*, Vol. 1.3 (3rd edn). Cambridge University Press, Cambridge.

Royston, J. P. (1991). Constructing time-specific reference ranges. *Statistics in Medicine*, **10**, 675–90.

Steel, S. A., Pearce, J. M., Nash, G., Christopher, B., Dormandy, J., and Bland, J. M. (1988). Maternal blood viscosity and uteroplacental blood flow velocity waveforms in normal and complicated pregnancies. *British Journal of Obstetrics and Gynaecology*, **95**, 747–52.

Thompson, M. L. and Theron, G. B. (1990). Maximum likelihood estimation of reference centiles. *Statistics in Medicine* **9**, 539–48.

Thompson, R. S., Trudinger, B. J., Cook, C. M., and Giles, W. B. (1988). Umbilical artery waveforms: normal reference values for A/B ratio and Pourcelot ratio. *British Journal of Obstetrics and Gynaecology*, **95**, 589–91.

van Vugt, J. M. G., Ruissen, C. J., Nienhuis, S. J., Hoogland, H. J., and de Haan, J. (1988). Comparison of blood velocity waveform indices recorded by pulsed Doppler and continuous wave Doppler in the umbilical artery. *Journal of Clinical Ultrasound*, **16**, 573–6.

Vyas, S., Nicolaides, K. H., Bower, S., and Campbell, S. (1990). Middle cerebral artery flow velocity waveforms in fetal hypoxaemia. *British Journal of Obstetrics and Gynaecology*, **97**, 797–803.

II CONTINUOUS WAVE DOPPLER ULTRASOUND

3. Signal acquisition and reporting results

Peter McParland and Malcolm Pearce

INTRODUCTION

The introduction of Doppler ultrasound to obstetrics initially promised measurement of actual blood flow which previously had relied on invasive techniques. However, volume flow measurements have not achieved widespread popularity: first, the technique is cumbersome; second, it requires pulsed wave equipment which is expensive; and finally, and most importantly, there is a large inherent error in measurements of volume flow. Attention has therefore turned to study of the maximum frequency envelope in an attempt to overcome the appreciable methodological errors inherent in quantitative flow measurement. This chapter aims to describe the technique in obtaining waveforms with continuous wave (CW) Doppler equipment and to identify the various factors that influence the waveform.

THE FLOW VELOCITY WAVEFORM

Terminology

The waveforms illustrated in Fig. 3.1 is obtained from the umbilical artery and vein in a normal pregnancy in the third trimester. As described in Chapter 1 (see Fig. 1.6), the vertical axis represents the Doppler-shifted frequencies whilst the horizontal axis is time. In addition, the grey scale of each pixel represents the number of targets that caused that particular Doppler-shifted frequency at that moment in time. This method of representing Doppler data is usually commonly known as a *Doppler sonogram*, or just a sonogram.

As Doppler-shifted frequencies are directly proportional to the velocity of the target, the sonogram also represents the change in velocities with time. For this reason, the sonogram is often referred to as a *flow velocity waveform*.

What the waveform represents

The shape of the waveform reflects the pulsatile nature of blood flow in an artery. Fetal cardiac contraction causes a force, in the form of pressure, to

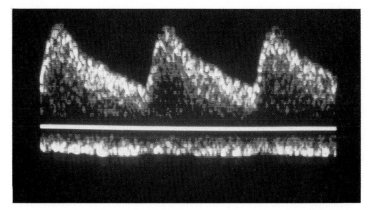

Fig. 3.1 Flow velocity waveform from the umbilical cord. The upper channel of the spectrum analyser shows the umbilical artery waveform and the lower channel shows the venous waveform. The colour scale of each individual pixel represents the number of targets moving with that particular velocity at that instant in time. The more yellow the colour scale, the greater the number of cells.

be applied to the red blood cells in the aorta and umbilical arteries. A high forward pressure gradient is generated and blood cells accelerate rapidly, producing the rising slope of the umbilical artery waveform (Fig. 3.1). The rate of acceleration depends on the density of the blood, the elasticity of the vessel wall, and the pressure of gradient generated (McDonald 1974). As the pressure moves away from the heart the gradient is reversed, acceleration ceases, the blood reaches its highest systolic velocity, and then decelerates resulting in the descending slope of the waveform. The velocity

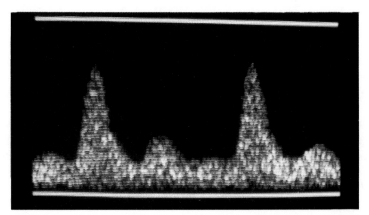

Fig. 3.2 Continuous wave recording from the brachial artery with the hand open.

at the end of diastole and the rate of deceleration are thought to reflect peripheral resistance.

Figure 3.2 is a CW recording from the brachial artery with the hand open, a situation that may be considered as representing low peripheral resistance. There is forward flow, represented by Doppler-shifted frequency in the upper channel of the spectrum analyser throughout the cardiac cycle. When the hand is closed and a fist is formed, the peripheral resistance increases. Figure 3.3 illustrates the brachial artery waveform in this situation. Doppler-shifted frequencies are absent from parts of diastole, representing cessation of blood flow at these times. If the peripheral resistance is even higher, then Doppler-shifted frequencies may be observed in the lower channel of the spectrum analyser. This is the normal situation in the external iliac artery with the patient at rest (Fig. 3.4).

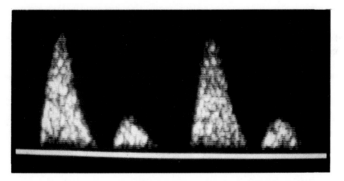

Fig. 3.3 Continuous wave recording from the brachial artery with the fist closed.

TECHNIQUE OF OBTAINING WAVEFORMS FROM THE UMBILICAL ARTERY

Equipment

Waveforms from the umbilical and uteroplacental circulation can be acquired with relatively simple CW equipment, which has the added advantage of being relatively cheap (about £7000). This essentially consists of a 2–4 MHz probe, a spectrum analyser, a loudspeaker, and a monitor for visual display. It may additionally have a recording device (usually an audio-tape recorder) or a computer disc system and a device for printing the waveforms such as a video printer.

Most simple CW equipment is little more than the Doppler heart-rate detector that obstetricians and midwives use to demonstrate the baby's heart beat to the mother. The main difference (and the reason for the

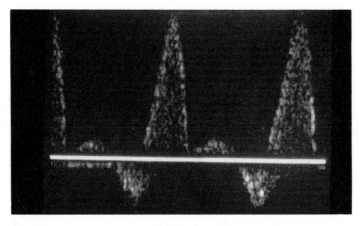

Fig. 3.4 Continuous wave recording from the external iliac artery with the patient at rest. This is a situation where the peripheral resistance is so great that flow is reversed, resulting in Doppler-shifted frequencies being recorded in the opposite channel.

added expense) is the presence of the spectrum analyser and the visual display. These, however, are essential for ensuring that the waveform is free from noise and uncontaminated by signal from other blood vessels, and for performing calculations.

Machine controls are usually very simple and consist of:

1. A sweep speed control. This determines the rate at which the waveforms cross the screen. A good starting point is 5 m/s.

2. A frequency range control. This determines the height of the waveform above the baseline and usually has four settings such as 2, 4, 8, and 16 kHz. The higher the frequency the lower the waveform. Four kilohertz is a good starting point.

3. The vessel wall (thump) filter control. This should be set to as low as possible, i.e. 50–65 Hz.

4. A control that sets the height of the baseline. If this is set so that the baseline is in the centre of the screen (see Fig. 3.10), both channels of the analyser can easily be seen. If, as in the uteroplacental circulation, there is unlikely to be a waveform in one channel then the baseline should be arranged so that the waveform fills most of the screen (see Fig. 3.11).

5. A gain control. Turning this up amplifies the Doppler-shifted signal.

6. A volume control for the loudspeaker.

7. A colour selector. This is purely a matter of personal preference. The choices are usually a grey scale, a red-orange scale, or a blue-green scale. The red-orange scale (on a black screen) is favoured by many operators because the contrast allows sharp waveforms.

8. A maximum frequency envelope follower. This draws a line around the maximum frequency outline (Fig. 3.5) and allows automatic, on-line calculations. However, it should not be employed until the operator is satisfied that the displayed waveform has a clear outline. Following automatic calculations, it should be possible to freeze the screen so that the chosen waveforms can be inspected for quality.

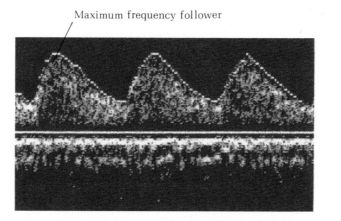

Maximum frequency follower

Fig. 3.5 Waveform from umbilical artery, illustrating the maximum frequency follower (the dotted white line).

Method

The initial description of obtaining umbilical artery flow velocity waveform (FVW) was by Fitzgerald and Drumm (1977), and the technique remains basically the same. The pregnant woman assumes a comfortable, semi-recumbent position. The abdomen may then be palpated to identify the fetal spine and limbs, as the umbilical cord is usually in close proximity to the limbs. A small amount of acoustic coupling gel is put on the maternal abdomen and the probe is applied. Very quickly the operator learns to recognize the typical signal from the umbilical artery (see Fig. 3.1). The signal is usually heard before it is visualized. Because the umbilical cord is usually surrounded by a pool of amniotic fluid, it is difficult to confuse its signal with that from other vessels.

Once the waveform is visible on the screen, small movements of the probe should be made so that the clearest maximum frequency outline is obtained. The waveform should be pure, in that it should be free from signals from other vessels. Alter the range setting such that the signal fills at least two-thirds of the channel and then alter the gain so that there is a sharp cut-off between the maximum frequency and the blank space above. If the machine has a maximum frequency follower, it should now be turned on. If not, the screen is frozen and calculations are made by means of cursers, a light pen, or a tracker ball. It is customary to attempt to display the umbilical vein in the opposite channel of the analyser. A steady signal (see Fig. 3.1) indicates fetal apnoea.

Problems

1. Failure to obtain any signal:
    (i) Check the machine is correctly set up and that all the connections are tight.
    (ii) Use real-time ultrasound to determine: (a) whether the baby is alive; and (b) the site of a loop of cord.

2. A contaminated signal
    (i) Contamination with maternal vessels is usually easy to recognize because of the slower maternal heart rate. Angling the probe will usually improve the signal: if not try a different spot on the uterus.
    (ii) Contamination of the artery with the venous signal. As the umbilical cord has coiled vessels, it is possible to record artery and vein in one channel with their waveforms superimposed on each other. The effect of this may be that the umbilical vein signal covers the diastolic component of the arterial FVW. Slight angulation will result in the vein appearing in the opposite channel.
    (iii) Recording both arteries—one in each channel. In virtually all cases the waveforms are identical, supporting the idea that on the placenta the umbilical arteries anastomose and then branch and are distributed to overlapping areas. The result of this is not invariable and there have been reports of obtaining two different waveforms in the same patient in association with extensive placental infarction (Trudinger *et al.* 1988).

Absence of end-diastolic frequencies

Absence of end-diastolic frequencies (AEDF) has serious clinical implications (for example, see McParland *et al.* 1990) and care must be taken to ensure that this finding is real. In Chapter 7, Fig. 7.1 illustrates AEDF, while Fig. 7.2 illustrates reversed frequencies in end-diastole. Artefactual AEDF may be due to:

1. A vessel wall filter that is set too high. Reduce the filter setting to its minimum position, usually 50–65 Hz. This will allow low-level Doppler-shifted frequencies to become apparent.

2. A high angle of insonation. Figure 3.6 illustrates the effect of changing the angle of insonation on the height of the waveform.

3. Fetal movement or breathing movement. This can cause marked changes in the umbilical artery waveform (see below). Fetal apnoea can be demonstrated by steady-state flow in the umbilical vein. Even if this is not recorded, with a little practice it is easy to recognize the changes in the waveform (Fig. 3.7).

AEDF may be confirmed as follows:

1. If only CW equipment is available, then a policy such as that adopted as St. George's Hospital is advisable. AEDF was reported only when umbilical artery recordings had been obtained from two different sites on the maternal abdomen, on two successive days.

2. If PW or duplex equipment is available, then record the signal from the descending fetal aorta (see Chapters 11 and 12). In almost all

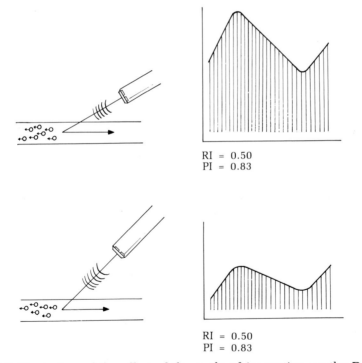

RI = 0.50
PI = 0.83

RI = 0.50
PI = 0.83

Fig. 3.6 Illustration of the effect of the angle of insonation on the Doppler waveform. The greater the angle between the beam and the vessel, the lower the resultant waveform. Note, however, that the indices do not change.

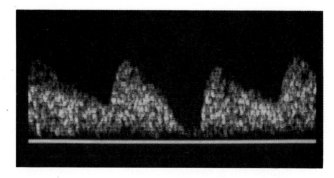

Fig. **3.7** Umbilical artery waveform recorded during fetal breathing movements.

cases where the umbilical artery shows AEDF, frequencies cannot be recorded in end-diastole in the aortic waveform.

Twins

Several groups have described the use of Doppler ultrasound in twin pregnancies. Most have utilized duplex equipment with pulsed Doppler and real-time ultrasound; thus the sample gate can be placed in the appropriate umbilical cord of the fetus under study. Several studies using CW have also been described. The methodology used by Farmakides *et al.* (1985) involved placing the Doppler transducer on the lateral half of the uterus to identify one of the twins. The second cord was then looked for on the other side of the uterus; although efforts were made to ensure that the Doppler probe was pointing in difficult directions, one cannot be sure which waveform belongs to which twin, and this method cannot be commended.

Thus it has been suggested that if CW equipment is to be used, it is necessary first to visualize the fetus to be studied with real-time ultrasound and to use this to guide the Doppler probe. The real-time machine can be used to observe fetal heart rate motion and is then matched with the audible signal from the umbilical artery (Giles *et al.* 1985). Problems may be encountered when both umbilical cords are close to each other *in utero* with similar heart rates.

ANALYSIS OF THE FLOW VELOCITY WAVEFORM

Almost all groups have reported indices based upon the maximum velocity envelope; the commonly used indices are illustrated in Figure 3.8. Using

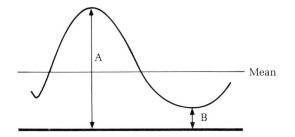

Fig. 3.8 Derivation of the indices commonly used to characterize the maximum frequency envelope. A, maximum systolic frequency; B, least diastolic frequency. A/B = A/B ratio (Stuart *et al.* 1980); A−B/A = resistance index (Pourcelot 1974); A−B/mean = pulsatility index (Gosling and King 1975).

this simplistic approach disregards much of the information that may be obtained from the sonogram, but has the following advantages:

1. The maximum frequency envelope is usually recorded even when the vessel is insonated in a non-uniform manner.

2. The maximum frequency envelope is not distorted by high-amplitude, low-frequency signals from the vessel walls.

3. The maximum frequency envelope is usually recognizable even with poor-quality signals such as those that may be obtained in the presence of oligohydramnios or excessive maternal obesity.

4. The indices are simple to calculate, especially the A/B ratio (commonly called the S/D ratio in the American literature) and the resistance index (RI).

Most of the literature of Doppler waveforms from the umbilical artery has reported on these indices and has then attempted to demonstrate correlations with pregnancy outcome measures. Thus, observation and statistics rather than actual fluid mechanics have provided the framework for interpretation of Doppler waveforms.

Choice of index

All three indices are very highly correlated (Thompson *et al.* 1986, 1988; Mulders *et al.* 1987: Pearce *et al.* 1988). The RI and the A/B ratio are related mathematically as follows:

$$A/B = 1/(1 - RI)$$

The pulsatility index (PI), unlike the A/B ratio and the RI, involves the whole waveform and not just the maximum and minimum points, and it has not been suggested that this index should yield more information and therefore be more useful. This has not been shown to date, and in the clinical setting it is unlikely that one index offers any clear advantage over the others. The accuracy of such simple analysis of FVWs can be improved if the chosen index is calculated over three to five consecutive cardiac cycles, with the mean value being used for further analysis.

Factors affecting the flow velocity waveform

Heart rate   If the heart rate slows, then the value of the end-diastolic frequency is likely to fall, giving a corresonding increase in A/B ratio, RI, and PI. Conversely, if the fetal heart rate accelerates, the end-diastolic frequencies may increase, thus lowering the A/B, RI, and PI. Several studies that address the relationship between fetal heart rate (FHR) and FVW have been published.

In the fetal circulation, Mires *et al.* (1987) reported a significant negative correlation ($r = -0.49$) between umbilical artery A/B ratio and instanta-neous FHR, and suggested that A/B ratios should be corrected for FHR even within the normal range (120–160 beats per minute (b.p.m)). Other studies, however, have suggested that umbilical artery A/B ratios are independent of FHR within the normal range (Thompson *et al.* 1986, 1988; Gagnon *et al.* 1988; Gudmundsson and Marsal 1988; Kofinas *et al.* 1989). However, the A/B ratio is likely to be lowered significantly in the presence of fetal tachycardia (> 160 b.p.m.) and elevated in the presence of fetal bradycardia (< 120 b.p.m.). Most authors do not make corrections for heart rate as the marked changes in the umbilical artery waveform that occur due to increased placental vascular resistance overshadow the small variation that occurs because of heart rate changes.

Fetal breathing movements   All healthy fetuses periodically exhibit breathing movements, including contraction of the diaphragm, inward movements of the thorax, and expansion of the abdominal wall (Marsal 1978). Such movements result in marked effects on the fetal circulation and thus affect the peak systolic and diastolic frequencies, in addition to alter-ing the length of the cardiac cycle (see Fig. 3.7). During the respiratory cycle, flow velocities in the umbilical artery show a reduction in both systolic peak and end-diastolic velocities on inspiration and an increase in expiration. This probably results from an opening of pulmonary vascular bed on inspiration with a consequent reduction in the ventricular output directed through the ductus and down the aorta. Indeed Doppler ultra-sonography has in fact been described as a method for detecting fetal breathing movements (Boyle *et al.* 1986). Because of this variation with fetal breathing movements, Doppler waveforms from the umbilical artery should be recorded only during fetal apnoea; to establish that the fetus is not breathing, a sequence of 15–20 cycles demonstrating a smooth non-undulating venous signal with identical arterial waveforms should be observed.

Blood viscosity   There appears to be minimal change in the umbilical artery A/B ratio with an increase in whole blood viscosity (Steel *et al.* 1989*b*), but any change that is observed is more marked at high shear rates (Giles and Trudinger 1986). In the maternal circulation, however, small changes in viscosity do not appear to influence the FVW (Steel *et al.* 1988*a*), suggesting that changes in vascular architecture are more important.

Behavioural states   There is now clear evidence for the existence of behavioural states in the human fetus in late pregnancy (Nijhuis *et al.* 1982). Four distinct states are described.

State 1F: The fetus is largely quiescent but regular, brief body movements—mostly startles—may occur. Eye movements are absent and the heart rate is stable, with a small oscillation band-width (less than 10 b.p.m.). Isolated accelerations may occur, but are strictly related to movements.

State 2F: There are frequent and periodic gross body movements—mainly stretches and retroflexion together with movements of the extremities. Eye movements are continually present. The heart rate shows a wider oscillation band-width (more than 10 b.p.m.), and there are frequent accelerations during movement.

State 3F: Gross fetal body movements are absent but eye movements are continually present. The heart rate is stable but with a wider oscillation band-width than seen in state 1F; there are no accelerations.

State 4F: There is vigorous continual activity—mainly trunk movements. Eye movements are continually present. The heart rate is unstable with large, long-lasting accelerations, frequently fused into a sustained tachycardia.

At 38 weeks' gestation, these states are observed 32, 42, 1, and 7 per cent of the time, respectively.

The relationship between aortic, umbilical, and carotid artery FVWs in states 1F and 2F in both normal and abnormal pregnancies has been investigated (van Eyck *et al.* 1985, 1986, 1987, 1988). Based on the marked changes in FHR patterns and incidence of fetal body movements between different behavioural states, it is likely that these changes are associated with alterations in fetal cardiovascular performance and peripheral resistance which may affect the FVW; therefore, Doppler studies should probably be performed in the absence of body movements to allow for direct comparison between studies.

Interestingly, small-for-gestational age (SGA) fetuses show no differences in the umbilical artery waveform (or the aortic or carotid waveforms) between states 1F and 2F. It is suggested that the redistribution of blood flow that is observed in SGA fetuses over-rides the changes that occur between behavioural states.

Comparison of CW and PW as methods of obtaining umbilical artery waveforms

Several studies have compared PW and CW Doppler ultrasonography and have demonstrated no differences in indices obtained from FVW of the umbilical artery (Brar *er al.* 1988; Mehalek *et al.* 1988; van Vugt *et al.* 1988) between the two methods.

Reproducibility

It is important with any investigation to be aware of the possible sources of variation. The hope is that the investigation varies markedly between the normal and the pathological cases but that there is little variation within these groups. Sources of variation are discussed in more detail in Chapter 2, together with the statistical means for analysing and reporting the variation.

Variation between operators in acquiring and reporting indices from the umbilical artery has been reported as insignificant by several authors (Reuwer *et al.* 1984; Nienhuis *et al.* 1988; Pearce *et al.* 1988). Many studies unfortunately report variation in terms of a coefficient of variation (CV), and in most cases the means by which this has been derived is not detailed. Such studies include those of Murills *et al.* (1987) and Maulik *et al.* (1989), who report an interobserver CV of about 10 per cent, and those of Murills *et al.* (1987) and Davies *et al.* (1990), which report an intraobserver CV of up to 12 per cent. These latter studies are hard to interpret but it appears to be justifiable to conclude that differences within or between observers do not significantly alter interpretation of umbilical artery Doppler-shifted waveforms.

UTEROPLACENTAL WAVEFORMS

There is less information available in the literature on uteroplacental FVWs. The original method described by Campbell *et al.* (1983) used a pulsed Doppler system. The common iliac artery was visualized where it bifurcates into the external and internal iliac arteries. With the Doppler transducer directed caudally, signals from the internal iliac were obtained. The FVW of the internal iliac artery shows continuous forward flow during diastole, with a deep notch in relation to closure of the aortic valve (Fig. 3.9). If the transducer was directed more medially, vessels in the lateral uterine wall could be identified. These vessels vary from 2 to 4 mm in diameter. It is uncertain as to whether these are the uterine artery or its first branch, the arcuate artery, and they are best referred to as utero-placental vessels. Doppler signals obtained in normal pregnancy typically show a pattern of low pulsatility with high end-diastolic frequencies (Fig. 3.10)

Anatomy of the uteroplacental circulation

As the FVWs from the uteroplacental circulation have a characteristic pattern, they can also be acquired using CW ultrasound. Interpretation of such waveforms, however, has proved more difficult than those from the umbilical artery and this is largely explained by the complexity of the uteroplacental circulation. Each uterine artery gives off approximately eight arcuate arteries that encircle the uterine surface and form anastomoses with the contralateral side. The arcuate arteries give off radial arteries which eventually lead to about 200 spiral arteries, which supply the inter-villous space. Waveforms can be obtained from virtually all over the uterus and presumably from all types of vessels. It is thus impossible to say with CW Doppler whether an individual waveform represents uterine, radial, arcuate, or spiral artery, and thus the waveforms are generally termed uteroplacental waveforms.

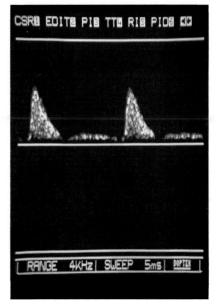

Fig. 3.9 (Left) Flow velocity waveform from the internal iliac artery.

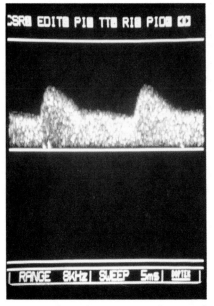

Fig. 3.10 Flow velocity waveform from a normal uteroplacental vessel.

Technique

With the woman in a comfortable semi-recumbent position, a little acoustic coupling gel is put on the maternal abdomen. Set the CW machine to a sweep speed of 5 m/s and a frequency range of 4 kHz, and turn the loudspeaker volume up until static noise is just audible.

Holding a 4 MHz CW probe vertically, imagine the point at which the iliac vessel crosses posterior to the uterus and then place the probe on this point. While listening to the loudspeaker output, the probe is angled until a signal is obtained. This will usually be from the external (see Fig. 3.4) or internal (see Fig. 3.9) iliac artery. The probe is gently slided medially until a waveform of very low pulsatility is heard. Small movements of the transducer, together with alterations in the gain, should then produce a waveform with a clear maximum frequency envelope. Turn on the maximum frequency follower or freeze the waveforms on the screen, and perform the required calculations as for the umbilical artery.

Problems

Most operators quickly learn the technique and can acquire waveforms from both sides of the uterus from 16 weeks' gestation to term. Maternal obesity may make signal acquisition impossible. Problems may arise as follows:

1. Failure to obtain a signal.

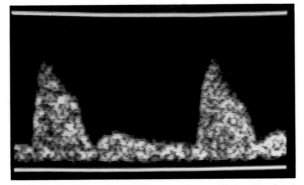

Fig. 3.11 Pathological uteroplacental waveform. Note the biphasic systolic deceleration slope which distinguishes this from an internal iliac artery waveform. There is also a deep dichrotic notch.

(i) If no signal at all is obtained, the machine settings and connections should be carefully checked.

(ii) Failure to locate a uteroplacental vessel. Relocate the iliac vessels and then angle the probe slightly in a caudal direction whilst sliding medially. If the probe is allowed to go too far medially, a signal from the umbilical artery is often obtained. If this is the case then the window between this signal and that from the iliac vessels is established and should be carefully searched. If failure does occur, the only resort is colour flow Doppler ultrasonography.

2. Failure to distinguish a pathological waveform from the internal iliac artery signal. Figure 3.11 illustrates a pathological uteroplacental waveform. It is readily distinguishable from the signal from the internal iliac artery (see Fig. 3.9) by the biphasic systolic deceleration slope.

3. Varying waveforms from different sites on the uterus. Most of the problems in interpretation of uteroplacental FVWs relate to the inability to define clearly which vessel is being insonated. In an attempt to overcome this problem, various groups have described the approximate site on the uterus from where the waveforms were obtained. Trudinger *er al.* (1985*a,b*) obtained FVWs from branches in the placental bed, having first located the placenta with real-time ultrasound. Where possible, the centre of the placental bed was examined. When the placenta was implanted posteriorly, a more peripheral part of the bed was recorded mid-way along the lateral uterine margin. Others have recorded measurements from the region of the right and left uterine arteries, which are then labelled placental side or non-placental side depending on their proximity to the placental bed (Pearce *et al.* 1988). This is a rather arbitrary designation as the placenta often covers a large area of the uterine surface and may be centrally placed.

It has been suggested that a large difference between the right and left uterine FVWs indicates that one artery is the dominant supplier to the placenta, and that this error in placentation may contribute to the development of pre-eclampsia and intra-uterine growth retardation (Schulman *et al.* 1987). This view has been challenged by Bewley *et al.* (1989), who recorded waveforms from four sites in the uterus: those acquired from the site where the uterine artery would be expected to be on either side,and also waveforms obtained from either side of the uterine fundus. The waveforms were further subclassified as placental or non-placental according to the site of the placenta. This group demonstrated that waveforms from the placental side of the uterus demonstrated a consistently lower RI than those obtained from the non-placental side. This work has been confirmed by Kofinas *et al.* (1988). This subject is dealt with further in Chapters 4 and 6.

REPORTING CW DOPPLER WAVEFORMS

Umbilical artery waveforms

The mean A/B ratio from three to five ideal waveforms should be reported, together with a comment as to whether the results lie within the data reference range that is in use within the department (see Chapter 4). However, evidence is accumulating that, in the absence of an acute event, it is very unlikely that end-diastolic frequencies will be lost within 1 week, so it may be sufficient to state whether end-diastolic frequencies are present or absent.

In cases with AEDF, the A/B ratio become infinity and the RI become unity. There is no evidence that the PI is of any use in these situations, so the findings should be reported in words: 'End-diastolic frequencies in the umbilical artery are absent' or 'There is reversal of end-diastolic frequencies'.

Uteroplacental waveforms

There is no standard method of reporting such waveforms but we (Pearce and McParland 1991) have suggested that both sides of the uterus should be examined and the waveforms reported as follows:

1. Uniform low resistance: waveforms from both sides of the uterus have a RI of less than 0.58.

2. Uniform high resistance: waveforms from both sides of the uterus have a RI of more than 0.58.

2. Mixed resistance pattern: one waveform (almost invariably that from the placental side) is of low resistance (RI < 0.58) while the waveform from the other side is of high resistance.

See Chapters 4 and 6 for further discussion and clinical applications.

REFERENCES

Brar, H. S., Medearis, A. L., DeVore, G. R., and Platt, L. D. (1988). Fetal umbilical velocimetry using continuous wave and pulsed-wave Doppler ultrasound in high-risk pregnancies: a comparison of systolic to diastolic rations. *Obstetrics and Gynecology*, **72**, 607–10.

Bewley, S., Campbell, S., and Cooper, D. (1989). Uteroplacental Doppler flow velocity waveforms in the second trimester. A complex circulation. *British Journal of Obstetrics and Gynaecology*, **96**, 1040–6.

Boyle, E. G., Davies, G. S., Gough, J. D., and Poore, E. R. (1986). Doppler ultrasound method for detecting human fetal breathing movements *in utero*. *British Medical Journal*, **i**, 17–18.

Campbell, S., Griffin, D. R., Pearce, J. M., Diaz-Recasens, J., Cohen-Overbeek, T. E., and Willson, K. (1983). New Doppler technique for assessing uteroplacental blood flow. *Lancet*, **i**, 675–7.

Davies, J. A., Lee, A., and Spencer, J. A. D. (1990). Variability of continuous wave Doppler flow velocity waveform indices from the umbilical artery. *Obstetrics and Gynecology*, **157**, 680–5.

Farmakides, G., Schulman, H., Saldan, L. R., Bracero, L. A., Fleischer, A., and Rochelson, B. (1985). Surveillance of twin pregnancy with umbilical arterial velocimetry. *American Journal of Obstetrics and Gynecology*, **153**, 789–92.

Fitzgerald, D. E. and Drumm, J. E. (1977). Non-invasive measurement of human fetal circulation using ultrasound: a new method. *British Medical Journal*, **2**, 1450–1.

Gagnon, R., Morrow, R., Ritchie, K., Hunse, C., and Patrick, J. 1988). Umbilical and uterine artery blood flow velocities after vibratory acoustic stimulation. *American Journal of Obstetrics and Gynecology*, **159**, 574–8.

Giles, W. B. and Trudinger, B. J. (1986). Umbilical cord whole blood viscosity and the umbilical artery velocity time waveforms: a correlation. *British Journal of Obstetrics and Gynaecology*, **93**, 466–70.

Giles, W. B., Trudinger, B. J., and Baird, P. J. (1985). Fetal umbilical artery flow velocity waveforms and placental resistance: pathological correlation. *British Journal of Obstetrics and Gynaecology*, **92**, 31–8.

Gosling, R. G. and King, D. H. (1975). Ultrasound angiology. In *Ultrasonic angiology in arteries and veins* (ed. A. Harcus and L. Adamson), pp. 61–98. Churchill Livingstone, Edinburgh.

Gudmundsson, S. and Marsal, K. (1988). Umbilical artery and uteroplacental blood flow velocity waveforms in normal pregnancy—a cross-sectional study. *Acta Obstetrica Gynecologica Scandinavica*, **67**, 347–54.

Kofinas, A. D., Penry, M., Greiss, F. C., Meis, P. J., and Nelson, L. H. (1988). The effect of placental location on uterine artery flow velocity waveforms. *American Journal of Obstetrics and Gynecology*, **159**, 1504–8.

Kofinas, A. D., Espeland, M., Swain, M., Penry, M., and Nelson, L. H. (1989). Correcting umbilical artery flow velocity waveforms for fetal heart rate is unnecessary. *American Journal of Obstetrics and Gynecology*, **160**, 704–7.

McDonald, D. A. (1974). *Blood flow in arteries* (2nd edn). Edward Arnold, London.

McParland, P., Steel, S., and Pearce, J. M. (1990). The clinical implications of absent or reversed end-diastolic frequencies in umbilical artery flow velocity waveforms. *European Journal of Obstetrics, Gynecology, and Reproductive Biology*, **37**, 15–23.

Marsal, K. (1978). Fetal breathing movements in man—characteristics and clinical significance. *Obstetrics and Gynecology*, **52**, 394–401.

Maulik, D., Yarlagadda, P., Youngblood, J. P., and Willoughby, L. (1989). Components of variability of umbilical arterial Doppler velocimetry—A prospective analysis, *American Journal of Obstetrics and Gynaecology*, **160**, 1406–12.

Mehalek, K. E., Berkowitz, G. S., Chitkara, U., Rosenberg, J. and Berkowitz, R. L. (1988). Comparison of continuous-wave and pulsed Doppler S/D ratios of umbilical and uterine arteries. *Obstetrics and Gynecology*, **72**, 603–6.

Mires, G., Dempster, J., Patel, N. B., and Crawford, J. W. (1987). The effect of fetal heart rate on umbilical artery flow velocity waveforms. *British Journal of Obstetrics and Gynaecology*, **94**, 665–9.

Mulders, L. G. M., Wijn, P. F. F., Jongsma, H. W., and Hein, P. R. (1987). A comparative study of three indices of umbilical blood flow in relation to prediction of growth retardation. *Journal of Perinatal Medicine*, **15**, 3–12.

Murills, A. J., Gorman, F., Bamford, P. N., Gazzard, V. M., and Keen, A. C. (1987). Reproducibility in umbilical artery blood velocity waveforms. In *Obstetric and neonatal blood flow*. Conference Proceedings, Vol. 2. Royal College of Surgeons, Biological Engineering Society, London.

Nienhuis, S. J., van Vugt, J. M., Hoogland, H. J., Ruissen, C. J., and de Haan, J. (1988). Interexaminer variability of fetal Doppler velocity waveforms. *Gynecology and Obstetric Investigation*, **25**, 152–7.

Nijhuis, J. G., Prechtl, H. F., Martin, C. B., and Bots, R. S. (1982). Are there behavioural states in the human fetus? *Early Development*, **6**, 177–95.

Pearce, J. M. and MacParland, P. (1991). Uteroplacental circulation. *Contemporary Reviews in Obstetrics and Gynaecology*, **3**, 6–12.

Pearce, J. M., Campbell, S., Cohen-Overbeek, T. E., Hackett, G. A., Hernandez, J., and Royston, J. P. (1988). References ranges and sources of variation for indices of pulsed Doppler flow velocity waveforms from the uteroplacental and fetal circulation. *British Journal of Obstetrics and Gynaecology*, **95**, 248–56.

Pourcelot, L. (1974). Applications cliniques de l'examen Doppler transcutane. In *Velocimetric ultrasonor Doppler* (ed. P. Peronneau), pp. 213–40. Inserm 7–11, October 34, Paris.

Reuwer, P. J., Nuyen, W. C., Beijer, H. J., *et al.* (1984). Characteristics of flow velocities in the umbilical arteries assessed by Doppler ultrasound. *European Journal of Obstetrics and Gynaecology*, **17**, 397–408.

Schulman, H., Ducey, J., Farmakides, G., and Fleischer, A. (1987). Uterine artery Doppler velocimetry: the significance of divergent systolic/diastolic ratios. *American Journal of Obstetrics and Gynecology*, **157**, 1539–42.

Steel, S. A., Pearce, J. M., Nash, G., Christopher, B., Dormandy, J., and Bland, J. M. (1988). Maternal blood viscosity and uteroplacental blood flow velocity waveforms in normal and complicated pregnancies. British Journal of Obstetrics and Gynaecology, **95**, 747–52.

Steel, S. A., Pearce, J. M., Nash, G., Christopher, B., Dormandy, J., and Bland, J. M. (1989). Correlation between Doppler flow velocity waveforms and cord blood viscosity. *British Journal of Obstetrics and Gynaecology*, **96**, 1168–72.

Stuart, B., Drumm, J., Fitzgerald, D. E., and Duignan, N. M. (1980). Fetal blood velocity waveforms in normal pregnancy. *British Journal of Obstetrics and Gynaecology*, **87**, 780–5.

Thompson, R. S., Trudinger, B. J., and Cook, C. M. (1986). A comparison of Doppler ultrasound waveform indices in the umbilical artery—1. Indices derived from the maximum velocity waveform. *Ultrasound in Medicine and Biology*, **12**, 835–44.

Thompson, R. S., Trudinger, B. J., and Cook, C. M. (1988). Doppler ultrasound waveform indices: A/B ratio, pulsatility index and Pourcelot ratio. *British Journal of Obstetrics and Gynaecology*, **95**, 581–8.

Trudinger, B. J. and Cook, C. M. (1988). Different umbilical artery flow velocity waveforms in one patient. *Obstetrics and Gynecology*, **71**, 1019–21.

Trudinger, B. J., Giles, W. B., and Cook, C. M. (1985*a*). Flow velocity waveforms in the maternal uteroplacental and fetal umbilical placental circulations. *American Journal of Obstetrics and Gynecology*, **152**, 155–63.

Trudinger, B. J., Giles, W. B., and Cook, C. M. (1985*b*). Uteroplacental blood flow velocity-time waveforms in normal and complicated pregnancy. *British Journal of Obstetrics and Gynaecology*, **92**, 39–45.

van Eyck, J., Wladimiroff, J. W., Noordam, M. J., Tonge, H. M., and Prechtl, H. F. R. (1985). The blood flow velocity waveform in the fetal descending aorta; its relationship to fetal behavioural states in normal pregnancy at 37–38 weeks, *Early Human Development*, **12**, 137–43.

van Eyck, J., Wladimiroff, J. W., Noordam, M. J., Tonge, H. M., and Prechtl, H. F. R. (1986). The blood flow velocity waveform in the fetal descending aorta; its relationship to behavioural states in the growth retarded fetus at 37–38 weeks of gestation. *Early Human Development*, **14**, 99–107.

van Eyck, J., Wladimiroff, J. W., Noordam, M. J., van den Wijngaard, J. A. G. W., and Prechtl, H. F. R. (1988). The blood flow velocity waveform in the fetal internal carotid and umbilical artery: its relation to fetal behavioural states in the growth retarded fetus at 37–38 weeks gestation. *British Journal of Obstetrics and Gynaecology*, **95**, 473–7.

van Eyck, J., Wladimiroff, J. W., van den Wijngaard, J. A. G. W., Noordam, M. J., and Precht, H. F. R. (1987). The blood flow velocity waveform in the fetal internal carotid and umbilical artery; its relation to fetal behavioural states in normal pregnancy at 37–38 weeks. *British Journal of Obstetrics and Gynaecology*, **94**, 736–41.

van Vugt, J. M. G., Ruissen, C. J., Nienhuis, S. J., Hoogland, H. J., and de Haan, J. (1988). Comparison of blood velocity waveform indices recorded by pulsed Doppler and continuous wave Doppler in the umbilical artery. *Journal of Clinical Ultrasound*, **16**, 573–6.

4. Doppler waveforms in normal pregnancy

Malcolm Pearce

INTRODUCTION

Chapter 3 describes the techniques of acquiring both umbilical artery and uteroplacental waveforms by means of continuous wave Doppler ultrasound equipment. This chapter discusses the results of such studies in normal preganancy.

UMBILICAL ARTERY WAVEFORMS

Introduction

As long ago as 1977, Fitzgerald and Drumm, using a combination of real-time imaging, pulsed wave and continuous wave Doppler ultrasound obtained signals from the umbilical cord. They demonstrated that reproducible signals were obtainable from both the umbilical artery and vein. The shape of the umbilical artery waveform changes during the course of pregnancy, with an increase in the diastolic component (Fig. 4.1) (Stuart *et al.* 1980).

Data reference ranges

Both longitudinal and cross-sectional data reference ranges have been established (Reuwer *et al.* 1984; Schulman *et al.* 1984, 1989; Erskine and Ritchie 1985; Trudinger *et al.* 1985*b*; Trudinger *et al.* 1985*c*; Gerson *et al.* 1987; Al-Ghazali *et al.* 1988; Gudmundsson and Marsal 1988; Pearce *et al.* 1988; Thompson *et al.* 1988; Hendricks *et al.* 1989).

All investigators have used a similar technique to obtain the flow velocity waveform. The Doppler probe is placed upon the maternal abdomen (with or without prior localization of the umbilical cord using real time ultrasound) and the umbilical artery waveform is recognized by its audible and visual signal (see Fig. 3.1). Table 4.1 lists the essential characteristics of each study.

Chapter 2 outlines the problems of establishing a data reference range. The studies in Table 4.1 may be criticized on the following grounds.

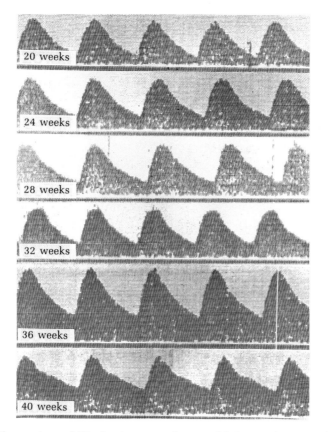

Fig. 4.1 Change in umbilical artery waveforms with increasing gestation. This is due mainly to an increase in the height of the diastolic frequencies. (Courtesy of Professor Brian Trudinger.)

Inappropriate sample selection   In theory, the sample selected should be representative of the whole pregnant population, but in practice the sample is often biased by the willingness of the patients to take part in the study—this is probably unavoidable. The sample should include healthy pregnant women, and whilst it is therefore reasonable to exclude women with diabetes or twins, women should not be excluded on data that are known only retrospectively, such as low birth-weight or pre-term delivery. The retrospective exclusion of such patients was reported in all studies listed in Table 4.1.

Cross-sectional versus longitudinal study   Longitudinal data are collected by authors who envisage carrying out serial studies on patients, looking

Table 4.1 Studies describing data reference ranges for umbilical artery waveforms

Reference	Method	No. of patients	Gestational range (weeks)	Comments
Reuwer *et al.* (1984)	PW/L	23	16–40	Mean PI ± SD in 2-weekly groups Large SD at <28 weeks
Schulman *et al.* (1984)	CW/?	89	15–41	Linear regression only from 25 weeks
Schulman *et al.* (1989)	CW/L	110	20–40	Mean ± SD in 2-weekly groups Large SD at <28 weeks
Trudinger *et al.* (1985)	CW/L	15	28–40	Mean ± SD in 2-weekly groups
Gerson *et al.* (1987)	PW/L	209	19–43	Mean ± SD in 4-weekly groups
Erskine and Ritchie (1985)	PW/L	15	16–40	Mean ± 2SD in 4-weekly groups Large SD at <24 weeks
Gudmundsson and Marsal (1988)	PW/L	125	20–42	Mean ± 2SD in 2-weekly groups Not smoothed
Al-Ghazali *et al.* (1988)	PW/C	271	16–42	5th, 50th, and 95th centiles—all data points shown
Pearce *et al.* (1988)	PW/L	34	16–40	Log transformation—all data points shown
Hendricks *et al.* (1989)	CW/C	590	12–44	Mean ± 1.96SD

Note: all studies appear to have retrospective exclusions.
C, cross-sectional; CW, continuous wave; L, longitudinal; PI, pulsatility index; PW, pulsed wave; SD, standard deviation.

for change. Such data should be plotted as the percentage fall in A/B ratio (or similar) with increasing gestation. Such charts do not exist for Doppler ultrasound indices, and studies that report longitudinal data in terms of raw indices are therefore flawed (see Chapter 2).

Schulman *et al.* (1984) do not state whether the study was longitudinal or cross-sectional, although their later study (Schulman *et al*. 1989) was clearly longitudinal involving monthly studies on 110 patients from 20 weeks' gestation to term. Studies by Trudinger *et al*. (1985*b*,*c*), Gerson *et al*., 1987, Pearce *et al*. 1988 Thompson *et al*. 1988, and Erskine and Ritchie 1985 are all longitudinal in nature. Hendricks *et al*. (1989) does not clearly state the type of study performed, although it appears also to be longitudinal.

Sample size   As stated in Chapter 2, in order to construct a reference range the data should change smoothly with gestation, represent the data at all gestational ages, and be as mathematically simple as possible. As the A/B ratio and resistance index are mathematically linked, only one data reference range should be derived and the other should be calculated.

Furthermore, the A/B ratio has been shown by several authors to be skewed (Thompson *et al*. 1988; Hendricks *et al*. 1989), but transformation of the resistance index produces an approximately normal distribution (Figs 4.2 and 4.3).

Before 18 weeks' gestation, end-diastolic frequencies are commonly not recordable (Fisk *et al*. 1988; Hendricks *et al*. 1989), so statistical manipulation of data is meaningless. In addition, all indices are highly skewed so that analysis by parametric data is not possible.

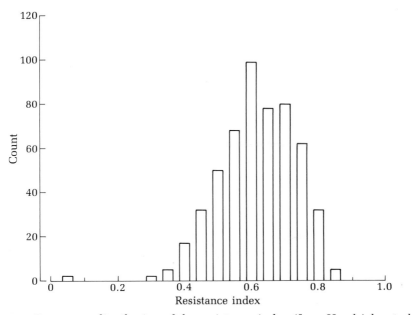

Fig. 4.2 Frequency distribution of the resistance index (from Hendricks *et al*. 1989).

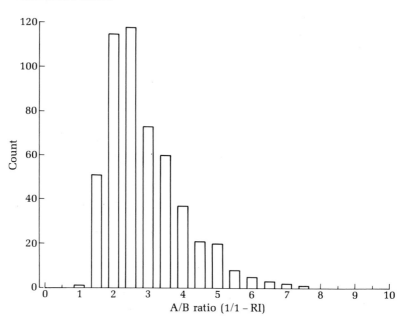

Fig. 4.3 Frequency distribution of the A/B ratio, derived from the resistance index (A/B = 1/1−RI) (from Hendricks *et al.* 1989).

The means for determining sample size for both cross-sectional and longitudinal data are given in Chapter 2. Most studies have too few patients.

Presentation Ideally, the lines representing the data reference range should be superimposed on all the data points so that the reader can judge the goodness of fit (see Fig. 2.7). There are few studies in which this is the case.

Studies that differ from clinical practice The method of acquiring and analysing the waveforms should be the same as that which is to be used clinically. Pearce *et al.* (1988) derived their data reference range after compensating for cardiac cycle length; this is not yet performed in clinical practice. The effects of heart rate on the A/B ratio are fully discussed in Chapter 3, but within physiological limits heart rate appears to have no significant effect on the A/B ratio.

Summary and recommendations

Presently, none of the available studies meets the criteria suggested in Chapter 2. The study by Hendricks *et al.* (1989) appears to be the least flawed: its disadvantages are that it uses longitudinal data and that retrospective exclusion of patients took place. Figure 4.4 illustrates the data reference range for the A/B ratio from these authors.

Figure 4.5 illustrates the mean change in A/B ratio with increasing gestation from several studies. All authors demonstrate a fall in A/B ratio with increasing gestation. This fall is almost entirely due to an increase in the diastolic component of the waveform, suggesting a fall in peripheral resistance. Trudinger *et al.* (1985*b*) believe this to be due entirely to the development of the umbilical arteriolar system with advancing gestation (see also Chapter 11). However, Pearce *et al.* (1988) demonstrated that after correcting for fetal heart rate the fall in the A/B ratio is not as great, and these authors believe that some of this change is due to the decrease in fetal heart rate that is observed with increasing gestation (Fig. 4.6).

UTEROPLACENTAL CIRCULATION

Introduction
The initial report of Doppler waveforms from the uteroplacental circulation (Campbell *et al.* 1983) followed a casual remark by the senior author. These authors used duplex real-time and pulsed Doppler ultrasound to obtain waveforms from vessels running through the myometrium. Having

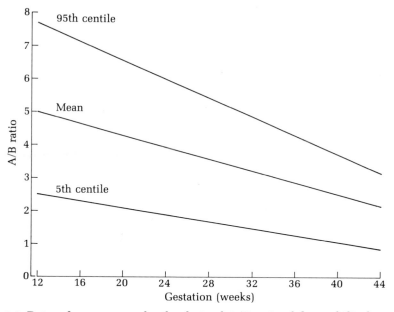

Fig. 4.4 Data reference range for the derived A/B ratio of the umbilical artery (modified from Hendricks *et al.* 1989).

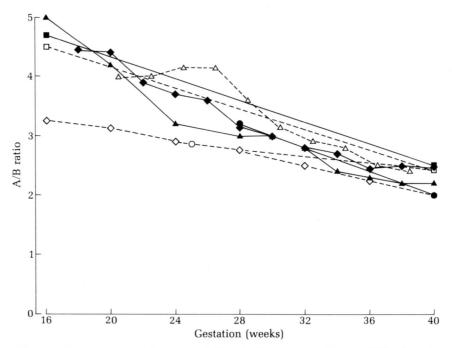

Fig. 4.5 Comparison of the mean A/B ratio from some of the published works. ○, Schulman *et al.* 1984; ▼, Erskine and Ritchie 1985; ●, Trudinger *et al.* 1985; □, Al-Ghazali, *et al.* 1988; ▽, Gudmundsson and Marsal 1988; ■, Hendricks *et al.* 1989; ◇, Pearce *et al.* 1988; ◆, Schulman *et al.* 1989.

recognized the typical waveform patterns, other authors obtained waveforms using continuous wave equipment. With either method, it is impossible to determine the precise vessel from which the waveform arises as the iliac-uterine-arcuate circulation lies in an area that is only 4 cm². For this reason, most authors refer to these waveforms as arising from the utero-placental circulation. Colour-coded Doppler ultrasound will allow precise localization of the vessel (see Chapter 6), but has yet to be fully evaluated.

Data reference ranges

Each uterine artery supplies four arcuate arteries, which, in turn, supply about 25 spiral arteries. Waveforms can thus be acquired from multiple sites on the uterus, a situation at least partially explored in the study by Bewley *et al.* (1989). Figure 4.7 illustrates the four sites used by Bewley, while Figure 4.8 is a cross-sectional study of the resistance index at these sites at between 16 and 26 weeks' gestation. The site demonstrating the lowest impedance is the placental arcuate artery.

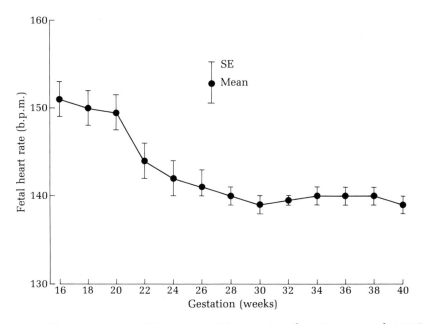

Fig. 4.6 Change in the fetal heart rate with gestation (from Pearce *et al.* 1988).

Currently, there is no standardization of the means of obtaining data reference ranges from the uteroplacental circulation, but Table 4.2 details the published studies.

Pearce *et al.* (1988) used pulsed Doppler ultrasound to recognize small vessels in the uterine wall, which they called arcuate arteries. The range gate of the pulsed Doppler equipment was then placed over the vessel, and therefore the source of the signal was visualized. In some cases, however, these authors state that the characteristic waveform was obtained without the vessel being visualized. Using this method Pearce *et al.* (1988) studied 34 women, retrospectively defined as normal, and after correcting for maternal heart rate (by use of the frequency index profile) reference ranges were defined for the placental and non-placental sides of the uterus (Fig. 4.9 and 4.10).

Trudinger *et al.* (1985*a*) described a simple method in which a continuous wave Doppler probe was aimed at the subplacental bed, which had previously been located with real-time ultrasound. Yet a third method was described by Schulman *et al.* (1986). The continuous wave Doppler probe was directed to the para-uterine areas of the lower uterine segment and then moved until the waveform, previously described from duplex studies, was identified. This is now the most popular method and has been used in screening studies (see Chapter 6).

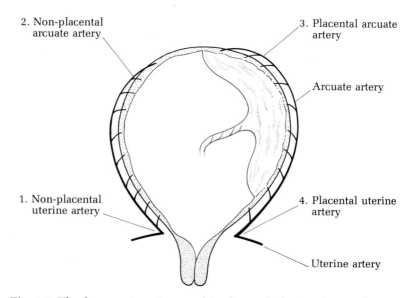

Fig. 4.7 The four uterine sites used in the study by Bewley *et al.* (1989).

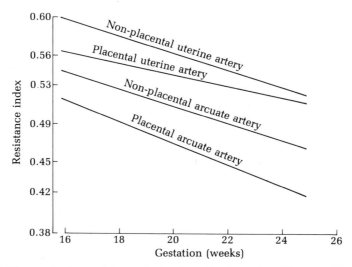

Fig. 4.8 Change in the resistance index from the four sites illustrated in Figure 4.7 (from Bewley *et al.* 1989).

Table 4.2 Published data reference ranges for waveforms from the uteroplacental circulation

Author	Doppler	Site(s)	Comments
Trudinger *et al* (1985*a*)	CW	SP	12 patients, 20–40 weeks Longitudinal Linear regression Negative correlation with gestational age*
Al-Ghazali *et al.* (1988)	PW	SP	271 patients, 16–40 weeks Cross-sectional No change with gestational age
McCowan *et al.* (1988)	CW	SP PU NPU	15 patients, 16–40 weeks Longitudinal Quadratic regression with no change after 26 weeks NPU > PU, SP = PU
Gudmundsson and Marsal (1988)	PW	SP	125 patients, 20–42 weeks Cross-sectional Linear regression Negative correlation with gestational age
Schulman *et al.* (1986)	CW	U	79 women, 14–40 weeks Cross-sectional Quadratic regression with no change after 26 weeks Average PU and NPU
Pearce *et al.* (1988)	PW	PU NPU	34 women, 16–40 weeks Longitudinal Quadratic regression with no change after 24 weeks NPU > PU

* Used the B/A ratio, giving a positive correlation with gestational age.
SP, subplacental; PU, placental uterine artery; NPU, non-placental uterine artery; U, uterine; CW, continuous wave; PW, pulsed wave.

The data reference ranges that have been published show considerable variation. Three studies demonstrate a fall in impedance in the second trimester that levels off in the third trimester (Schulman *et al.* 1986; McCowan *et al.* 1988; Pearce *et al.* 1988), whereas two studies show a continuing fall throughout the last two trimesters (Trudinger *et al.* 1985*a*; Al-Ghazali *et al.* 1988).

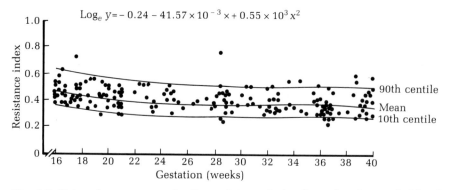

Fig. 4.9 Data reference range for the resistance index from the placental side of the uterus with increasing gestation (from Pearce *et al.* 1988).

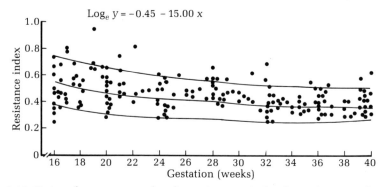

Fig. 4.10 Data reference range for the resistance index from the non-placental side of the uterus with increasing gestation (from Pearce *et al.* 1988).

When reviewing these publications it is important to consider the site of origin of the uteroplacental waveforms. Two studies have emphasized that waveforms from the non-placental side of the uterus demonstrate higher resistance indices than those obtained from the placental side (Kofinas *et al.* 1988; Lieberman *et al.* 1988).

Conclusion

From the little available evidence, it appears that there is a fall in the impedance in the uteroplacental circulation in early pregnancy and that little or no change is seen in the resistance index, from either side of the uterus after 26 weeks' gestation. At present, the use of a single figure for the upper limit of the data reference range, for example 0.58 for resistance index, seems appropriate.

REFERENCES

Al-Ghazali, W., Chapman, M. G., and Allan, L. D. (1988). Doppler assessment of the cardiac and uteroplacental circulations in normal and complicated pregnancies. *British Journal of Obstetrics and Gynaecology*, **95**, 575–80.

Bewley, S., Campbell, S., and Cooper, D. (1989). Uteroplacental Doppler flow velocity waveforms in the second trimester: a complex circulation. *British Journal of Obstetrics and Gynaecology*, **96**, 1040–6.

Campbell, S., Griffin, D. R., Pearce, J. M. F., Diaz-Recasens, J., Cohen-Overbeek, T. A., and Willson, K. (1983). New Doppler technique for assessing uteroplacental bloodflow. *Lancet*, **i**, 675–7.

Erskine, R. L. A. and Ritchie, J. W. K. (1985). Umbilical artery blood flow characteristics in normal and growth retarded fetuses. *British Journal of Obstetrics and Gynaecology*, **92**, 605–10.

Fisk, N. M., MacLachlan, N., Ellis, C., Tannirandorn, Y., Tonge, H. M, and Rodeck, C. H. (1988). Absent end-diastolic frequencies in first trimester umbilical artery. *Lancet*, **ii**, 46.

Fitzgerald, D. E. and Drumm, J. E. (1977). Non-invasive measurement of human fetal circulation using ultrasound: a new method. *British Medical Journal*, **2**, 1450–1.

Gerson, A. G., Wallace, D. M., Stiller, R. J., Pauls, D., Weiner, S., and Bolognese, R. J. (1987). Doppler evaluation of umbilical venous and arterial blood flow in the second and third trimesters of normal pregnancy. *Obstetrics and Gynecology*, **70**, 622–6.

Gudmundsson, S. and Marsal, K. (1988). Umbilical artery and uteroplacental blood flow velocity waveforms in normal pregnancy—a cross-sectional study. *Acta Obstetrica et Gynecologica Scandinavica*, **67**, 347–54.

Hendricks, S. K., Sorensen, T. K., Wang, K. Y., Bushnell, J. M., Segiun, E. M., and Zingheim, R. W. (1989). Doppler umbilical artery waveform indices—normal values from fourteen to forty-two weeks. *American Journal of Obstetrics and Gynecology*, **161**, 761–5.

Kofinas, A. D., Penry, M., Greiss, F. C., Meis, P. J., and Nelson, L. H. (1988). The effect of placental localisation on uterine artery flow velocity waveforms. *American Journal of Obstetrics and Gynecology*, **159**, 1504–8.

McCowan, L. M., Ritchie, K., Mo, L. Y., Bascom, P. A., and Sherrett, H. (1988). Uterine artery flow velocity waveforms in normal and growth retarded pregnancies. *American Journal of Obstetrics and Gynecology*, **158**, 499–504.

Pearce, J. M. F., Campbell, S., Cohen-Overbeek, T. A., Hackett, G., Hernandez, J., and Royston, J. P. (1988). Reference ranges and sources of variation for indices of pulsed Doppler flow velocity waveforms from the uteroplacental and fetal circulation. *British Journal of Obstetrics and Gynaecology*, **95**, 248–56.

Reuwer, P. J. H. M., Bruinse, P., Stoutenbeek, P., and Haspels, A. A. (1984). Doppler assessment of the fetoplacental circulation in normal and growth retarded fetuses. *European Journal of Obstetrics, Gynecology, and Reproductive Biology*, **18**, 199–205.

Schulman, H., Fleischer, A., Stern, W., Farmakides, G., Jagani, N., and Blattner, P. (1984). Umbilical velocity wave ratios in human pregnancy. *American Journal of Obstetrics and Gynecology*, **148**, 985–90.

Schulman, H., Fleischer, A., Farmakides, G., Bracero, L., Rochelson, B., and Grubfeld, L. (1986). Development of the uterine artery compliance in pregnancy as detected by Doppler ultrasound. *American Journal of Obstetrics and Gynecology*, **155**, 1031–6.

Schulman, H., Winter, D., Farmakides, G., Ducey, J., Guzman, E., Coury, E., and Penny, B. (1989). Pregnancy surveillance with Doppler velocimetry of uterine and umbilical arteries. *American Journal of Obstetrics and Gynecology*, **160**, 192–60

Stuart, B., Drum, J., Fitzgerald, D. E., and Duignan, N. M. (1980). Fetal blood flow velocity waveforms in normal pregnancy. *British Journal of Obstetrics and Gynaecology*, **87**, 780–5.

Thompson, R. C., Trudinger, B. J., Cook, C. M., and Giles, W. B. 1988). Normal values for umbilical artery waveform indices. *British Journal of Obstetrics and Gynaecology*, **95**, 589–91.

Trudinger, B. J., Giles, W. B., and Cook, C. M. (1985a). Uteroplacental blood flow velocity-time waveforms in normal and complicated pregnancy. *British Journal of Obstetrics and Gynaecology*, **92**, 39–45.

Trudinger, B. J., Giles, W. B., Cook, C. M., Bombardieri, J., and Collins, L. (1985b). Fetal umbilical artery flow velocity waveforms and placental resistance: clinical significance. *British Journal of Obstetrics and Gynaecology*, **92**, 23–30.

Trudinger, B. J., Giles, W. B., and Cook, C. M. (1985c). Flow velocity waveforms in the maternal uteroplacental and fetal umbilical circulations. *American Journal of Obstetrics and Gynecology*, **152**, 155–63.

5. Umbilical artery Doppler ultrasonography as a screening tool

Jim Dornan and Bryan Beattie

INTRODUCTION

Most of the current screening tests that are accepted as beneficial or routine have not been subjected to rigorous evaluation. Before the widespread introduction of a new technology such as Doppler ultrasonography, we should determine its value in an objective manner, unbiased by investigators' enthusiasm. This chapter evaluates the currently available evidence for using Doppler velocimetry from the umbilical artery as a screening test in pregnancies at no clinical identifiable perinatal risk.

SCREENING TESTS AS THEY AFFECT THE CLINICIAN

The properties of screening tests can be found in Chapter 2, which should be read before this chapter. Many properties of screening tests, however, are mainly useful to those evaluating the test and to epidemiologists, but here we wish briefly to discuss those aspects of the test that affect the clinician. There are two main questions that need to be asked:

1. Should this particular pregnant woman have the test?
2. How do I interpret the results for this particular woman?

The test property that is most commonly used to help answer this question is the positive predictive value (PPV). The PPV is best considered as the chance of having the disorder sought if the screening test result is positive. For example, if the PPV of Doppler ultrasonography as a predictor of a small-for-gestational age (SGA) infant was 10 per cent, women with an abnormal test result would only have a 1 in 10 chance of giving birth to an SGA infant.

The PPV, however, varies according to the prevalence of the condition in the population studied; the PPV is higher as the condition sought becomes more common. This means that the reported PPV may be different from that in the local population. For instance, a test that is useful at distinguishing those women who will have a SGA infant in a population where 50 per cent of women are affected (a high-risk population) may be of no value where only 5 per cent of the population is affected (low-risk population). This either means that the test has to be evaluated on the local population or that the test properties have to be re-calculated, given the prevalence in the local population.

One approach to this problem is to use the likelihood ratio (LR). The LR for a test is the number of individuals affected/ number of unaffected individuals. The LR allows the clinician to determine the PPV and negative predictive value (NPV) for a particular woman if the prevalence of the outcome in the local population or in the risk group to which the woman belongs is known. The LR can be used both in the situation where the test result is classified as normal or abnormal, and where the test is assessed using different cut-off points. This latter circumstance is more useful in the clinical situation because individuals are at varied risk levels for the condition even before testing (prior probability). For example, assume that a hypertensive patient has a 50 per cent chance of delivering an SGA infant because of her hypertension. We now apply an antenatal screening test that has an LR for a positive test of 0.4 and for a negative test of 0.3. We can easily derive the woman's post-test probability from the nomogram shown in Fig. 5.1, where this example is worked. If the test is positive her post-test probability now rises to 81 per cent, whereas if the test is negative it falls to 24 per cent.

The problem of choosing outcome measures

Using perinatal death as an outcome measure requires extremely large studies because the event is rare. Perinatal morbidity is difficult to quantify and there is currently no 'gold standard' outcome measure of morbidity against which to judge test results. Birth-weight and indices that reflect intra-uterine nutritional status and hypoxia are therefore reported by many authors.

UMBILICAL ARTERY DOPPLER VELOCIMETRY IN LOW-RISK PREGNANCIES

Introduction

The data for this review were obtained from a literature search using Medline (1980–90) and the *Oxford Database of Perinatal Trials* (Chalmers 1990) in order to identify published, unpublished, and ongoing studies that assessed the value of umbilical artery velocimetry in pregnancies with no clinically identifiable perinatal risk. Investigators of ongoing or completed, unpublished trials were contacted to determine whether the data were

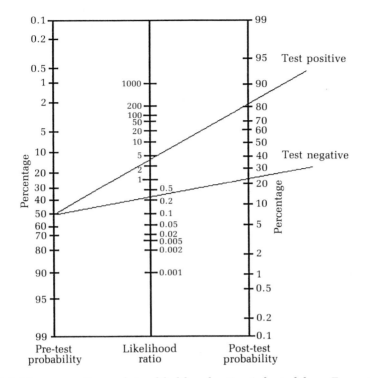

Fig. 5.1 Nomogram for applying likelihood ratios (adapted from Fagan 1975).

available for inclusion, in order to try to prevent a publication bias. In one study (Beattie and Dornan 1989), data not included in the publication were made available for this review.

Five published prospective studies were identified (Beattie and Dornan 1989; Hanretty *et al.* 1989; Sijmons *et al.* 1989; Schulman *et al.* 1989; Newnham *et al.* 1990). In one of the studies (Schulman *et al.* 1989), the clinicians were not blind to the Doppler results so this study was not considered further. There were no published, randomized, controlled trials assessing the effectiveness of screening in a low-risk population, although we are aware of one in progress J. P. Neilson (personal communication, 1990). Table 5.1 summarizes the details of the five studies.

Patients and methods

All studies used different Doppler ultrasound equipment, different testing intervals, varying definitions of abnormal test results, and different outcome measures. Tables 5.2–5.6 attempt to summarize the results, and means have been calculated for some test properties to allow overall conclusions to be drawn.

Table 5.1 Details of studies assessing umbilical artery doppler velocimetry in low-risk pregnancies

Study	Blinded study	Gestation at testing (weeks)	Definition of an abnormal test result	Outcome measures
Beattie and Dornan (1989)	Yes	28, 34, 38 28, 34, 38 28, 34, 38	PI > P90 AB > P90 RP > P90	Birth-weight < P10 Birth-weight < P5 Ponderal index < P10 Ponderal index < P2.3 Skinfold thickness < P5 MAC/HC < P5 Apgar score @ 1 min < 7 Apgar score @ 5 min < 7 Cord artery pH < 7.2 Cord haematocrit > 65 Fetal distress

Newnham et al. (1990)	Yes	18, 24	AB > 6	Birth-weight < P10
		28	AB > 4.88	Apgar score @ 5 min < 7
		34	AB > 3.91	Cord artery pH < 7.2
				Fetal distress
Sijmons et al. (1989)	Yes	28	PI > 1.46	Birth-weight < P10
		34	PI > 1.27	Birth-weight < P2.3
				Ponderal index < P10
				Ponderal index < P2.3
Hanretty et al. (1989)	Yes	26–30	AB > 4.11	Birth-weight < P10
		34–36	AB > 3.86	Apgar score @ 1 min < 6
				Apgar score @ 5 min < 6
				Neonatal intensive care unit
				Pregnancy-induced hypertension
Schulman et al. (1989)	No	—		Details not evaluated in this review

AB, A/B ratio; HC, head circumference; MAC, mid-arm circumference; P, per centile; PI, pulsatility index; RP, resistance index.

Table 5.3 Test properties for umbilical artery Doppler velocimetry using birth-weight < 5th centile for gestational age as the outcome measure

Reference	n	Prevalence (%)	Gestation (weeks)	Test cut-off	Sensitivity	Specificity	PPV	NPV	LR+	LR−
Beattie and Dornan (1989)	2097	5.0	28	PI > 1.73	0.28	0.89	0.11	0.97	2.5	0.8
Hanretty et al. (1989)	344	5.5	26–30	AB > 4.11	0.11	0.95	0.11	0.95	2.1	0.9
Beattie and Dornan (1989)	2091	5.0	28	AB > 4.29	0.31	0.90	0.12	0.97	3.1	0.8
Beattie and Dornan (1989)	2091	5.0	28	RP > 0.76	0.14	0.94	0.09	0.96	2.3	0.9
Mean		5.1	28		0.21	0.92	0.11	0.96	2.5	0.9
Beattie and Dornan (1989)	2036	5.1	34	PI > 1.28	0.32	0.89	0.12	0.97	2.9	0.8
Beattie and Dornan (1989)	2034	5.1	34	AB > 3.44	0.40	0.84	0.11	0.97	2.5	0.7
Hanretty et al. (1989)	344	4.7	34–36	AB > 3.86	0.06	0.95	0.06	0.95	1.2	1.0
Beattie and Dornan (1989)	2034	5.1	34	Rp > 0.70	0.33	0.88	0.12	0.97	2.8	0.8
Mean		5.0	34		0.28	0.89	0.10	0.97	2.4	0.8
Beattie and Dornan (1989)	1597	4.6	38	PI > 1.17	0.31	0.86	0.09	0.97	2.2	0.8
Beattie and Dornan (1989)	1597	4.6	38	AB > 3.00	0.30	0.89	0.11	0.97	2.7	0.8
Beattie and Dornan (1989)	1597	4.6	38	RP > 0.66	0.40	0.82	0.09	0.97	1.9	0.8
Mean		4.6	38		0.34	0.86	0.10	0.97	2.3	0.8

PPV, positive predictive value; NPV, negative predictive value; LR+, likelihood ratio with an abnormal test; LR−, likelihood ratio with a normal test; AB, A/B ratio; PI, pulsatility index; RP, resistance index.

Table 5.2 Test properties for umbilical artery Doppler velocimetry using birth-weight < 10th centile for gestational age as the outcome measure

Reference	n	Prevalence (%)	Gestation (weeks)	Test cut-off	Sensitivity	Specificity	PPV	NPV	LR+	LR−
Newnhan et al. (1990)	516	9.9	18	AB > 6.0	0.29	0.74	0.11	0.91	1.1	1.0
Newnhan et al. (1990)	268	7.1	24	AB > 6.0	0.11	0.96	0.17	0.93	2.6	0.9
Sijmons et al. (1989)	394	22.6	26–30	PI > 1.46	0.17	0.95	0.50	0.80	3.4	0.9
Beattie and Dornan (1989)	2097	10.0	28	PI > 1.73	0.20	0.92	0.21	0.91	2.3	0.9
Beattie and Dornan (1989)	2091	10.0	28	AB > 4.29	0.22	0.91	0.22	0.91	2.6	0.9
Newnham et al. (1990)	470	9.1	28	AB > 4.88	0.19	0.96	0.30	0.92	4.2	0.9
Beattie and Dornan (1989)	2091	10.0	28	RP > 0.76	0.19	0.92	0.22	0.91	2.4	0.9
Mean		12.3	28		0.19	0.93	0.29	0.89	3.0	0.9
Sijmons et al. (1989)	394	22.6	32–36	PI > 1.27	0.22	0.94	0.53	0.81	3.9	0.8
Beattie and Dornan (1989)	2036	10.2	34	PI > 1.28	0.22	0.92	0.23	0.91	2.6	0.9
Beattie and Dornan (1989)	2034	10.2	34	AB > 3.44	0.22	0.91	0.24	0.91	2.5	0.9
Newnham et al. (1990)	445	8.1	34	AB > 3.91	0.17	0.95	0.23	0.93	3.4	0.9
Beattie and Dornan (1989)	2034	10.2	34	RP > 0.70	0.21	0.92	0.23	0.91	2.7	0.9
Mean		12.3	34		0.21	0.93	0.29	0.89	3.0	0.9
Beattie and Dornan (1989)	1597	9.1	38	PI > 1.17	0.27	0.93	0.26	0.93	3.5	0.8
Beattie and Dornan (1989)	1597	9.1	38	AB > 3.00	0.20	0.94	0.24	0.92	3.1	0.9
Beattie and Dornan (1989)	1597	9.1	38	RP > 0.66	0.23	0.93	0.23	0.92	3.1	0.8
Mean		9.1	38		0.23	0.93	0.24	0.92	3.2	0.8

PPV, positive predictive value; NPV, negative predictive value; LR+, likelihood ratio with an abnormal test; LR−, likelihood ratio with a normal test; AB, A/B ratio; PI, pulsatility index; RP, resistance index.

Table 5.4 Test properties for umbilical artery Doppler velocimetry

Reference	n	Prevalence (%)	Gestation (weeks)	Test cut-off	Sensitivity	Specificity	PPV	NPV	LR+	LR−	Outcome measure
Sijmons et al. (1989)	352	4.3	26–30	PI > 1.46	0.20	0.94	0.13	0.96	3.4	0.9	Ponderal index < 2.3rd centile for gestational age
Sijmons et al. (1989)	330	3.3	32–36	PI > 1.27	0.27	0.92	0.10	0.97	3.2	0.8	
Beattie and Dornan (1989)		2.3		Any	Not significant (P > 0.05)						
Newnham et al. (1990)	342	9.9	18	AB > 6.0	0.26	0.74	0.10	0.9	1.0	1.0	(NS)
Newnham et al. (1990)	232	9.4	24	AB > 6.0	0.08	0.96	0.17	0.91	2.0	1.0	Fetal hypoxia*
Newnham et al. (1990)	404	9.2	28	AB > 4.88	0.12	0.95	0.19	0.92	2.2	0.9	
Newnham et al. (1990)	384	8.8	34	AB > 3.91	0.15	0.95	0.23	0.92	3.1	0.9	
Hanretty et al. (1989)	344	26.5	26–30	AB > 4.11	0.07	0.95	0.33	0.74	1.4	1.0	Pregnancy induced hypertension
Hanretty et al. (1989)	374	28.1	34–36	AB > 3.86	0.06	0.96	0.33	0.72	1.3	1.3	

* Apgar score < 7 at 1 min, cord artery pH < 72, operative delivery for fetal distress or abnormal fetal heart rate trace.
PPV; positive predictive value; NPV, negative predictive value; LR+, likelihood ratio with an abnormal test; LR−, likelihood ratio with a normal test; NS, test not statistically significant.

Table 5.5 Prevalence of observed cases of absent end-diastolic velocity (AEDF) at different gestations

Reference	Cases	n	Prevalence (%)	Gestation (weeks)	Filter
Newnham *et al.* (1990)	135	518	26.0	18	280 Hz
Newnham *et al.* (1990)	11	268	4.0	24	280 Hz
Schulman *et al.* (1989)	5	255	2.0	26–36	?
Sijmons *et al* (1989)	0	470	0.0	26–30	200 Hz
Beattie and Dornan (1989)	6	2097	0.03	28	200 Hz
Hanretty *et al.* (1989)	6	357	1.7	26–30	200 Hz
Sijmons *et al.* (1989)	0	445	0.0	32–36	200 Hz
Beattie and Dornan (1989)	2	2036	0.01	34	200 Hz
Hanretty *et al.* (1989)	6	395	1.5	34–36	200 Hz

Prevalence of AEDF from pooled data at 26–30 weeks = 0.41 per cent (12/2924).
Prevalence of AEDF from pooled data at 32–36 weeks = 0.28 per cent (8/2876).

Table 5.6 Pregnancy outcome following the observation of absent end-diastolic velocity (AEDF) after 28 weeks' gestation

Reference	26–30 weeks' gestation	34–36 weeks' gestation	SGA*	Hypoxia†	Mortality
Hanretty *et al.* (1989)	AEDV	—	AGA	No	Alive
	AEDV	—	AGA	No	Alive
	AEDV	—	SGA	No	Alive
	AEDV	AB = 2.3	AGA	No	Alive
	AEDV	AEDV	AGA	No	Alive
	AB = 1.92	AEDV	AGA	No	Alive
	AB = 4.27	AEDV	AGA	Yes	Alive
	ND	AEDV	AGA	No	Alive
	ND	AEDV	SGA	No	Alive
Beattie and Dornan (1989)	AEDV		AGA	—	Still birth
	AEDV	AEDV	AGA	—	Still birth
	AEDV	AEDV	SGA	No	Alive
	AEDV	Normal	AGA	No	Alive
	AEDV	Normal	AGA	No	Alive
	AEDV	Normal	AGA	No	Alive

* < 5th percentile (P5) birth-weight for gestational age; † 1- or 5-min Apgar score < 7.
AB, A/B ratio; AGA, appropriate for gestational age; SGA, small for gestational age.

The largest study to date was conducted over a 12-month period in Belfast, and recruited 2097 unselected patients from an antenatal population of a tertiary referral centre. Most of the pregnancies had no identifiable perinatal risk: the unit also serves a large catchment area for routine obstetric services. The study population represented 62 per cent of the antenatal pregnancies for August 1987 to July 1988, and was comparable to the unscreened population for factors known to be associated with the birth of small-for-gestational age infants. Waveforms were obtained by means of a Doptek 9000 CW spectrum analyser (Doptek Ltd, Chichester, UK) utilizing a 4 MHz probe and a vessel wall filter set at 200 Hz. The A/B ratio, pulsatility index (PI), and resistance index (RI) were determined at 28, 34, and 38 weeks' gestation. The clinicians were blind to the results of the Doppler study. An abnormal test result was declared when the value exceeded the 90th percentile at that particular gestation.

Modern neonatal nutritional indices and birth-weight centiles were used to define intra-uterine growth retardation. Small for gestational age (SGA) was defined for the purposes of this study as an eventual birth-weight of less than the fifth centile using the charts of Gardner and Pearson (1971), although data on infants of less than the tenth centile is also reported. The prevalence of SGA in the study was 104 out of 2097 (5 per cent), thus suggesting that the population is similar to that in much of the UK.

Other additional measures of neonatal nutritional status were made, such as the ponderal index, midarm circumference: head circumference ratio (MAC:HC), and triceps and subscapular skinfold thickness measurement (Georgieff *et al.* 1986; Patterson and Pouliot 1987; Whitelaw 1977). Acute fetal hypoxia was determined by an Apgar score of less than 7 at 1 min and an umbilical cord pH of less than 7.2, whilst an elevated umbilical cord artery haematocrit of more than 65 per cent was selected as a measure of chronic hypoxia. Operative delivery for fetal distress was also noted.

Newnham *et al.* (1990) examined 535 pregnancies of medium risk at 18, 24, 28, and 34 weeks' gestation. He used as a cut-off level for the S/D (A/B) ratio of > 6, > 6, 4.88, and 3.91 at these four gestations, respectively, based upon the 95th percentiles determined from 271 pregnancies that subsequently had a normal outcome. They averaged the S/D ratio from three cardiac cycles, acquiring the waveforms by means of a Medasonics SP25A spectrum analyser, using a 280-Hz high-pass filter. Fetal hypoxia was clinically determined by an obstetrician not involved in the study. Operative delivery for fetal distress, an abnormal cardiotocograph, a cord pH of less than 7.2., and a 5-min Apgar score of less than 7 were all used as the criteria for an abnormal outcome. Intra-uterine growth retardation, was defined in this study, as a corrected birth-weight as less than the 10th centile for gestational age. By using receiver operator characteristic (ROC) curves these authors were able to evaluate their results using different cut-off levels, and they reported 516 women.

Sijmons *et al.* (1989) and Briunse *et al.* (1989) have published the results of prospective studies using the PI from the umbilical artery waveforms as a screening tool for the delivery of an SGA or nutritionally deprived fetus. They used an Alvar 4-MHz pulsed Doppler device with subsequent off-line waveform analysis by means of a Doptek 9000 spectrum analyser (Doptek, UK Ltd). The PI was averaged over five cardiac cycles at 26–30 and 32–36 weeks' gestation. They determined that the PI was abnormal if it had a value of more than the 95th centile of a data reference range derived from a previous study of 70 normal pregnancies. The 95th centile was reported as 1.46 and 1.27 at 28 and 34 weeks, respectively.

These authors recruited 400 unselected patients and chose as outcome measures SGA, defined as a birth-weight of less than the 10th centile, and also the 2.3rd centile together with a low Ponderal index. The prevalence of SGA (birth-weight of less than the 10th centile) in the Dutch population was high at 22 per cent, which the authors attributed to a large population of cigarette smokers. This, however, indicates that the results from this study should not be considered as being representative of an unselected low-risk population.

Hanretty *et al.* (1989) evaluated both the uteroplacental and umbilical circulations in 543 unselected pregnancies in a low-risk Scottish popula-tion. They screened the women at 26–30 and 34–36 weeks, utilizing an angioscan with a 4 MHz continuous wave probe. They reported the A/B ratio and chose as their cut-off value the 95th centile derived from a pilot study carried out on 150 normal pregnancies, reporting values of 4.11 and 3.86 at 26–30 and 34–46 weeks, respectively. Outcome measures were SGA (less than the 5th centile), the incidence of pregnancy-induced hyper-tension, admission to the neonatal intensive care unit, and an Apgar score of less than 7 at 1 min.

Results

Two groups (Beattie *et al.* 1987; Newnham *et al.* 1990) have addressed the frequency distribution of the waveform indices and have shown that they are positively skewed (Fig. 4.3). These authors made allowances for this by use of non-parametric statistics (Beattie *et al.* 1987) or logarithmic transfor-mations (Newnham *et al.* 1990). The results of the individual studies are summarized in Tables 5.2–5.6

The sensitivity of umbilical artery Doppler velocimetry is clearly un-acceptably low for all outcome measures studied; this appears to be true for all indices and at all gestational ages. For example, the overall mean sensitivity for the prediction of SGA (birth-weights less than the 10th centile) was only 23 per cent (Table 5.2), i.e. the test overlooked 77 per cent of such infants.

Clinically, obstetricians use tests to increase their certainty that a women has (or does not have) the disorder that is being sought. Review of the tables indicates that Doppler velocimetry only slightly increases the prior probability. For example, the calculated means of the predictive value of a positive test (PPV) in Table 5.2 indicate that the risks of delivering an SGA infant increase from a background rate of 12.3 per cent, to 29 per cent at gestations of 28 or 34 weeks. Similarly, the probability of a normal outcome increases only slightly from a background risk of 87.7 per cent (1 − prevalence) to 89 per cent (predictive value of a negative test, NPV) at 28 and 34 weeks' gestation.

From Table 5.4 it can be seen that even when the extremes of birthweight are considered (less than the 2.3rd centile), although the sensitivity increases to up to 42 per cent with a likelihood ratio of up to 5.8 suggesting a considerably increased risk if the test is positive, there is little or no reduction in risk if the test is negative (LR of up to 1.0).

In the Belfast study, the poor sensitivity of the technique to predict delivery of an SGA infant is apparent from Table 5.3. Figure 5.2 shows an ROC curve for the A/B ratio obtained from the umbilical artery waveforms at 34 weeks' gestation. There is a typical marked reduction in the specificity as the threshold is reduced (the percentile cut-off point is lowered) in order to try to improve the sensitivity.

Poor nutritional status as defined by a low Ponderal index (Table 5.4) is also poorly predicted by Doppler velocimetry. The Belfast study (Beattie and Dornan 1989) failed to demonstrate a significant relationship between an abnormal Doppler test result and a poorly nourished baby.

The poor predictive value of Doppler velocimetry is probably explained by the heterogeneous causes for smallness. However, because a low Ponderal index is believed to indicate intra-uterine malnutrition consequent upon placental insufficiency, it was anticipated that a high proportion of this group would have abnormal Doppler studies. This was clearly not the case.

Fetal hypoxia, defined by multiple criteria, was used as the outcome measure in one study (Newnham *et al.* 1990). The maximum sensitivity of Doppler velocimetry was 26 per cent, but the probability of developing fetal hypoxia varied little with the test result. Whilst abnormal results from Doppler velocimetry were significantly associated with SGA, and especially so if there was superimposed hypoxia, only a weak association was found with hypoxia alone. Retrospective analysis of the Belfast data, using the same criteria for defining fetal hypoxia, failed to show any relationship with abnormal Doppler findings.

Hanretty *et al.* (1989) evaluated both umbilical artery and uteroplacental

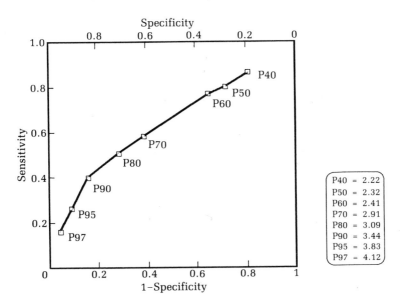

Fig. 5.2 A receiver operator characteristic (ROC) curve which evaluates the effect of changing the cut-off percentiles (P) for the A/B ratio of the umbilical artery waveform obtained at 34 weeks' gestation.

waveforms as a screening test for pregnancy-induced hypertension. The prevalence was up to 28 per cent, but the waveforms predicted only 7 per cent of these affected individuals. This contrasts sharply with larger studies on uteroplacental waveforms (see Chapter 6).

Results based upon absent end-diastolic frequencies

The diastolic component of the umbilical artery waveform usually increases as gestation increases (see Fig. 4.1, p. 82). Absence of end-diastolic frequencies (AEDF) is an ominous sign associated with a high risk of perinatal death and handicap (see Chapter 7). Pooled data from the screening studies suggest a prevalence of 0.4 per cent at 26–30 weeks' gestation and of 0.3 per cent at 32–36 weeks' gestation (Table 5.5).

The results were not known to the clinicians, so the pregnancies were managed along standard clinical lines. Table 5.6 shows that the outcome was varied. Overall, 16 pregnancies were complicated by AEDF in the studies reported by Beattie and Dornan (1989) and Hanretty *et al.* (1989). These resulted in two stillbirths, three SGA infants, and one hypoxic infant, but in ten normal pregnancies. AEDF in a low-risk population therefore does not seem to carry the same serious significance as observed in high-risk populations (McParland *et al.* 1990).

CONCLUSION

It is clear from this review that Doppler velocimetry from the umbilical artery is not a useful technique for screening low-risk pregnancies. Fetal growth is a complex process, involving alteration of the genetic growth potential of the fetus by the circulatory and nutritive properties of the placenta. The fact that Doppler examines only the circulatory properties of these components may explain some of its limitations. In addition, it seems that the fetal circulation is often protected until late in the disease process (see Chapter 8), which may explain the better results achieved by screening with uteroplacental waveforms (see Chapter 6).

The infrequent finding of AEDF in a low-risk population is difficult to interpret, and screening for this finding in a low-risk population cannot be justified.

Table 5.7 lists the criteria that are necessary before a screening test is implemented. Table 5.8 answers the criteria for Doppler velocimetry, the last two points being conclusive.

Table 5.7 Criteria for implementation of a screening programme (Grant and Mohide 1982)

1. The condition sought should be an important health problem.

2. The natural history of the condition, including development from latent to overt stages, should be adequately understood.

3. The condition should have an identifiable latent period of an early symptomatic phase during which intervention is possible.

4. A suitable screening test should be available.

5. The test should be acceptable to those tested.

6. There should be a satisfactory diagnostic test with an agreed policy of case definition.

7. There should be an effective management for patients with the recognized condition.

8. The search for the condition should be a continuing process.

9. The resources needed for diagnosis and treatment should be available.

10. The costs incurred as a result of finding cases should be economically balanced in relation to possible expenditure on an alternative programmer or on medical care as a whole.

Table 5.8 Application of criteria for introduction of Doppler ultrasonography as a screening programme using the criteria specified in Table 5.7

1. *Yes:* IUGR and its fetal and neonatal metabolic and hypoxic consequences certainly are a major health problem in perinatal medicine. They are associated with a high risk of intra-uterine death, neonatal mortality, and neurological damage.

2. *Yes:* Placental insufficiency is thought to develop from its latent stage which precedes fetal compromise to one in which IUGR, fetal hypoxia, and even intra-uterine death may occur.

3. *Yes:* There is certainly a symptomatic stage in the fetus with intra-uterine malnourishment, poor growth, and biophysical evidence of fetal hypoxia. Intervention in the form of early delivery, oxygen therapy, or low-dose aspirin may have a role. Improved end-diastolic waveforms and perinatal outcome have been reported in published studies already (Trudinger 1988).

4. *No:* Doppler ultrasonography is not a suitable screening tool in low-risk pregnancies.

5. *Yes:* The test is acceptable to the patient. It causes no discomfort to the patient and is non-invasive, quick, and easily applied.

6. *Yes:* Diagnostic tests such as Biophysical Profile Scoring can be applied to the fetus at risk of intra-uterine hypoxia. Estimated fetal weights on ultrasound examination will identify the IUGR fetus with low birth-weight for gestational age. Regular biophysical fetal assessment would therefore seem an appropriate approach to surveillance of the fetus identified as being at risk. Case definition can be based on biophysical profile scores and estimated fetal weight, although intra-uterine indices of nutrition status such as MAC/HC are undergoing evaluation in Belfast.

7. *Yes:* Effective management by close surveillance, early delivery, and potentially the use of aspirin therapy may improve outcome. Antenatal diagnosis may also allow delivery in an appropriate centre with proper neonatal surveillance for the known metabolic consequences of IUGR.

8. *Yes:* The Doppler technique can be applied at any stage throughout the second and third trimesters on a repeated basis.

9. *No:* As it stands to date, the identification of some 10 per cent of the antenatal population as being in an at-risk group and requiring intensive biophysical fetal surveillance would considerably burden the health-care system, especially when one considers that some 70 per cent of IUGR fetuses would still be missed and the effectiveness for treatment has not yet been proven.

Table 5.8 (Continued)

---

10. No: The poor performance of the screening test and the unproven value
of any intervention cannot justify its introduction when there are
simpler, cheaper alternatives such as measurement of symphysis fundal
height (Rosenberg *et al.* 1982) or more sensitive tests such as
ultrasound fetometry (Neilson *et al.* 1984).

IUGR, intra-uterine growth retardation; MAC, mid-arm circumference; HC, head circumference.

REFERENCES

Beattie, R. B. and Dornan, J. C. (1989). Antenatal screening for intrauterine growth retardation using umbilical artery Doppler ultrasound. *British Medical Journal*, **298**, 631–5.

Beattie, R. B., Dornan, J. C., and Thompson, W. (1987). Intrauterine growth retardation: prediction of fetal distress by Doppler ultrasound. *Lancet*, **ii**, 974.

Bruinse, H. W., Sijmons, E. A., and Reuwer, P. J. H. M. (1989). Clinical value of screening for fetal growth retardation by Doppler ultrasound. *Journal of Ultrasound in Medicine*, **8**, 207–9.

Chalmers, I. (1990). *Oxford Database of Perinatal Trials*. Version 1.1, Issue 3. Oxford University Press, Oxford.

Fagan, T. J. (1975). Nomogram for Bayes' theorem. *New England Journal of Medicine*, **293**, 257.

Gairdner, D. and Pearson, J. (1971). A growth chart for premature and other infants. *Archives of Disease in Childhood*, **46**, 783–7.

Georgieff, M. K., Sasanow, S. R., Mammel, M. C., and Pereira, G. C., (1986). Midarm circumference/head circumference ratios for identification of symptomatic LGA, AGA and SGA newborn infants. *Journal of Pediatrics*, **2**, 316–21.

Grant, A. and Mohide, P. (1982). Screening and diagnostic tests in antenatal care. In *Effectiveness and satisfaction in antenatal care* (ed. M. Enkin and I. Chalmers), pp. 22–59. Spastics International Medical Publications, William Heinemann Medical Books, London.

Hanretty, K. P., Primrose, M. H., Neilson, J. P., and Whittle, M. J. (1989). Pregnancy screening by Doppler uteroplacental and umbilical artery waveforms. *British Journal of Obstetrics and Gynaecology*, **96**, 1163–7.

McParland, P., Steel. S. A., and Pearce, J. M. (1990). The clinical implications of absent or reversed end-diastolic frequencies in umbilical artery flow velocity waveforms. *European Journal of Obstetrics and Gynaecology*, **37**, 15–23.

Newnham, J. P., Lyn, L., Patterson, R. N., James, I. R., Diepveen, D. A., and Reid, S. A. (1990). An evaluation of the efficacy of Doppler flow velocity waveforms analysis as a screening test in pregnancy. *American Journal of Obstetrics and Gynecology*, **162**, 403–10.

Neilson, J. P., Munjana, S. P., and Whitfield, C. R. (1984). Screening for small for dates fetuses: a controlled trial. *British Medical Journal*, **289**, 1179–80.

Patterson, R. M. and Pouliot, M. R. (1987). Neonatal morphometrics and perinatal outcome: who is growth retarded? *American Journal of Obstetrics and Gynecology*, **3**, 691–3.

Rosenberg, K., Grant, J. M., Tweedie, J., Atchinson, G., and Gallagher, F. (1982). Measurement of fundal height as a screening test for fetal growth retardation. *British Journal of Obstetrics and Gynaecology*, **89**, 447–50.

Schulman, H., Winter, D., Farmakides, G., *et al.* (1989). Pregnancy surveillance with Doppler velocimetry of uterine and umbilical arteries. *American Journal of Obstetrics and Gynecology*, **160**, 192–6.

Sijmons, E. A., Reuwer, P. J. H. M., van Beek, E., and Bruinse, H. W. (1989). The validity of screening for small-for-gestational age and low-weight-for-length infants by Doppler ultrasound. *British Journal of Obstetrics and Gynaecology*, **96**, 192–6.

Trudinger, B. J., Cook, C. M., Thompson, R., Giles, W. B., and Connelly, A. (1988). Low dose aspirin therapy improves fetal weight in umbilical-plancental insufficiency. *Lancet*, **2**, 214–15.

Whitelaw, A. (1977). Subcutaneous fat measurement as an indication of nutrition of the fetus and newborn. In *Nutrition and metabolism of the newborn* (ed. H. K. A. Visser), pp. 131–43. Symposium proceedings. Nijhoff, Holland.

6. The application of continuous wave screening to the uteroplacental circulation

Susan Bewley and Sarah Bower

INTRODUCTION

Although pre-eclampsia (PET) and intra-uterine growth retardation (IUGR) are major causes of maternal and perinatal mortality and morbidity, the conditions are poorly defined and the underlying pathology is ill understood. There is a hypothesis that they are both manifestations of failed trophoblastic invasion and 'uterine ischaemia'. The disease is exhibited in mothers as PET, with its associated mortality and morbidity, and in the fetus as growth retardation, which may be accompanied by hypoxia, neonatal brain damage, and perinatal mortality. Morphological studies have suggested a failure of trophoblastic invasion as a common underlying cause (Brosens *et al*. 977; Khong *et al*. 1986), and this may be manifested in early pregnancy as an increased resistance to flow in the uteroplacental circulation as measured by Doppler ultrasound (McParland and Pearce 1988). The animal model of repetitive embolization of the ewe uterine circulation gives support to this concept of an underlying maternal abnormality (Clapp *et al*., 1980, 1982). Embolization led to increased uterine vascular resistance and decreased uterine blood flow, as well as growth retardation of the fetus and changes in umbilical blood flow and resistance.

The assumption on which Doppler screening is based is that the fall of uteroplacental flow velocity waveform (FVW) resistance indices by 22–24 weeks' gestation represents the second wave of trophoblastic invasion, and that the uteroplacental FVW reflects the depth of trophoblastic invasion. Thus, Doppler indices of the second trimester uteroplacental circulation might predict third trimester complications.

DIFFICULTIES OF INSONATING THE UTEROPLACENTAL CIRCULATION

There are inherent difficulties in insonating the uteroplacental circulation, which will be described first before evaluating the screening work to date.

Anatomical obstacles

There are two major differences between the vessels of the uteroplacental circulation and the majority of the fetal vessels studied so far: their size and complexity.

The uteroplancental tree is a complicated branching structure (Itskovitz *et al.* 1980) (see Fig. 6.1), and investigators have not reached unanimous agreement about which part to study and whether one part reflects the whole network—let alone whether theirs is the relevant measure when it comes to screening. It may well be that different disease processes arise from, or are reflected in, different parts of the tree. It is simple to comprehend that what goes on in the trunk, branches, and twigs of a tree will affect the foliage (or oxygenation of the fetal cotyledons) differentially. Thus, some investigators have studied the uterine artery near its origin (Schulman *et al.* 1986), some the arcuates arteries in the lateral wall (Campbell *et al.* 1983), some the subplacental vasculature (Trudinger *et al.* 1985), and some have tried to devise overall measures (Bewley *et al.* 1989).

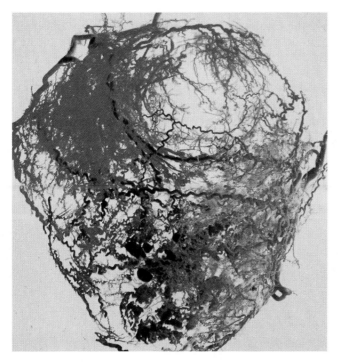

Fig. 6.1 Polymer injection of the pregnant uterine arteries demonstrating the three-dimensional anatomy of the uteroplacental circulation.

Physiological variability

The physiological variability and changes in response to stresses and disease have been less extensively investigated in the maternal than in the fetal circulation. Flow velocity waveforms are thought not to be influenced from day to day, nor by time of day, meals, smoking, or external vibratory acoustic stimulation (Gagnon *et al.* 1988; Hastie *et al.* 1988; Morrow *et al.* 1988; Pearce *et al.* 1988) but to be affected by maternal heart rate and exercise (Mulders *et al.* 1988; Morrow *et al.* 1989). Nevertheless, the instability of the circulation makes accurate and reproducible measurements in screening difficult.

This variability has led to much wider coefficient of variation measurements for uterine FVWs than for fetal FVWs, ranging from 6 to 15 per cent (Long *et al.* 1988; Stabile *et al.* 1988). Two extreme examples of this potentially wide variation are illustrated in Figs 6.2 and 6.3. In the first, there is a large beat-to-beat variation with sinus arrhythmia as the mother breathes, and in the second, a woman with a non-palpable Braxton Hicks' contraction develops a high-resistance FVW, and eventually even reverse flow, over a period of 3 min. These difficulties with reproducibility can lead to initial disappointment and disillusion.

So, before the results of the screening studies are established, the efforts of the examiner may be hampered by the very nature of the circulation under study.

Continuous wave versus pulsed or colour Doppler ultrasound

As far as the size of uteroplacental vessels goes, there have been claims that, using duplex pulsed wave (PW) equipment, uterine or arcuate arteries are visible with ultrasonography, but, as the pictures in Fig. 6.4 eloquently demonstrate, even when a double-walled object is seen it may not be the artery (shown as a red flash) using colour Doppler ultrasound. Thus,

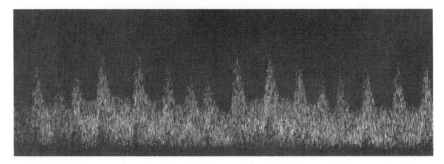

Fig. 6.2 Flow velocity waveforms from a uteroplacental artery demonstrating sinus arrhythmia.

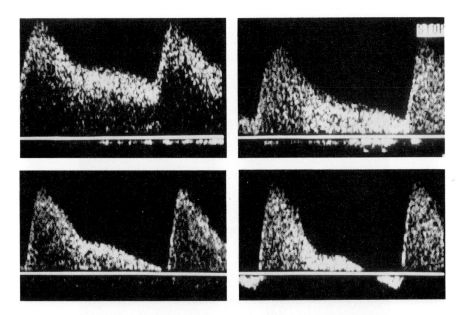

Fig. 6.3 Flow velocity waveforms from a uteroplacental artery at 26 weeks. The top left-hand panel is the waveform at rest and the remaining panels demonstrate the changes that occurred during a Braxton Hicks' contraction, that the woman was not aware of and which lasted for 3 min. There is a gradual diminution in frequencies in end-diastole and the development and reverse flow.

although PW ultrasonography with a range gate may demonstrate the exact depth of insonation, it does not necessarily visualize the vessels accurately, and so there is no convincing reason to advocate its use for the uteroplacental circulation.

Continuous wave (CW) has the advantages of cost, manouvrability of the probe (as there is no linear array), and smaller machine size (Fig. 6.5). In any case, CW and PW ultrasound have shown consistent results (Mehalek *et al.* 1988), so for screening CW has to be preferred. As it is impossible to determine which vessel produces the signal with CW, the signals are best described as coming from a uteroplacental vessel.

Colour flow is a very recent innovation and, as explained above, shows very well the limitations of conventional PW ultrasound for studying the uteroplacental circulation. Branches can be followed all over the uterus and under the placenta. It has the potential eventually to measure velocity, volume, and pressure gradients. It has given us remarkable pictures of the uterine vessels (Fig. 6.6) and has improved accuracy when compared with PW ultrasound (Arduini *et al.* 1990). Initial results suggest that it may

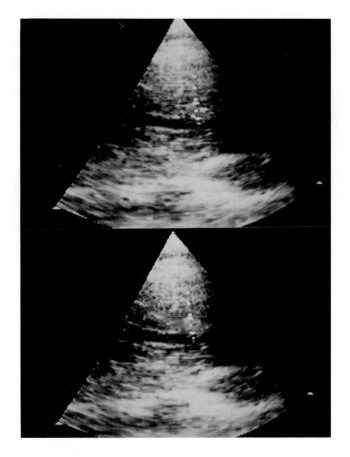

Fig. 6.4 Pulsed images of the lateral uterine wall. The top panel shows a double-walled vessel that appears to be a vessel. When colour flow Doppler ultrasound is turned on (lower panel), the flash of colour does not correspond with what was felt to be a vessel.

have a useful role as a secondary screening test to CW Doppler ultrasound screening (see below).

Does the FVW index matter?

Although the Americans and Australians have tended to use S/D ratios (or A/B ratios) (Stuart *et al*. 1980), there is a preference in the UK to use the resistance index, RI (Pourcelot 1974). There is a direct relationship of S/D to RI and one can easily be converted to the other, using the formula $RI = 1 - 1/(S/D)$, but, in view of the fact that they are inversely related, if one is

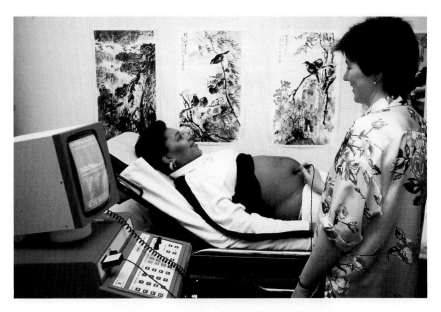

Fig. 6.5 An illustration of the convenience of the Doptek continuous wave ultrasound equipment.

normally distributed the other cannot be (Thompson *et al.* 1988). For choosing screening cut-offs and for analysis, it is preferable to have a normally distributed variable. In a normal pregnant population, RI is normally distributed (Bewley *et al.* 1989)

The pulsatility index (PI) (Gosling and King 1975) has not generally been used in the uteroplacental circulation, because there are huge variations and errors in its measurement (Ruissen *et al.* 1988). Also, the normal FVWs on the maternal side have a simple shape (Fig. 6.7 (a)) and so PI is not so appropriate. None of the screening studies reviewed used PI and there is no pressing reason why they should.

It may be that there is information in the waveform shape that is lost in the simpler measures. There has been a suggestion that a notch is more predictive than RI alone in cases of high α-fetoprotein without fetal abnormality (Aristodou *et al.* 1990).

SCREENING RESULTS

Bearing the considerable difficulties of uteroplacental insonation in mind, sense can be made of the disparate results that the screening studies have

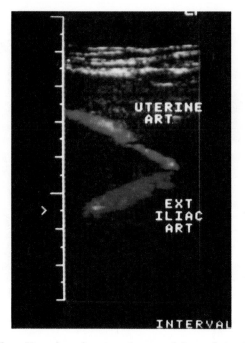

Fig. 6.6 Colour flow Doppler ultrasound map of the pelvic side-wall, demonstrating the internal iliac artery and its branch, the uterine artery.

revealed so far. Although at least seven Doppler studies screening for these complications have been reported (Campbell *et al.* 1986; Arduini *et al.* 1987; Hanretty *et al.* 1989; Schulman *et al.* 1989; Jacobson *et al.* 1990; Newnham *et al.* 1990; Steel *et al.* 1990), they produced widely varying results and presently no unifying conclusion can be drawn.

There are a variety of possible explanations for the big discrepancies between the studies, largely related to wide differences in technique; some used CW, others PW ultrasound. They have used varying and different definitions of PET, IUGR, and poor pregnancy outcome, as well as combining the outcome in unique ways. Sometimes there appears to have been a strange selection of 'unselected' patients and choice of cut-off since abnormal FVWs were found in from 2.8 per cent (Hanretty *et al.* 1989) to 37 per cent (Steel *et al.* 1988) of the population.

There were differences in the normal ranges and selection processes. Abnormality was sometimes based on the worst FVW (Campbell *et al.* 1986; Arduini *et al.* 1987), an average (Schulman *et al.* 1986), or even the best FVW (Hanretty *et al.* 1989). Some studies had a large percentage of subjects with failed recordings or who were lost to follow-up. Those women who ended their pregnancies as an emergency elsewhere, whose

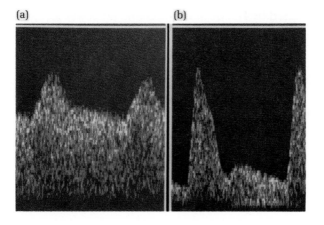

Fig. 6.7 Flow velocity waveforms from a uteroplacental artery: (a) low resistance pattern; (b) high resistance pattern.

notes were sequestered at some point, or who moved may have been a different group than those with known outcomes. Many studies did not assess outcome in a blind way, separate from knowledge of the test result.

General populations

Early optimism

Campbell *et al.* (1986) reported a single study performed at 16–18 weeks' gestation of consecutive attenders for a booking ultrasound scan. The results were concealed from the clinicians. Eighty-five per cent (126/149) of the cases were available for analysis. A cut-off of RI = 0.58 from either side of the uterus was used to define an abnormal FVW. This value represented two standard deviations from the mean of a normal range of FVWs that had been transformed by a computer program called a frequency index profile (FIP). However, 40 per cent (50 women) of this apparently unselected group had an RI above the 95th centile of the normal range.

The criteria for definition of abnormality were: (1) pregnancy-induced hypertension (PIH): systolic blood pressure > 30 or diastolic blood pressure: > 15 with proteinuria or generalized oedema (as defined by Chesley 1978); (2) IUGR: a birth-weight < 10th centile corrected for sex and parity; and (3) birth asphyxia: where all three features of abnormal non-stress test antepartum cardiotocograph (CTG), scalp, or cord venous pH > 7.2 and 5-min Apgar score > 7 were present.

Of these women with abnormal FVWs, 10 developed PIH (two accompanied by IUGR and one by an intrauterine death, IUD), 10 pregnancies were complicated by IUGR alone, and one fetus was asphyxiated at birth. Of the 76 with normal FVWs, five developed PIH (one accompanied by IUGR) and five pregnancies were complicated by IUGR alone. A total of 31 women developed PIH, growth retardation or asphyxia in labour, giving the test a sensitivity and specificity of 68 per cent and 69 per cent, respectively. The positive and negative predictive values were 42 per cent and 87 per cent, respectively.

With 15 per cent of subjects lost to follow-up and a high complication rate of 25 per cent in the remainder, it seems that the study group may not have been randomly selected and representative. With such a high prevalence of disease, the predictive values would be expected to drop when the test was applied to a truly 'normal' pregnant population (Grant and Mohide 1982).

Some entirely negative results

Hanretty *et al.* (1989) reported a study of the uteroplacental circulation on 543 unselected women in the antenatal clinic at 26–30 or 34–36 weeks' gestation. There were 357 women in the earlier group and 395 in the later group, whilst 209 women appeared in both. The results were not available to the clinicians. The CW transducer was moved until uteroplacental FVWs representing the lowest resistance were obtained. No satisfactory FVW could be obtained from 18 and 19 per cent or cases, respectively, in the two groups. An A/B ratio of 2.07 (RI = 0.52) or 2.0 (RI = 0.5) was used for the definition of abnormal at the two gestation periods, representing values over the 95th centile of another pilot study of 150 patients. Results showed that 6.5 and 2.8 per cent of the pregnancies in the two groups had abnormal uteroplacental FVWs.

The criteria for definition of abnormality were: (1) PIH: a blood pressure $\geq 140/90$ if the obstetrician arranged for further investigation of treatment; and (2) small for gestational age (SGA): a birth-weight of less than the 5th centile of a locally derived database. They also compared the prematurity, Caesarean section, instrumental delivery, elective delivery, low Apgar, and special-care baby unit admission rates.

No significant differences in the percentage of women who developed complications in the normal or abnormal groups were found. Recruitment at an antenatal clinic may have biased collection in favour of high-risk pregnancies. Forty-six per cent of women were admitted or investigated during the pregnancy, 25 per cent developed PIH, 24 per cent of pregnancies were delivered electively, and 36 per cent had instrumental deliveries. With more than an 18 per cent failure rate to obtain recordings, the study group may have become biased even if the subjects had been randomly selected initially. The method of FVW collection was not from a defined site, and was designed to find low resistance, not high or even standard, FVWs. There was an eccentric definition of PIH and no break-down of the hypertension by severity or the presence of proteinuria.

Schulman *et al.* (1989) have reported a screening study using CW ultra-sound of both the uterine and umbilical arteries. Studies were performed on 255 women (46 per cent of potential participants) at monthly intervals from 20 weeks' gestation. Nine women (3.5 per cent) had an average 26-week uterine RI > 0.62, which was considered abnormal. Seven of the nine had IUGR, PIH, or PET (no definitions given) giving the test a positive predictive value of 78 per cent. Those who had volunteered for the study had higher risk scores than non-volunteers. Results were given to both the women and clinicians. No women appear to have been lost to follow-up.

Relation of subplacental FVWs to hypoxia

Newnham *et al.* (1990) have reported a study of 615 women who were recruited from a public antenatal clinic and scanned at 18, 24, 28, and 34 weeks' gestation using CW Doppler, with PW ultrasound to confirm un-usual or abnormal FVWs. Results were not revealed to the women or clinicians. An S/D of more than the 95th centile for normal pregnancy was considered abnormal.

The criteria used for abnormality were: (1) IUGR: a birth-weight below the 10th centile; and (2) fetal hypoxia: a determination made arbitrarily and retrospectively by an obstetrician, including the factors of operative delivery for abnormal CTG, a 5-min Apgar score or less than 7, and an umbilical artery pH < 7.2, if these were not thought to be the result of birth difficulties after birth.

Of the 615, 34 did not consent to participate in the trial, 33 were excluded for gestational age of more than 20 weeks, twins, language difficulties, being non-pregnant, or having a fetal abnormality. A further 13 delivered elsewhere and delivery details were incomplete, leaving 535 pregnancies for analysis. The population had a prevalence of 7 per cent with APH, 13.5 per cent with PIH (of which 6.5 per cent had proteinuria, 9.5 per cent SGA, and 8.6 per cent with fetal hypoxia (all but one case judged to be intrapartum).

A significant correlation was observed between uteroplacental S/D at 24 weeks' gestation and fetal hypoxia. Uteroplacental S/D was not significantly correlated with fetal hypoxia at any other gestational age, nor with SGA or other complications, including PET, at any gestation. At 24 weeks an abnormal S/D predicted fetal hypoxia with a sensitivity of 24 per cent and a specificity of 94 per cent (prevalence 9.9 per cent of the 253 results available at that gestation).

These results contrast with those of other workers, as the correlation was confined to hypoxia, but the explanation may lie in the site of insonation.

The technique of Trudinger *et al.* (1985) was used, where FVWs are collected from beneath the placenta.

Resolution? Many correlations but poor predictive properties

A class-sectional study of 977 women was performed by Bewley *et al.* (1991), recruited from the booking ultrasound clinic at 16–24 weeks' gestation. The RI in the uteroplacental circulation was measured by CW Doppler ultrasound. Women were recruited consecutively when attending for their routine booking scan at 16–24 weeks' gestation. No results were revealed to the subjects or the clinicians. No action was taken on the basis of any readings. The test was performed with the observer unbiased to clinical information or a history of previous complications.

Continuous wave signals were collected from four fixed sites on the uterus, left and right 'arcuate' and left and right 'uterine' (Bewley *et al.* 1989) (Fig. 6.8). A different methodology was employed in that an overall averaged RI was calculated. This had the highest correlation with birthweight, suggesting that it gave an indication of the whole uterine circulation.

The average RI, from the four sites was called AVRI and this was related to gestational age by regression analysis. A value above the 95th centile of AVRI is referred to as AVRI 95. There was no marked difference in the screening parameters of AVRI and the worst RI, although the best RI (i.e. the lowest value) was useless.

The medical diagnoses of outcome were made by three independent obstetricians. The criteria for definition of abnormality were: (1) hypertension: two recordings of diastolic blood pressure $\geq$ 90 mmHg 4 h apart, or

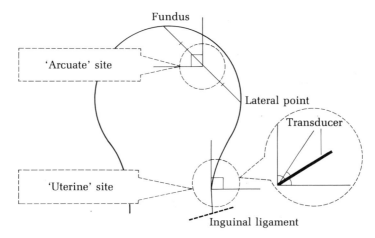

Fig. 6.8 Varying insonation sites used by Bewley *et al.* (1989).

one reading of $\geq$ 110 mmHg at any stage of pregnancy (Davey and MacGillivray 1988); (2) PIH: hypertension appearing for the first time or more than 20 weeks, subdivided into proteinuric ($>$ 150 mg/24h, or $> +$ on dipstick urine testing) or non-proteinuric; (3) severe proteinuric PIH: a diastolic blood pressure $\geq$ 110 mmHg and proteinuria $>$ 500 mg/24h or $\geq + +$ on dipstick (and a rise of $\geq$ 30/35 mmHg if hypertension was present at less than 20 weeks); (4) antepartum haemorrhage (APH): divided into abruption, if there was proven retroplacental clot, and other causes; (5) fetal loss or IUD: the death of a fetus between the blood-flow screening scan and delivery (excluding termination of pregnancy); (6) operative delivery for fetal distress (ODFD): as defined by the operator, and (7) SGA. Actual birth-weight was expressed as a number of standard deviations from the mean expected weight for gestation, and babies were considered SGA (under the 3rd, 5th, and 10th centiles) if they were $> 1.96, >$ 1.65, or > 1.28 standard deviations from the mean, respectively.

Statistical analysis was performed in 925 cases, the remainder being excluded for a variety of reasons. Outcome losses were small and data were available for 96.5 per cent (943/977) of the population. The 14 twin pregnancies were excluded from the screening analysis.

To define the risk to any particular pregnancy of developing complications, the outcomes were also amalgamated into two groups. 'Any' complication included all pregnancies with SGA $<$ 10th centile, PIH, antepartum haemorrhage (APH), IUD, or ODFD. 'Severe' complications represented severest disease and a more stringent definition of abnormal; SGA $<$ 3rd centile or severe proteinuric PIH or placental abruption or IUD. Women with 'severe' complications were also included in the 'any' group.

Pregnancies with high AVRI values had a higher incidence of PET abruption, SGA babies, and fetal or perinatal loss. Uteroplacental Doppler ultrasonography can pick up differences between normal and abnormal pregnancies, and distinguish a certain pathological process, but the overlap is too great for accurate prediction. As a demonstration of this, Fig. 6.9 shows the mean AVRI for a variety of conditions. There is a difference in the second trimester between pregnancies destined to develop abruption rather than placental praevia, proteinuric rather than non-proteinuric PIH, and neonatal complications rather than none. This suggests that there may be a unifying aetiology picked up by Doppler ultrasound that leads to some of the cases of APH, some of the cases of PIH, and some of the small babies. Also, by subdividing the complications, it can be seen how important and difficult the definition of outcome is when there is no better gold standard for comparison. However, Fig. 6.9 also shows the overlap between the groups that makes the predictive values poor. So, there is something in the uteroplacental circulation but it is elusive and inaccurate at present.

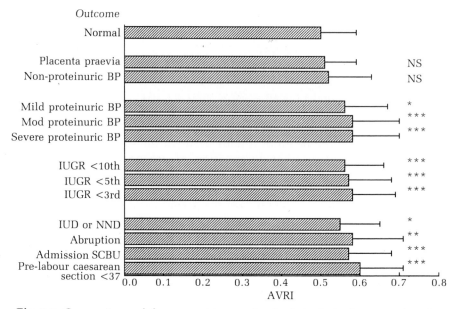

Fig. 6.9 Comparison of the mean (+ one standard deviation) averaged resistance index (AVRI) in normal and complicated pregnancies. BP, blood pressure (hypertension); IUGR, intra-uterine growth retardation; IUD, intra-uterine death; NND, neonatal death; SCBU, special-care baby unit; C/S, caesarean section; NS, not significant. ***p ≤ 0.005; **p ≤ 0.01; p ≤ 0.05.

The screening characteristics of the study are shown in Table 6.1. When the AVRI was above the 95th centile for gestation, the overall risk of pregnancy complications was 67 per cent, and the risk of a severe complication was 25 per cent. However, the sensitivity of the test for these complications was only 13 and 21 per cent, respectively. The screening results were low, even though the top 5 per cent of the screening tests contained 15–33 per cent of each complication, and an individual's relative risk increased by up to 9.8 times. Any individual woman's risk of having complications was multiplied several times by having a high AVRI. Cut-off point above the 95th centile for gestation was thought to be suitable for abnormality, and although the sensitivities are low at this cut-off point, the specificities are high. Using the original cut-off point of 0.58 gave sensitivities comparable to the other papers although the specificities were much lower. Even with a cut-off point of 0.58, Campbell *et al.* (1986) defined 30 per cent of the population as abnormal. The AVRI index is made up of arcuate and uterine vessels, so more of the population would be defined as abnormal.

The predictive values were high when the test result was very high. Thus, in the AVRI group, a woman had a 25 per cent chance of a very serious

Table 6.1 Prediction of different separate complications using Doppler test AVRI 95 as the cut-off point for abnormality

Outcome	Prevalence (%)	Sensitivity (%)	Specificity (%)	PPV (%)	NPV (%)	n
Intra-uterine death	1.3	25	94	6	99	925
Abruption	0.9	38	95	6	99	922
Proteinuric	3.8	24	96	17	97	903
SGA < 3rd centile	3.2	20	95	12	97	913
SGA < 10th centile	12.8	15	96	35	88	913
Any complication	30.2	13	97	67	72	912
Severe complication(s)	7.0	21	95	25	94	889

AVRI 95, averaged resistance index > 95th centile for gestational age; SGA, small-for-gestational age; PPV, positive predictive value; NPV, negative predictive value.

complication, and a 67 per cent chance of one probably requiring investigation or admission to hospital. So, the test identifies a high-risk group of women. This may be acceptable for collecting a group for research purposes and for any individual woman who could have increased surveillance or antenatal care, but in routine practice the majority of women with disease would be missed. False reassurance can lull the woman and the clinician into complacency and can form the basis for litigation for missed disease.

Different screening characteristics in different groups
There are suggestions that changing the exact application might make the test useful. Comparing tests performed at less than 20 weeks' and more than 20 weeks' gestation showed an improvement in sensitivity for severe complications of pregnancy, from 14 to 27 per cent. There was a marked difference in the sensitivity of the test in predicting severe proteinuric hypertension between Caucasian and Afro-Caribbean women, 8 per cent as opposed to 46 per cent. There are racial differences in PET, although they are not apparent at 16–24 weeks' gestation. This might suggest that in Afro-Caribbean women, PET is more severe, with higher AVRI values, and therefore more disease is correctly predicted. Alternatively, more hypertension in Caucasians is labelled PET when it is not associated with abnormal maternal circulations and may be essential hypertension. The World Health Organization (WHO) has found that, in the second trimester, there are similar blood pressures between races despite very different incidences of PIH later (WHO 1988). The Doppler screening test was more accurate than an obstetric risk score (Adelstein and Fedrick 1978) in the prediction of problems. The screening test was similar when used in

primigravid or multigravid populations, although there was a difference in the sensitivity for SGA at less than the 10th centile, 19 versus 9 per cent.

Screening in high-risk populations

There is a suggestion emerging that the Doppler ultrasound test works better in certain groups, such as primigravidae or Afro-Caribbeans, hence the need to study the possible value of screening in high-risk populations.

Good predictions if high risk of PIH

Arduini *et al.* (1987) studied a group of 60 women at high risk of developing PIH. Thirty-eight (63 per cent) had previous PIH, 15 (25 per cent) had previous PET, four (7 per cent) renal disease, and three (5 per cent) had collagen disease. Readings were taken from the lateral uterine wall using PW ultrasound on a single occasion at 18–20 weeks' gestation. An RI > 0.57 was considered abnormal and the authors did not indicate whether the results were concealed from the clinicians. All 60 pregnancies were followed up.

The criterion for definition of abnormality was: PIH, two blood pressure readings > 140/90 mmHg 4 h apart. Of the 20 (33 per cent) women with abnormal FVWs, 14 developed PIH, whereas 8 out of 32 with normal FVWs developed PIH. The breakdown of results was only given for PIH. For PIH alone the test has a sensitivity and specificity of 64 and 84 per cent, respectively. The positive and negative predictive values were 70 and 80 per cent, with a prevalence of 37 per cent. The predictive values are very high as this is a high-risk population.

Doppler less predictive than uric acid and abdominal circumference

Jacobson *et al.* (1990) performed a study recruiting 93 women from a high-risk antenatal clinic. Pulsed wave ultrasound was used to obtain a mean RI of two FVWs from the left and right lateral uterine walls at 20 and 24 weeks' gestation. These were not related to placental side but considered higher and lower values, and were not used for management. An abnormal value was RI ≥ 0.58 for the higher reading and RI ≥ 0.50 for the lower. The criteria for abnormal outcome were: (1) IUGR: birth-weight less than the 10th centile for gestation and sex; (2) PET: hypertension with proteinuria or hyperuricaemia; (3) hypertension: a rise in diastolic blood pressure of > 25 mmHg if the baseline diastolic pressure was > 90 mmHg, and a rise of > 15 mmHg if the baseline was > 90 mmHg; (4) proteinuria: ≥ 500 mg/24h disappearing after delivery; and (5) hyperuricaemia: final plasma ≥ 0.35 mmol/l. Not surprisingly, in view of the selection, the study group had a high rate of complications: 29 per cent developed pre-eclampsia (of which 9.7 per cent was proteinuric), 18.3 per cent had

IUGR, and 14 per cent were delivered due to severe maternal or fetal compromise.

When signals were unobtainable, the majority had poor outcomes, so absent FVWs were considered abnormal. The 'worse', or higher, RI was found to be more discriminating than the lower value. Abnormal FVWs at 24 weeks predicted: (a) PET with a sensitivity of 44 per cent and positive predictive value of 33 per cent; (b) proteinuric PET with values of 67 per cent and 17 per cent; (c) IUGR with values of 71 per cent and 33 per cent; and (d) delivery due to severe maternal or fetal compromise with values of 77 per cent and 28 per cent, respectively. As the complications worsened, the predictions improved. Although the authors found that a 20-week FVW, but not 20-week abdominal circumference (AC), was significantly associated with IUGR, they did not provide a comparison of FVW, AC and uric acid at 20 weeks. They still managed to conclude that a rise in uric acid was the best predictor of PET and that fetal AC was the best predictor of IUGR. A comparison was made of the 24-week uteroplacental FVW with uric acid and fetal AC. High RI was the most sensitive indicator, but positive predictive values were lower and there was a high false-positive rate. This study had more stringent definitions than others and the results are similar to those of Campbell *et al.* (1986) and Arduini *et al.* (1987)

Good predictions of hypertension in primigravidae

Steel *et al.* (1988, 1990) screened only primigravidae for prediction of hypertensive diseases of pregnancy. A CW ultrasound study of primigravidae only was made at 18–20 weeks, and repeated at 24 weeks if the result was abnormal. The results were not made available to the clinicians. In the preliminary report, 200 out of 252 (79 per cent) cases were available for analysis, and this rose to 1014 out of 1198 (85 per cent) by the end of the study. However, failure to attend at 24 weeks was considered one reason for exclusion. Because only those with abnormal results were recalled, this may have biased the analysis.

An unspecified number of 'waveforms on either side of the uterus' was obtained and if any had an RI > 0.58 the test was considered abnormal. In the pilot study (Steel *et al.* 1988), 75 women (37 per cent) were found to have abnormal waveforms at 18–20 weeks, but this had fallen to 21 (11 per cent) by 24 weeks' gestation.

The criteria for abnormality were: (1) hypertension: a blood pressure of more than 140/90 mmHg, recorded for the first time in late pregnancy, on two occasions more than 4 h apart; and (2) SGA: a fetal abdominal circumference measurement of less than two standard deviations from the mean or, in the absence of a third trimester scan, a birth-weight of less than the 10th centile. Proteinuria was defined as greater than 300 mg/24 h or greater than $++$ on dipstick testing. SGA was further subdivided into symmetrical or asymmetrical on the basis of the ultrasonic head/abdominal circumference ratio.

The results are illustrated in Table 6.2, although there are marked difference between the groups some 48 per cent of the women with abnormal Doppler waveforms had a normal pregnancy outcome. Figure 6.10 shows the distribution of the worst RI obtained from women who subsequently

Table 6.2 Pregnancy outcome based on waveform analysis at 24 weeks' gestation (from Steel *et al.* 1990)

Outcome	Normal waveforms	Abnormal waveforms	*p*
Number	896	118	
Hypertension (%)	45 (5)	29 (25)	< 0.001
Proteinuric hypertension (%)	7 (0.8)	12 (10)	< 0.001
Hypertension with intrauterine growth retardation (%)	0	15 (13)	< 0.001
Onset of hypertension			
< 37 weeks	6 (0.7)	18 (15)	< 0.001
< 34 weeks	3 (0.4)	13 (11)	< 0.001
Maximum blood pressure (mmHg)			
Systolic > 160	11 (1)	13 (11)	< 0.001
Diastolic > 110	8 (0.9)	13 (11)	< 0.001
Need for hypotensive agents (%)			
Oral only	2 (0.2)	3 (2.5)	0.007
Intravenous	1 (0.1)	6 (5)	< 0.001
Gestation at onset of labour (%)			
< 37 weeks	1 (0.1)	21 (18)	< 0.001
< 34 weeks	1 (0.1)	9 (8)	< 0.001
Intra-uterine growth retardation (%)			
Symmetrical	18 (2)	4 (3)	NS
Asymmetrical	28 (3)	23 (20)	< 0.001
Birth-weight			
< 50th centile	28 (3)	21 (18)	< 0.001
< 10th centile	65 (7)	32 (27)	< 0.001
Perinatal death and deaths before discharge (%)			
Still births	8 (0.9)	3 (3)	NS
Neonatal deaths	2 (0.2)	2 (2)	NS
Total	10 (1)	5 (4)	0.03

NS, not significant.

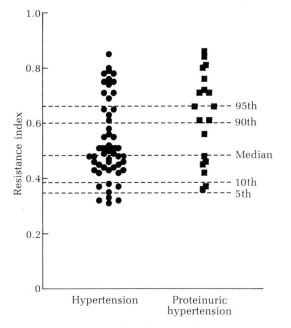
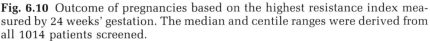

Fig. 6.10 Outcome of pregnancies based on the highest resistance index measured by 24 weeks' gestation. The median and centile ranges were derived from all 1014 patients screened.

became hypertensive. Steel *et al.* (1990) described a dose effect for women with RI results above the 90th centile, in that the worse the RI the worse the pregnancy outcome.

Conclusion   There appear to be subpopulations of pregnant women who may benefit from Doppler screening of the uteroplacental circulation.

APPRAISAL OF SCREENING RESULTS

Putting all the studies together (Table 6.3) suggests that the results from CW Doppler ultrasonography from the uteroplacental circulation are too poor to justify its routine use.

The reasons for the overlap in the results from the uteroplacental circulation may be summarized as follows:

1. The test is known to have low reproducibility.
2. Even if the test were more accurate, it may be that the uteroplacental circulation is not static.

3.   The definitions of the outcome variables are inadequate.

4.   All outcome variables represent a heterogeneous mixture of under-lying pathologies.

A false-positive test may result from attempts to overcome inadequate placentation. The placenta may be able to redistribute blood locally away from underperfused segments, so protecting fetal growth. A loss of one-third of the villous parenchyma can occur without effect on fetal growth (Fox 1983). In some cases delivery may occur before the development of pre-eclampsia or before a growth-retarded fetus dies. There may be a greater overlap of normal and abnormal waveforms at early gestations, and in some cases minimum placental resistance may not have been achieved by 24 weeks' gestation.

A false-negative result might arise during sampling of a very large circulation or if there is a mixed population of vessels (Steel *et al.* 1990). Abnormal pregnancies may suffer from greater variation or instability. Abnormal waveforms may possibly arise later in pregnancy after the screening test has been performed. Cases of early onset pre-eclampsia may be due to underlying renal disease and as such may have a normal circulation.

RECENT DEVELOPMENTS

Colour flow imaging

The results of screening with CW ultrasound suggest that it may be success-ful in recognizing the severer forms of pregnancy complications, especially in high-risk groups such as primigravidae. The false-positive rate of approx-imately 50 per cent has led some authors to suggest that such women should be subjected to colour flow Doppler ultrasonography in order accurately to identify the uterine artery. Waveforms can then be acquired by pulsed Doppler ultrasound. Figure 6.6 demonstrates the ease with which colour flow mapping can identify the uterine artery.

In a recent study at King's College Hospital in London (Bower 1991, unpublished data) a two-stage screening procedure was employed as follows:

(1) A total of 2437 women were screened by means of CW Doppler waveforms from both sides of the uterus at 20 weeks' gestation. This is a rapid and cheap procedure (Bewley *et al.* 1991). An abnormal result was considered as a RI > 0.58 from either side of the uterus, or the presence of a dichrotic notch. At 20 weeks, 15 per cent of the population had an abnormal result.

(2) Women with an abnormal result were asked to attend for colour flow mapping and pulsed Doppler studies at 24 weeks' gestation, and, if these were abnormal, again at 26 weeks' gestation. At 24 weeks, 5.4 per cent of women had abnormal findings, and this figure fell to 4.1 per cent at 26 weeks' gestation.

Outcome was available on 2190 women and of these:

1. Nine per cent developed PIH (6.5 per cent were non-proteinuric and 2.5 per cent were proteinuric).
2. SGA infants with a birth-weight of less than the 5th centile were delivered by 4.1 per cent of the women.

Table 6.4 illustrates the results. The sensitivity and positive predictive value for screening for proteinuric hypertension are higher than values reported from CW ultrasound studies (a maximum of 63 per cent sensitivity and a 13 per cent positive predictive value (Steel *et al.* 1990), and this is maximal by 26 weeks' gestation. The results for non-proteinuric hypertension are much poorer than those reported from CW ultrasound studies, which were awful. This strongly suggests a different aetiology for the two conditions. Screening for SGA is poor and the results are very similar to those obtained with CW Doppler ultrasound.

Figure 6.11 illustrates the different waveform characteristics and their distribution in the 41 patients with proteinuric hypertension. Thus, it can be seen that the presence of a dichrotic notch is a better predictor than just an abnormal RI.

A RANDOMIZED CONTROLLED TRIAL OF SCREENING AND INTERVENTION

The final test of a screening test should be a randomized controlled trial (RCT). This can either be an RCT to determine the benefits and hazards, or an RCT to look at the screening combined with some form of intervention. The St. George's Hospital group (Steel *et al.* 1988, 1990; McParland 1990) have recognized the poor predictive value of CW waveforms from the uteroplacental circulation but have pointed out that it is useful in that it recognizes: (i) 60 per cent of all cases of proteinuric hypertension; and (ii) 90 per cent of cases of proteinuric hypertension associated with small babies.

The recent suggestion (Wallenburg and Rotmans 1987; Beaufils *et al.* 1988) that low-dose aspirin may prevent PIH set the scene for an intervention study. Primigravid women with abnormal waveforms were randomized at 24 weeks' gestation to receive either 75 mg aspirin per day or

Table 6.3 Essential features of published screening studies

	Campbell et al. (1986)	Arduini et al. (1987)	Hanretty et al. (1989)	Schulman et al. (1989)
Method	PW	PW	CW	CW
Vessel	Arcuate lateral wall	Arcuate lateral wall	Anywhere on uterus	Uterine mean of two
Recruitment	Consecutive	At risk of PIH multiparous women	Antenatal clinic	
Gestation (weeks)	16–18	18–20	26–30	20+ (4-weekly)
Blindness				
Clinician	Yes	?	Yes	No
Patient	?		?	No
Analysis	?	?	?	?
Number (after exclusions)	149	60	357	556
Available	126	60	291	255
Percentage lost to follow-up		0	19 (failed tests)	255

Abnormal FVW	RI > 0.58	RI > 0.57	Lowest A/B >95th centile	A/B > 2.6 @ 26 weeks
Percentage with abnormal FVW	25	30		
IUGR	<10th	<10th	—	—
PIH (mmHg)	>140/90	>140/90	>140/90	
Other	Fetal distress			
Sensitivity (%)	68	64		
Specificity (%)	69	84		
PPV	42	70		78
NPV	87	80		

CW, continuous wave; PW, pulsed wave; FVW, flow velocity waveform; IUGR, intra-uterine growth retardation; PPV, positive predictive value; NPV, negative predictive value; PIH, pregnancy-induced hypertension; SD, standard deviation; UP bed, uteroplacental bed.

Table 6.3 (continued)

	Newnham et al. (1990)	Jacobson et al. (1990)	Steel et al. (1990)	Bewley et al. (1991)
Method	CW	PW	CW	CW
Vessel	Up bed	Lateral wall	Both sides of uterus	Mean of four fixed of sites
Recruitment			Primiparous at scan	Routine ultrasonography
Gestation (weeks)	18+ (4-weekly)	20 and/or 24	Two-stage (18 and 24)	16–24
Blindness				
Clinician	Yes	Yes	Yes	Yes
Patient	Yes	?	?	Yes
Analysis	Yes	Yes	?	Yes
Number (after exclusions)	615 (94.5%)	93	1198 1114	1014 977

Available	535		1014	925
Percentage lost to follow-up			9	3.5
Abnormal FVW	A/B > 95th centile	RI > 0.58	RI > 0.58	RI for gestation; < 9th centile
Percentage with abnormal FVW			12	5
IUGR	< 10th centile		AC < 2 SDs 5th, 10th centile	< 3rd/5th/10th centiles
PIH (mmHg)	> 140/90		> 140/90 + protein	Differing severity + protein
Other	Hypoxia			Abruption
Sensitivity (%)	24	44–77	18–100	9–38
Specificity (%)	94		89–91	94–96
PPV		17–33	3–27	6–67
NPV				88–99

Table 6.4 Prediction of pregnancy outcome from colour flow and pulsed Doppler ultrasonography

	Sensitivity (%)	Specificity (%)	PPV	NPV
Proteinuric PIH				
20 weeks	76	86	13	99
24 weeks	76	96	35	99
26 weeks	74	97	44	99
Non-proteinuric hypertension				
20 weeks	15	86	7	94
24 weeks	3	94	4	93
26 weeks	0	95	0	92
SGA*				
20 weeks	45	87	13	97
24 weeks	36	95	27	97
26 weeks	36	97	36	97

* Birth-weight less than 5th centile; PIH, pregnancy-induced hypertension; SGA, small for gestational age; PPV, positive predictive value; NPV, negative predictive value.

placebo. Table 6.5 illustrates the results. The placebo group had a similar outcome to the previous study from this group (Steel *et al.* 1990; see Table 6.2). Overall, the incidence of PIH was halved, but this did not reach statistical significance. However, the complications of hypertension were rarer and tended to come on much later in pregnancy. Of the four perinatal deaths in this study, the baby that died in the aspirin group was the result of a cord accident in labour; it occurred in a well grown infant (3.97 kg). The three deaths in the placebo group were in infants born between 25 and 28 weeks' gestation weighing 300–800 g, and in all cases delivery was necessary because of maternal hypertensive disease.

Many other potential treatments have been suggested for preventing and treating PIH and SGA, including bedrest (Laurin and Persson 1987), oxygen administration (Nicolaides *et al.* 1987), and nifedipine (Lindow *et al.* 1988). Doppler ultrasonography provides a means of identifying at-risk pregnancies so that these therapies can be assessed.

CONCLUSION

The uterine circulation is a very complex branching structure. Waveforms from this circulation are affected by the position of the placenta, the

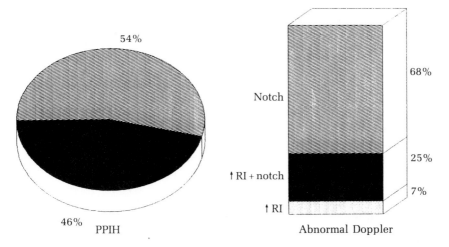

Fig. 6.11 Different pulsed waveform characteristics of the 363 women identified as abnormal by continuous wave Doppler ultrasound. The distribution of these characteristics in 41 women with proteinuric, pregnancy-induced hypertension (PPIH) is shown in the pie chart.

rotation of the uterus, which vessel is insonated, and probably several maternal factors.

Intra-uterine death, proteinuric hypertension, placental abruption, and SGA babies are associated with abnormal waveforms in early pregnancy, well before the development of symptoms or signs of the disease. These results lend support to the concept of a single pathology affecting the uteroplacental circulation, with differing clinical presentations. Most outcome measures studied have heterogeneous causes, but the increasingly high predictions of the more severe forms of disease strongly suggest that Doppler waveforms are recognizing pregnancies complicated from reduced uterine blood supply, perhaps secondary to inadequate trophoblast invasion (p. 206).

Screening by CW Doppler ultrasound is easy, cheap, convenient, quick, and reliable. Its accuracy, however, does not justify its introduction for all pregnant women. Screening by colour flow and pulsed Doppler ultrasound is probably not practical for all women because it is expensive and time consuming. The recent suggestion that the false-positive rate of CW Doppler ultrasonography may be reduced by colour flow and PW Doppler ultrasonography has promise.

When applied to high-risk groups, such as primigravidae and perhaps Afro-Caribbean women, CW Doppler ultrasonography may have a place in recognizing a group that may be amenable to intervention. The single randomized controlled trial that has been reported is very promising.

Table 6.5 Pregnancy outcome (from McParland *et al.* 1990)

Outcome measure	Placebo group	Aspirin group	p
Pregnancy-induced hypertension (n (%))	13 (25)	6 (13)	NS
Proteinuric hypertension (n (%))	10 (19)	1 (2)	< 0.02
Onset of hypertension before 37 weeks (n (%))	9 (17)	0	< 0.01
Gestation at delivery (weeks (SD))	38.7 (3.9)	39.5 (2.1)	NS
Birth-weight (g (SD))	2954 (852)	3068 (555)	NS
Number of infants (n (%))			
< 2500 g	13 (25)	7 (15)	NS
< 1500 g	4 (8)	0	NS
< 5th centile	7 (14)	7 (14)	NS
Blood loss at delivery (ml (SD))	358 (228)	289 (188)	NS
Perinatal deaths	3	1	NS

NS, not significant, SD, standard deviation.

REFERENCES

Adelstein, P. and Fedrick, J. (1978). Antenatal identification of women at increased risk of being delivered of a low birth weight infant at term. *British Journal of Obstetrics and Gynaecology*, **85**, 8–11.

Arduini, D., Rizzo, G., Romanini, C., and Mancuso, S. (1987). Uteroplacental blood flow velocity waveforms as predictors of pregnancy-induced hypertension. *European Journal of Obstetrics, Gynecology, and Reproductive Biology*, **26**, 335–41.

Arduini, D., Rizzo, G., Boccolini, M. R., Romanini, C., and Mancuso, S. (1990). Functional assessment of uteroplacental and fetal circulations by means of color Doppler ultrasonography. *Journal of Ultrasound Medicine.* **9**, 249–53.

Aristodou, A., van den Hof, M. C., Campbell, S., and Nicolaides, K. (1990). Uterine artery Doppler in the investigation of pregnancies with raised maternal serum alpha-fetoprotein. *British Journal of Obstetrics and Gynaecology*, **97**, 431–5.

Beaufils, M., Uzan, S., Donsimoni, R., and Colau, J. C. (1988). Prevention of pre-eclampsia by early antiplatelet therapy. *Lancet*, **i**, 840–2.

Bewley, S., Campbell, S., and Cooper, D. (1989). Uteroplacental Doppler flow velocity waveforms in the second trimester. A complex circulation. *British Journal of Obstetrics and Gynaecology*, **96**, 1040–6. *Erratum* (1990). *British Journal of Obstetrics and Gynaecology*, **97**, 214.

Bewley, S., Cooper, D., and Campbell, S. (1991). Doppler investigation of uteroplacental blood flow resistance in the second trimester: a screening study for pre-eclampsia and intrauterine growth retardation. *British Journal of Obstetrics and Gynaecology*, **88**, 871–9.

Brosens, I., Dixon, H. G., and Robertson, W. B. (1977). Fetal growth retardation and the arteries of the placental bed. *British Journal of Obstetrics and Gynaecology*, **84**, 656–63.

Campbell, S., Diaz-Recasens, J., Griffin, D. R., *et al.* (1983). New Doppler technique for assessing uteroplacental blood flow. *Lancet*, **i**, 675–7.

Campbell, S., Pearce, J. M. F., Hackett, G., Cohen-Overbeek, T., and Hernandez, C. (1986). Qualitative assessment of uteroplacental blood flow: early screening test for high-risk pregnancies. *Obstetrics and Gynecology*, **68**, 649–53.

Chesley, L. (1978). *Hypertensive disorders of pregnancy*, pp. 9–11. Appleton-Century-Crofts, New York.

Clapp, J. F., Szeto, H. H., Larrow, R., Hewitt, J., and Mann, L. I. (1980). Umbilical blood flow response to embolization of the uterine circulation. *American Journal of Obstetrics and Gynecology*, **138**, 60–5.

Clapp, J. F., McLaughlin, M. K., Larrow, R., Farnham, J., and Mann, L. I. (1982). The uterine haemodynamic response to repetitive unilateral vascular embolization in the pregnant ewe. *American Journal of Obstetrics and Gynecology*, **144**, 309–18.

Davey, D. A. and MacGillivray, I. (1988). The classification and definition of the hypertensive disorders of pregnancy. *American Journal of Obstetrics and Gynecology*, **158**, 892–8.

Fox, H. (1983). Placental pathology. In *Progress in obstetrics and gynaecology*, Vol. 3. (ed. J. Studd), pp. 47–56. Churchill Livingstone, Edinburgh.

Gagnon, R., Morrow, R., Ritchie, K., Hunse, C., and Patrick, J. (1988). Umbilical and uterine blood flow velocities after vibratory acoustic stimulation. *American Journal of Obstetrics and Gynecology*, **159**, 574–8.

Gosling, R. G. and King, D. H. (1975). Ultrasonic angiology. In *Arteries and veins* (ed. A. W. Harcus and L. Adamson), pp. 61–98. Churchill Livingstone, Edinburgh.

Hanretty, K. P., Primrose, H., Neilson, J. P., and Whittle, M. J. (1989). Pregnancy screening by Doppler uteroplacental and umbilical artery waveforms. *British Journal of Obstetrics and Gynaecology*, **96**, 1163–7.

Hastie, S. J., Howie, C. A., Whittle, M. J., and Rubin, P. C. (1988). Daily variability of umbilical and lateral uterine wall artery blood velocity waveform measurements. *British Journal of Obstetrics and Gynaecology*, **95**, 571–4.

Itskovitz, J., Lindebaum, E. S., and Brandes, J. M. (1980). Arterial anastamosis in the pregnant human uterus. *Obstetrics and Gynecology*, **55**, 67–71.

Jacobson, S-L., Imhof, R., Manning, N., *et al* (1990). The value of Doppler assessment of the uteroplacental circulation in predicting preeclampsia of intrauterine growth retardation. *American Journal of Obstetrics and Gynecology*, **162**, 110–14.

Khong, T. Y., de Wolf, F., Robertson, W. B., and Brosens, I. (1986). Inadequate maternal vascular response to placentation in pregnancies complicated by pre-eclampsia and by small-for-gestational age infants. *British Journal of Obstetrics and Gynaecology*, **93**, 1049–59

Laurin, J. and Persson, P. H. (1987). The effect of bedrest in hospital on fetal outcome in pregnancies complicated by intra-uterine growth retardation. *Acta Obstetrica et Gynecologica Scandinavica*, **66**, 407–11.

Lindow, S. W., Davies, N., Davey D. A., and Smith, J. A. (1988). The effect of sublingual nifedipine on uteroplacental blood flow in hypertensive pregnancy. *British Journal of Obstetrics and Gynaecology*, **95**, 1276–81.

Long, M. G., Price, M., and Spencer, J. A. D. (1988). Uteroplacental perfusion after epidural analgesia for elective caesarean section. *British Journal of Obstetrics and Gynaecology*, **95**, 1081–2.

McParland, P. and Pearce, J. M. (1988). Doppler blood flow in pregnancy. *Placenta* **9**, 427–50.

McParland, P., Pearce, J. M., and Chamberlain, G. V. P (1990). Doppler ultrasound and aspirin in the recognition and prevention of pregnancy-induced hypertension. *Lancet*, **335**, 1552–5.

Mehalek, K. E., Berkowitz, G. S., Chitkara, U., Rosenberg, J., and Berkowitz, R. L. (1988). Comparison of continuous-wave and pulsed Doppler S/D ratios of umbilical and uterine arteries. *Obstetrics and Gynecology*, **72**, 603–6.

Morrow, R. J., Ritchie, J. W. K., and Bull, S. B. (1988). Maternal cigarette smoking: the effects on umbilical and uterine blood flow velocity. *American Journal of Obstetrics and Gynecology*, **159**, 1069–71.

Morrow, R. J., Ritchie, J. W. K., and Bull, S. B. (1989). Fetal and maternal hemodynamic responses to exercise in pregnancy assessed by Doppler ultrasonography. *American Journal of Obstetrics and Gynecology*, **160**, 138–40.

Mulders, L. G. M., Jongsma, H. W., Wijn, P. F. F., and Hein, P. R. (1988). The uterine artery blood flow velocity waveform: reproducibility and results in normal pregnancy. *Early Human Development*, **17**, 55–70.

Newnham, J. P., Patterson, L. L., James, I. R., Diepeveen, D. A., and Reid, S. E. (1990). An evaluation of the efficacy of Doppler flow velocity waveform analysis as a screening test in pregnancy. *American Journal of Obstetrics and Gynecology*, **162**, 403–10.

Nicolaides, K. H., Campbell, S., Bradley, R. J., Bilardo, C. M., Soothill, P. W., and Gibb, D. (1987). Maternal oxygen therapy for intrauterine growth retardation. *Lancet*, **i**, 942–5.

Pearce, J. M., Campbell, S., Cohen-Overbeek, T., Hackett, G., Hernandez, J., and Royston, J. P. (1988). References ranges and sources of variation for indices of pulsed Doppler flow velocity waveforms from the uteroplacental and fetal circulation. *British Journal of Obstetrics and Gynaecology*, **95**, 248–56.

Pourcelot, L. (1974). Applications clinique de l'examen Doppler transcutane. In *Velocimetric ultrasonor Doppler*, INSERM, No. 34, (ed. P. Peronneau), pp. 213–40. Paris.

Ruissen, C. J., van Vugt, J. M. G., and de Haan, J. (1988). Variability of PI calculations. *European Journal of Obstetrics, Gynecology, and Reproductive Biology*, **27**, 213–20.

Schulman, H., Fleischer, A., Farmakides, G., Bracero, L., Rochelson, B., and Grunfeld, L. (1986). Development of uterine artery compliance in pregnancy as detected by Doppler ultrasound. *American Journal of Obstetrics and Gynecology*, **155**, 1031–6.

Schulman, H., Winter, D., Farmakides, G., *et al*, (1989). Pregnancy surveillance with Doppler velocimetry of uterine and umbilical arteries. *American Journal of Obstetrics and Gynecology*, **160**, 192–6.

Stabile, I., Bilardo, C., Panella, M., Campbell, S., and Grudzinskas, J. G. (1988). Doppler measurements of uterine blood flow in the first trimester of normal and complicated pregnancies. In *Trophoblast research*, Vol. 3, (ed. P. Kaufmann and R. K. Miller), pp. 301–7. Plenum Publishing Corporation, New York.

Steel, S. A., Pearce, J. M., and Chamberlain, G. V. (1988). Doppler ultrasound of the uteroplacental circulation as a screening test for severe pre-eclampsia with intra-uterine growth retardation. *European Journal of Obstetrics, Gynecology, and Reproductive Biology*, **28**, 279–87.

Steel, S. A., Pearce, J. M., McParland, P., and Chamberlain, G. V. P. (1990). Early Doppler ultrasound screening in prediction of hypertensive disorders of pregnancy. *Lancet*, **i**, 1548–51.

Stuart, B., Drumm, J., Fitzgerald, D. E., and Duignan, N. M. (1980). Fetal blood velocity waveforms in normal pregnancy. *British Journal of Obstetrics and Gynaecology*, **87**, 780–5.

Thompson, R. S., Trudinger, B. J., and Cook, C. M. (1988). Doppler ultrasound waveform indices: A/B ratio, pulsatility index and Pourcelot ratio. *British Journal of Obstetrics and Gynaecology*, **95**, 581–8.

Trudinger, B. J., Giles, W. B., and Cook, C. M. (1985). Uteroplacental blood flow velocity–time waveforms in normal and complicated pregnancy. *British Journal of Obstetrics and Gynaecology*, **92**, 39–45.

Wallenburg, H. C. S. and Rotmans, N. (1987). Prevention of recurrent idiopathic fetal growth retardation by low-dose aspirin and dipyridamole. *American Journal of Obstetrics and Gynecology*, **157**, 1230–5.

World Health Organization, International Collaborative Study of Hypertensive Disorders of Pregnancy. (1988). Geographic variation in the incidence of hypertension in pregnancy. *American Journal of Obstetrics and Gynecology*, **158**, 80–3.

7. The application of umbilical artery studies to complicated pregnancies

Alfred Ng and Brian Trudinger

INTRODUCTION

As illustrated in Chapter 4, (Fig. 4.1) the resistance to blood flow in the umbilical arteries decreases progressively with increasing gestation. Abnormal umbilical artery flow velocity waveform (FVW) patterns include reduced, absent (Fig. 7.1) and even reversed diastolic frequencies (Fig. 7.2). When expressed in terms of the indices applied to the maximum frequency envelope of the waveform, an increase in arterial resistance is associated with an increase in the A/B (S/D) ratio or pulsatility index (PI) and an increase in the resistance index (RI), which tends towards unity.

Umbilical artery FVWs identify the presence of a vascular lesion within the placenta, the presence of placental vascular insufficiency (see Chapter 11). The effect of this on the fetus is determined both by the degree of vascular insufficiency and its duration. Numerous studies have now shown a strong association between abnormal FVWs and adverse fetal outcome (Trudinger *et al.* 1985*a*; Schulman 1987; Anyaegbunam *et al.* 1988; Berkowitz *et al.* 1988; Farmakides *et al.* 1988; Divon *et al.* 1989*a*; Lowery *et al.* 1990; Maulik *et al.* 1990).

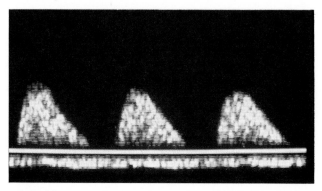

Fig. 7.1 Umbilical artery flow velocity waveforms showing absent end-diastolic frequencies (AEDF).

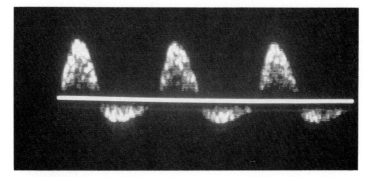

Fig. 7.2 Umbilical artery flow velocity waveforms showing reversed frequencies in end-diastole.

THE SMALL-FOR-GESTATIONAL AGE FETUS

Many studies have examined the role of umbilical artery FVWs in the prediction of fetuses that are small for gestational age (SGA) (Table 7.1). Umbilical artery FVWs are less sensitive in the prediction of SGA fetuses than sonographic fetal biometry or the use of ultrasonographically derived fetal weight estimates (Table 7.2).

The current role for Doppler velocimetry appears to be in those fetuses already identified as small on the basis of real-time ultrasonic biometry. Doppler testing discriminates small fetuses stressed by umbilical, placental constraint from those small fetuses that are constitutionally small and are not suffering from such constraint. Small fetuses that have normal Doppler FVWs do not appear to be at risk antenatally (Burke *et al.* 1990). The converse, however, is that small fetuses with abnormal Doppler FVWs are at increased risk of perinatal death, antepartum and intrapartum fetal distress, operative delivery for fetal distress, admission to the neonatal intensive care unit, and prolonged duration of hospitalization (Trudinger *et al.* 1985a; Laurin *et al.* 1987; Reuwer *et al.* 1987; 1989; Rochelson *et al.* 1987a, b; Dempster *et al.* 1989).

As the umbilical artery FVWs deteriorate to reduced, absent, and reversed end-diastolic flow, there is a graded correlation with the risk and severity of fetal compromise (McParland *et al.* 1991). In a recent review (Thompson *et al.* 1988) of the clinical outcome of 2178 high-risk patients who had undergone umbilical artery FVW studies, as the waveforms became more abnormal there was increasing evidence of growth failure as indicated by a fall in the mean birth-weight centile (Table 7.3). Perinatal mortality and morbidity rates exhibited a positive correlation with the degree of abnormality in the umbilical artery FVWs, with the worst outcome occurring in patients with absence of end-diastolic frequencies

Table 7.1 Prediction of SGA fetuses in high-risk pregnancies

Reference	Prevalence (%)	n	Criteria*	Sensitivity (%)	Specificity (%)	PPv (%)	NPV (%)
Fleischer et al. (1985)	17	189	S/D ≥ 3	78	83	49	95
	31	52	S/D ≥ 3	87	81	66	94
Arduini et al. (1987)	31	75	PI	61	73	50	81
Marsal and Persson (1988)	74	72	AEDF	60	95	97	45
Berkowitz et al. (1988)	25	385	S/D ≥ 3	55	92	73	—
Gaziano et al. (1988)	21	250	S/D ≥ 4	79	66	21	96
Divon, et al. (1988)	35	127	S/D ≥ 3	49	94	81	77
Dempster et al. (1989)	40	205	S/D ≥ 95th centile	41	82	61	68
Lowery et al. (1990)	47	146	S/D ≥ 3	65	66	24	92

* Diagnostic cut-off level for prediction of SGA fetuses. SGA, small for gestational age; PPV, positive predictive value; NPV, negative predictive value; S/D, systolic/diastolic ratio of the umbilical artery flow velocity waveforms; AEDF, absent end-diastolic frequencies; PI, pulsatility index.

Table 7.2 Comparison between sonographic and umbilical flow velocity waveform prediction of small-for-g fetuses

	Berkowitz et al. (1988)		Gaziano et al. (1988)		Divon et al. (1989a)		Chambers et al. (1989)	
Prevalence (%)	25		21		35		58	
Methods	A/B	EFW	A/B	EFW	A/B	EFW	RI	AC
Criteria	≥3	<10th centile	≥4	<10th centile	>3	<10th centile	>2SD	>SD
Sensitivity (%)	55	76	79	43	49	87	29	73
Specificity (%)	92	80	66	98	94	87	—	73
PPV (%)	73	60	21	77	81	78	77	84
NPV (%)	—	—	96	94	77	92	52	67

A/B, systolic/diastolic ratio of the umbilical artery; EFW, sonographically estimated fetal weight; RI, resistance index; PPV, positive predictive value; NPV, negative predictive value; SD, standard deviation; AC, ultrasonically measured, fetal, abdominal circumference.

Table 7.3 Outcome characteristics

		Result of last umbilical artery FVW study			
	Whole group	< 95th centile	95–99th centile	> 99th centile	AEDF
No. of patients	2178	1650 (76%)	193 (9%)	239 (11%)	96 (4%)
Delivery					
Gestational age	37.7	38.3	37.6‡	35.8§	31.1§
Labour planned					
Spontaneous	790	691 (42%)	56 (29%)	35 (15%)	8 (8%)‖
Induced	818	642 (39%)	86 (45%)	85 (36%)	5 (5%)‖
Elective caesarean	570	317 (19%)	51 (26%)	119 (50%)	83 (86%)‖
Labour outcome					
Vaginal	1371	1145	122	95	9
Emergency caesarean	237	188	20	25	4
Neonate					
Birth-weight (g)	2875	3097	2713§	2148§	1198§
Length (cm)	47.8	48.8	47§	44.2§	37.6§
Ponderal index	26.0	26.4	25.9	24.6§	21.8§
Centile weight (mean)	36.2	41.9	27.0§	15.1§	9.0§
SGA infants					
<10th centile	588 (27%)	293 (18%)3	73 (38%)	144 (60%)	78 (81%)‖
<5th centile	389 (18%)	165 (10%)	44 (23%)	111 (46%)	69 (72%)‖

Apgar scores				
1 min ≤ 6	531 (24%)	335 (20%)	53 (27%)	78 (33%)	65 (68%)‖
5 min ≤ 6	131 (6%)	62 (4%)	16 (8%)	27 (11%)	26 (27%)‖
Admission NICU	548	303	45	113	87‖
NICU stay					
Mean no. of days	18.5	10.0	18.9*	25.0§	43.7§
Perinatal deaths					
Fetal deaths	21	8	4	3	6
Neonatal deaths					
Day 0–7	38	16	4	9	9
Day 8–28	10	2	0	0	8
PNM rate	31.7	15.8	41.5	50.2	239.6‖
Corrected PNM	18.2	7.9	21.2	13.0	206.5‖
Major fetal anomaly					
Total no.	61	27	9	16	9‖
Survived first 28 days	81	14	5	7	5
Not surviving (including still births)	30 (6)	13 (2)	4 (1)	9 (2)	4 (1)

Results are shown as number (percentage of grouping) unless otherwise stated.
Differences significant in comparison to the normal (<95th centile) grouping are shown (analysis of variance with Bonferroni multiple comparisons): *p < 0.05; †p < 0.01; ‡p < 0.001; §p < 0.0001; ‖p < 0.0001, χ^2 statistic for categorical data.
FVW, flow velocity waveforms; AEDF, absent end-diastolic frequencies; SGA, small for gestational age; NICU, neonatal intensive care unit; PNM rate, perinatal mortality rate per 1000 total births; corrected PNM rate corrected for fetal anomaly.

(AEDF), confirming previous studies (Erskine and Ritchie 1985; Reuwer *et al.* 1987; Rochelson *et al.* 1987*a*; Divon *et al.* 1989*b*); McParland *et al.* 1991).

Biochemical analysis on umbilical venous blood samples obtained by cordocentesis and at elective caesarean section also suggest a graded relationship between the umbilical artery indices and the degree of fetal acidaemia and hypoxia, with absence of diastolic flow being most predictive of abnormal blood gas results (Ferrazzi *et al.* 1988; Nicolaides *et al.* 1988; Tyrrell *et al.* 1989; Bilardo *et al.* 1990). When the cardiac output was studied on fetuses with AEDF, an increase in right ventricular output was found. It has been suggested that this reflects redistribution of blood flow to achieve preferential perfusion of the cranial vessels (see Chapter 14). This gives further support to the idea that fetal deprivation is a consequence of the placental lesion detected by umbilical artery FVWs (Reed *et al.* 1987).

HYPERTENSIVE DISEASE OF PREGNANCY

In hypertensive disorders of pregnancy, umbilical artery FVWs appear to be predictive of adverse fetal outcome (Ducey *et al.* 1987; Cameron *et al.* 1988; Trudinger *et al.* 1990). Changes in Doppler waveforms from the umbilical artery predate changes in the cardiotocograph (non-stress test) or biophysical profile.

The incidence of maternal thrombocytopenia was found to be higher in patients with abnormal Doppler waveforms (Duvey *et al.* 1987), suggesting that there may be a correlation between the severity of the hypertension and the incidence of placental vascular lesions. In a series of 95 severely hypertensive women with proteinuria, an abnormal A/B ratio (S/D ratio) was present in two-thirds of cases (Trudinger *et al.* 1990). No relationship was observed between the duration of hypertension and the umbilical artery waveforms. Fetal mortality and morbidity rates were significantly associated with the presence of an abnormal umbilical artery waveform but not with the duration of hypertension. In several patients, abnormal umbilical artery waveforms were detected before the hypertensive process was apparent, raising the possibility that the placental vascular lesion precedes the clinical signs of hypertension.

MULTIPLE PREGNANCY

In uncomplicated twin and triplet pregnancies, the umbilical artery FVWs show the same progressive decrease in the A/B ratio (S/D ratio) as seen in singleton pregnancies (Giles *et al.* 1988, 1990; Neilson *et al.* 1989).

Abnormal umbilical artery FVWs predict SGA fetuses and those with an adverse outcome (Nimrod *et al.* 1987; Giles *et al.* 1988, 1990). As in singleton pregnancies, the umbilical artery flow studies appear to identify the fetus with umbilical placental vascular insufficiency. Not all SGA fetuses can be predicted by Doppler ultrasonography (Cameron *et al.* 1988), but the use of the difference in the A/B (S/D) ratio between the twin members appears to improve the detection of discordant growth (Farmakides *et al.* 1985; Saldana *et al.* 1987; Divon *et al.* 1989*b*). However, serial studies of each twin are necessary to identify continuing, concordant growth.

Disagreements exist regarding the umbilical artery flow patterns in the twin–twin transfusion syndrome (Farmakides *et al.* 1985; Giles *et al.* 1985, 1991; Pretorius *et al.* 1988). Significant twin transfusion is suspected when there exists discordant ultrasound measurements of fetal size, umbilical cord diameter, and amniotic fluid volume between members of the twin pair but concordant umbilical artery FVWs. The presence of normal resistance in the umbilical placental circulation led to the suggestion that umbilical waveforms should be normal, and this has been observed in clinical practice (Giles *et al.* 1991).

Even though Doppler waveforms are a useful addition to the real-time ultrasound suspicion of twin transfusion syndrome, they appear to have little or no place in the management of such pregnancies.

The value of Doppler waveforms in twin pregnancy lies in the early recognition of the fetus at risk. This was illustrated in a comparative study in which the perinatal mortality rate was examined before and after the introduction of a Doppler screening protocol (Giles *et al.* 1988). A total of 172 twin pairs, in which both fetuses were alive after 28 weeks' gestation, were studied. There was a significant reduction in the total perinatal mortality rate after the introduction of the Doppler studies. Doppler information did not lead to increased intervention: the gestational age at delivery and the caesarean section rates were comparable between the two groups. The authors felt that Doppler ultrasonography recognized a high-risk subgroup of twin pregnancies who required more intensive fetal surveillance.

THE LUPUS SYNDROME

A variety of recurrent adverse pregnancy outcomes including recurrent spontaneous abortion, SGA, unexplained intra-uterine death, and pre-eclampsia has been associated with the presence of antiphospholipid antibodies in the mother (Reece *et al.* 1990). These include the lupus anticoagulant and anticardiolipin antibody. Such mothers may be known to have systemic lupus erythematosus (SLE) or other autoimmune phenomena, but in others the obstetric manifestations may be the only clinical feature.

Fetal deterioration is predicted by the development of an abnormal umbilical artery waveform, and some authors have suggested that this is all that is required for pregnancy surveillance (Trudinger *et al*. 1988*a*), but others disagree (see Chapter 8). Umbilical artery waveforms undoubtedly have a major role in pregnancy surveillance when the fetus is shown to be small on real-time ultrasound biometry, but waveforms from the utero-placental circulation appear to be more predictive. Some women with SLE have antiR$_0$ antibodies which are associated with congenital heart block, and this is easily recognized by umbilical artery waveforms (see also Chapter 14).

MAJOR FETAL ANOMALY

A major concern over any antenatal test, but in particular cardiotocography (non-stress tests), is their failure to detect fetuses with major anomalies. Such fetuses are very likely to demonstrate antenatal signs of fetal distress and this may lead to an inappropriate delivery by Caesarean section. A high incidence of abnormal umbilical artery FVWs have been reported amongst fetuses with major anomalies. An increased A/B (S/D) ratio has been observed in fetuses with trisomy 13, 18, and 21 (Trudinger and Cook 1985; Rochelson *et al*. 1990) and other major structural abnormalities (Trudinger and Cook 1985; Meizner *et al*. 1987; Sherer *et al*. 1989; Gaziano *et al*. 1990). The placentae of fetuses with autosomal trisomies exhibit a significant reduction in the tertiary villus small arterial vessel count (Rochelson *et al*. 1990).

In summary, the finding of an abnormal umbilical artery waveform (especially AEDF) in a symmetrical SGA or a normally grown fetus should raise the possibility of a major structural anomaly, more so if the utero-placental waveforms are normal (see Chapter 8). This should lead to a detailed study of fetal anatomy, a search for structural markers suggestive of chromosomal abnormalities (Benecereff 1991), and consideration of karyotyping.

POST-DATES PREGNANCY

This problem has been addressed by only three studies to date, with conflicting results. Rightmire and Campbell (1987) and Guidetti *et al*. (1987) reported a poor correlation between various measures of fetal compromise and umbilical artery FVWs. The mathematical model of the placental vascular tree predicts that the larger the placental size the greater is the fraction of the vascular tree that needs to be obliterated to cause a detectable increase in the A/B (S/D) ratio (Thompson and Trudinger 1991). This, combined with the supposedly greater susceptibility of the mature fetus to the effects of hypoxia, may explain the poor correlation between various measures of fetal compromise and the umbilical artery FVWs.

Recently, Pearce and McParland (1991) have published a large observational study on more than 500 women with post-dates pregnancies. All pregnancies had their gestational age confirmed by real-time ultrasound fetal biometry in the first half of pregnancy. There were no fetal deaths and only 11 fetuses developed fetal distress in the first stage of labour. Doppler ultrasonography was more sensitive than standard methods of fetal surveillance at predicting fetal distress in the first stage (Table 7.4). The authors reported a very low incidence of abnormal uteroplacental waveforms in this group and suggested that the reason for the development of an abnormal umbilical circulation it is not hypoxic ischaemia of the intervillous space but aging of the fetal vessels that leads to an increased

Table 7.4 (a) The predictive value and efficiency of tests for fetal distress in the first stage of labour (from Pearce and McParland 1991)

			Predictive value	
Test	Sensitivity	Specificity	Positive	Negative
NST	55%	98%	35%	99%
AEDF	91%	100%	91%	100%
AF < 3 cm	82%	99%	60%	100%
AEDF and AF < 3 cm	100%	99%	61%	100%

(b) Comparison of antenatal tests for their ability to predict fetal distress using the kappa statistic (from Pearce and McParland 1991)

Outcome measure	NST	AEDF	AF < 3 cm	AEDF + AF < 3 cm
Fetal distress				
First stage	0.41	0.91	0.68	0.75
Second stage	0.05	0.29	0.39	0.43
Apgar scores < 5				
1 min	0.11	0.17	0.09	0.28
5 min	0.03	0.07	0.37	0.32

NST, non-stress test; AEDF, absent end-diastolic frequencies in the umbilical artery; AF, amniotic fluid column.

umbilical artery resistance pattern. With the very low incidence of adverse fetal outcome reported in this study, a multi-centre trial would be required to investigate the value of Doppler waveforms in post-dates pregnancies.

A CLINICAL STRATEGY FOR FETAL SURVEILLANCE

Umbilical artery waveforms recognize a vascular pathology in the placenta, and it is believed that this lesion leads to fetal compromise. The severity of the umbilical placental vascular insufficiency is reflected in the spectrum of abnormality of the waveforms. Although the risk of fetal compromise increases as the degree of Doppler abnormality increases, there is no cut-off level at which fetal morbidity starts to appear, and many therefore suggest that it is unreasonable to equate any particular value of the resistance ratios with the need for clinical intervention. There always exists a need to seek and quantitate evidence of fetal compromise by direct fetal testing.

The approach to the clinical use of Doppler waveforms from the umbilical artery is based upon two assumptions for which there is good evidence, namely:

1. Doppler-defined placental vascular abnormality precedes significant fetal deprivation.
2. Biophysical measures of fetal welfare, such as cardiotocography (non-stress test), biophysical profile, and ultrasonic fetal biometry, quantify the degree of fetal compromise.

Comparative studies of Doppler and biophysical testing have been reported. Using a perinatal asphyxia defined as an operative delivery for fetal distress, a low 5-min Apgar score, or admission to a neonatal intensive care unit as an outcome measure, abnormal Doppler findings were similar in their predictive power to an abnormal cardiotocograph (non-stress test) although an abnormal Doppler result had a greater sensitivity (Trudinger *et al*. 1986). The association of an abnormal cardiotocograph with abnormal Doppler findings selects a group with a very high mortality rate (Farmakides *et al*. 1988; Pearce *et al*. 1991). Similar conclusions can be drawn from comparative studies of Doppler waveforms and the presence of oligo-hydramnios (Lombardi *et al*. 1989).

Comparisons between fetal biometry and Doppler have been dealt with above (see Table 7.2). However, it is again worth stressing that biometry is the more sensitive technique for detecting SGA, although Doppler waveforms are more sensitive in discriminating the truly stressed fetus. Serial biometry and Doppler measurements in the constitutionally small, unstressed fetus demonstrate progressive fetal growth and a gradual decrease in the A/B (S/D) ratio as the placental vasculature expands. Doppler assessment is used to determine which small fetuses are truly at risk and in need of intensive fetal surveillance.

This appraoch can be summarized as follows:

1. Is the pregnancy high risk? This decision is based on clinical history and examination, perhaps supported by the ancillary aids of fetal movement counting and symphysis fundal height measurements.

2. Is there placental pathology that threatens the fetus? The presence of significant placental vascular pathology is inferred from the finding of abnormal Doppler waveforms from the umbilical artery.

3. How sick is the fetus? The extent to which the fetus is affected by direct fetal assessment utilizing fetal biometry, the biophysical profile, and fetal heart rate monitoring.

4. Is delivery of the fetus indicated? Currently, delivery is indicated if the risk of intra-uterine death or damage exceeds that of delivery. Therapies aimed at improving the intra-uterine environment are now being investigated, and this may influence the decision to deliver the patients.

FINAL PERSPECTIVES

Randomized, controlled trials

The above approach represents a rational utilization of Doppler waveforms from the umbilical artery in the clinical management of high-risk pregnancies. Three randomized, controlled trials of the availability of Doppler information all showed a decrease in intrapartum operative deliveries for fetal distress in the absence of an increased rate of premature obstetric delivery (Trudinger *et al.* 1987; Pearce *et al.* 1992; Tyrell *et al.* 1991). This indicates improved obstetric decision-making based on knowledge from the Doppler waveforms. The truly compromised fetus was better identified for close surveillance and appropriately timed delivery. The study by Pearce *et al.* (1992) demonstrated a statistical difference in perinatal and early infant mortality rates when action was taken based on the additional knowledge obtained from Doppler waveforms (see also Chapter 8). Conversely, all three studies showed a lack of intervention in the small fetus with normal waveforms with no short-term evidence of harm.

Antenatal therapy

Early detection of placental vascular lesions before significant fetal compromise has reflected the possibility of using Doppler umbilical artery studies to guide specific therapies aimed at halting or reversing the placental lesion. Platelet-associated thromboxane has been implicated in the pathogenesis of placental vascular obliteration (Mak *et al.* 1984; Trudinger *et al.* 1989; Wilcox *et al*). In a randomized controlled trial, soluble aspirin (150 mg/day) was administered to women whose pregnancies were complicated by an umbilical artery A/B (S/D) ratio of more than the 95th centile. The aspirin-treated pregnancies yielded infants with mean birth-weights that were 25 per cent heavier than those in the placebo group. There was also an increase in head circumference and in placental weights in the aspirin-treated group. The improvement was limited to patients with abnormal A/B (S/D) ratios but in whom end-diastolic frequencies were still recordable. Aspirin had no noticeable effect on fetuses with AEDF in the umbilical artery (Trudinger *et al.* 1988*b*). This suggests that the pathological disease process may be modified or delayed by low-dose aspirin if Doppler ultrasonography can recognize the process at an early stage.

REFERENCES

Angaegbunam, A., Langer, O., Brustman, L., Damus, K., Halpert, R., and Merkatz, I. R. (1988). The application of uterine and umbilical artery velocimetry to the antenatal supervision of pregnancies complication by sickle haemoglobino-pathies. *American Journal of Obstetrics and Gynecology*, **159**, 544–7.

Arduini, D., Rizzo, G., Romanini, C., and Mancuso, S. 1987). Fetal blood flow velocity waveforms as predictors of growth retardation. *Obstetrics and Gynecology*, **70**, 7–10.

Benecereff, B. (1991). Ultrasonic structural markers of chromosomal abnormalities. *Journal of the International Society for the Study of Ultrasound in Obstetrics and Gynaecology*, **1**, 24–30.

Berkowitz, G. S., Mehalek, K. E., Chitkara, U., Rosenberg, J., Cogswell, C., and Berkowitz, R. L. (1988). Doppler umbilical velocimetry in the prediction of adverse outcome in pregnancies at risk of intrauterine growth retardation. *Obstetrics and Gynecology*, **71**, 742–6.

Bilardo, C. M., Nicolaides, K. H., and Campbell, S. (1990). Doppler measurements of fetal and uteroplacental circulations: relationships with umbilical venous blood gases measured at cordocentesis. *American Journal of Obstetrics and Gynecology*, **162**, 115–20.

Burke, G., Stuart, B., Crowley, P., Scanaill, S. N., and Drumm, J. (1990). Is intrauterine growth retardation with normal umbilical artery blood flow a benign condition? *British Medical Journal*, **300**, 1044–5.

Cameron, A. D., Nicholson, S. F., Nimrod, C. A., Harder, J. R., and Davies, D. M. (1988). Doppler waveforms in the fetal aorta and umbilical artery in patients with hypertension in pregnancy. *American Journal of Obstetrics and Gynecology*, **158**, 339–45.

Chambers, S. E., Hoskins, P. R., Haddad, N. G., Johnstone, F. D., McDicken, W. N., and Muir, B. B. (1989). A comparison of fetal abdominal circumference measurements and Doppler ultrasound in the prediction of small-for-dates and fetal compromise. *British Journal of Obstetrics and Gynaecology*, **96**, 803–8.

Dempster, J., Mires, G. J., Patel, N., and Taylor, D. J. (1989). Umbilical artery velocity waveforms: poor association with small-for-gestational age babies. *British Journal of Obstetrics and Gynaecology*, **96**, 692–6.

Divon, M. Y., Girz, B. A., Lieblich, R., and Langer, O. (1989*a*). Clinical management of the fetus with markedly diminished umbilical artery end-diastolic flow. *American Journal of Obstetrics and Gynecology*, **161**, 1523–7.

Divon, M. Y., Girz, B. A., Sklar, A., Guidetti, D. A., and Langer, O. (1989*b*). Discordant twins—a prospective study of the diagnostic value of real time ultrasonography combined with umbilical artery velocimetry. *American Journal of Obstetrics and Gynaecology*, **161**, 757–60.

Divon, M. Y., Guidetti, D. A., Braverman, J. J., Oberlander, E., Langer, O., and Merkatz, I. R. (1988). Intrauterine growth retardation—a prospective study of the diagnostic value of real-time sonography combined with umbilical artery flow velocimetry. *Obstetrics and Gynecology*, **72**, 611–14.

Ducey, J., Schulman, H., Farmakides, G., *et al.* (1987). A classification of hypertension in pregnancy based on Doppler velocimetry. *American Journal of Obstetrics and Gynecology*, **157**, 680–5.

Erskine, R. L. A. and Ritchie, J. W. K. (1985). Umbilical artery blood flow characteristics in normal and growth-retarded fetuses. *British Journal of Obstetrics and Gynaecology*, **92**, 605–10.

Farmakides, G., Schulman, H., Saldana, L. R., Bracero, L. A., Fleischer, A., and Rochelson, B. (1965). Surveillance of twin pregnancy with umbilical arterial velocimetry. *American Journal of Obstetrics and Gynecology*, **153**, 789–92.

Farmakides, G., Schulman, H., Winter, D., Ducey, J., Guzman, E., and Penny, B. (1988). Prenatal surveillance using nonstress testing and Doppler velocimetry. *Obstetrics and Gynecology*, **71**, 184–7.

Ferrazzi, E., Pardi, G., Bauscaglia, M., *et al.* (1988). The correlation of biochemical monitoring versus umbilical flow velocity measurement of the human fetus. *American Journal of Obstetrics and Gynecology*, **159**, 1081–7.

Fleischer, A., Schulman, H., Farmakides, G., Bracero, L., Blattner, P., and Randolph, G. (1985). Umbilical artery velocity waveforms and intrauterine growth retardation. *American Journal of Obstetrics and Gynecology*, **151**, 502–5.

Gaziano, E., Know, E., Wager, G. P., Bendel, R. P., Boyce, D. J., and Olsen, J. (1988). The predictability of the small-for-gestational age infant by real time ultrasound derived measurements combined with pulsed Doppler umbilical artery velocimetry. *American Journal of Obstetrics and Gynecology*, **158**, 1431–9.

Gaziano, E. P., Knox, E., Wagner, G. P., Bendel, R. P., and Olson, J. D. (1990). Pulsed Doppler umbilical artery waveforms: significance of elevated umbilical artery systolic/diastolic ratios in the normally grown fetus. *Obstetrics and Gynecology* **75**, 189–93.

Giles, W. B., Trudinger, B. J., and Cook, C. M. (1985). Fetal umbilical artery flow velocity-time waveforms in twin pregnancies. *British Journal of Obstetrics and Gynaecology*, **92**, 490–7.

Giles, W. B., Trudinger, B. J., Cook, C. M., and Connelly, A. (1988). Umbilical artery flow velocity waveforms and twin pregnancy outcome. *Obstetrics and Gynecology*, **72**, 894–7.

Giles, W. B., Trudinger, B. J., Cook, C. M., and Connelly, A. J. (1990). Umbilical artery waveforms in triplet pregnancies. *Obstetrics and Gynecology*, **75**, 813–6.

Giles, W. B., Trudinger, B. J., Cook, C. M., and Connelly, A. J. (1991). Umbilical artery studies in the twin-twin syndrome. *Obstetrics and Gynecology*, (in press).

Guidetti, D. A., Divon, M. Y., Cavalieri, R. L., Langer, O., and Merkatz, I. R. (1987). Fetal umbilical artery flow velocimetry in postdates pregnancies. *American Journal of Obstetrics and Gynecology* **157**, 1521–3.

Laurin, J., Marsal, K., Persson, P., and Lingman, G. (1987). Ultrasound measurement of fetal blood flow in predicting fetal outcome. *British Journal of Obstetrics and Gynaecology*, **94**, 940–8.

Lombardi, S. J., Rosemond, R., Ball, R., Entman, S. S., and Boehm, F. H. (1989). Umbilical artery velocimetry as a predictor of adverse outcome in pregnancies complicated by oligohydramnios. *Obstetrics and Gynecology*, **74**, 338–41.

Lowery, C. L., Henson, B., Wan, J., and Brumfield, C. G. (1990). A comparison between umbilical velocimetry and standard antepartum surveillance in hospitalized high-risk patients. *American Obstetrics and Gynecology*, **162**, 710–4.

McParland, P., Steel, S. A., and Pearce, J. M. (1991). The clinical implications of absent or reversed end-diastolic frequencies in the umbilical artery flow velocity waveforms. *European Journal of Obstetrics and Gynaecology and Reproductive Biology*, **37**, 15–23.

Mak, K. K. W., Gude, N. M., Walters, W. A. W., and Boura, A. L. A. (1984). Effects of vasoactive autocoids on the human umbilical–fetal vasculature. *British Journal of Obstetrics and Gynaecology*, **91**, 99–106

Marsal, K. and Persson, P. (1988). Ultrasonic measurement of fetal blood velocity waveforms as a secondary diagnostic test for intrauterine growth retardation. *Journal of Clinical Ultrasound*, **16**, 239–44.

Maulik, D., Yarlagadda, P. Youngblood, J. P., and Ciston, P. (1990). The diagnostic efficacy of the umbilical arterial systolic/diastolic ratio as a screening tool: a prospective blinded study. *American Journal of Obstetrics and Gynecology*, **162**, 1518–25.

Meizner, I., Katz, M., and Lunenfeld, E. (1987). Umbilical and uterine flow velocity waveforms in pregnancies complicated by major fetal anomalies. *Prenatal Diagnosis*, **7**, 491–6.

Neilson, J. P., Danskin, F., and Hastie, S. J. (1989). Monozygotic twin Pregnancy: diagnostic and Doppler ultrasound studies. *British Journal of Obstetrics and Gynaecology*, **96**, 1413-18.

Nicolaides K. H., Bilardo, C. M., Soothill, P. W., and Campbell, S. (1988). Absence of end diastolic frequencies in the umbilical artery: a sign of fetal hypoxia and acidosis. *British Medical Journal*, **297**, 1026–7.

Nimrod, C., Davies, D., Harder, J., et al. (1987). Doppler ultrasound in the prediction of fetal outcome in twin pregnancies. *American Journal of Obstetrics and Gynecology*, **156**, 402–6.

Pearce, J. M. and McParland, P. (1991). A comparison of Doppler flow velocity waveforms, amniotic fluid columns and non-stress tests as a means of monitoring postdates pregnancies. *Obstetrics and Gynecology*, **77**, 204–8.

Pearce, J. M., Campbell, S., Smith, P., and Gamsu, H. (1992) A randomised, controlled trial of Doppler waveforms from the uteroplacental and fetoplacental circulation. *British Journal of Obstetrics and Gynecology*, (in Press).

Pretorins, D. H., Manchester, D., Parker, S., and Nelson, T. R. (1988). Doppler ultrasound of twin transfusion syndrome. *Journal of Ultrasound in Medicine*, **7**, 117–24.

Reece, E. A., Gabrielli, S., Cullen, M. T., Zheng, X. Z., Hobbins, J. C., and Harris, E. N. (1990). Recurrent adverse pregnancy outcome and antiphospholipid antibodies. *American Journal of Obstetrics and Gynecology* **163**, 162–9.

Reed, K. L., Anderson, C. F., and Shenker, L. (1987). Changes in intracardiac Doppler flow velocities in fetuses with absent umbilical artery diastolic flow. *American Journal of Obstetrics and Gynecology*, **157**, 774–9.

Reuwer, P. J. H., Sijmons, E. A., Rietman, G. W., van Tiel, M. W. M., and Bruinse, H. W. (1987). Intrauterine growth retardation: prediction of perinatal distress by Doppler ultrasound. *Lancet*, **ii**, 415–8.

Rightmire, D. A. and Campbell, S. (1987). Fetal and maternal Doppler blood flow parameters in postterm pregnancies. *Obstetrics and Gynecology*, **69**, 891–4.

Rochelson, B., Schulman, H., Farmakides, G., *et al.* (1987*a*). *American Journal of Obstetrics and Gynecology*, **156**, 1213–18.

Rochelson, B. L., Schulman, H., Fleischer, A., *et al.* (1987*b*). The clinical significance of Doppler umbilical artery velocimetry in the small for gestational age fetus. *American Journal of Obstetrics and Gynecology*, **156**, 1223–6.

Rochelson, B., Kaplan, C., Guzman, E., Arato, M., Hansen, K., and Trunca, C. (1990). A quantitative analysis of placental vasculature in the third trimester fetus with autosomal trisomy. *Obstetrics and Gynecology* **75**, 59–63.

Saldana, L. R., Eads, C., and Schaefer, T. R. (1987). Umbilical blood waveforms in fetal surveillance of twins. *American Journal of Obstetrics and Gynecology*, **157**, 712–15.

Sherer, D. M., Armstrong, B., Shah, Y. G., Metlay, L. A., and Woods, J. R. Jr. (1989). Prenatal sonographic diagnosis, Doppler velocimetry umbilical cord studies and subsequent management of an acardiac twin pregnancy. *Obstetrics and Gynecology* **74**, 472–5.

Schulman, H. (1987). The clinical implications of Doppler ultrasound analysis of the uterine and umbilical arteries. *American Journal of Obstetrics and Gynecology*, **156**, 889–93.

Thompson, R. S. and Trudinger, B. J. (1991). Doppler waveforms and the umbilical placental circulation: an investigation of a mathematical model. *Ultrasound in Medicine and Biology*, (in Press).

Thompson, R. S., Trudinger, B. J., and Cook, C. M. (1988). Doppler ultrasound waveform indices: *AB ratio, pulsatility index and Pourcelot ratio. British Journal of Obstetrics and Gynaecology*, **85**, 581–8.

Trudinger, B. J. and Cook, C. M. (1985). Umbilical and uterine artery flow velocity waveforms in pregnancy associated with major fetal abnormality. *British Journal of Obstetrics and Gynecology*, **92**, 666–70.

Trudinger, B. J. and Cook, C. M. (1990). Doppler umbilical and uterine flow velocity waveforms in severe pregnancy hypertension. *British Journal of Obstetrics and Gynaecology*, **97**, 142–8.

Trudinger, B. J., Giles, W. B., Cook, C. M., Bombardieri, J., and Collins, L. (1985*a*). Fetal umbilical artery flow velocity waveforms and placental resistance: clinical significance. *British Journal of Obstetrics and Gynaecology*, **92**, 23–30.

Trudinger, B. J., Giles, W. B., and Cook, C. M. (1985*b*). Flow velocity waveforms in the maternal uteroplacental and fetal umbilical placental circulation. *American Journal of Obstetrics and Gynecology*, **92**, 155–63.

Trudinger, B. J., Cook, C. M., Jones, L., and Giles, W. B. (1986). A comparison of fetal heart rate monitoring and umbilical artery waveforms in the recognition of fetal compromise. *British Journal of Obstetrics and Gynaecology*, **93**, 171–5.

Trudinger, B. J., Cook, C. M., Giles, W. B., Connelly, A., and Thompson, R. S. (1987). Umbilical artery flow velocity waveforms in high-risk pregnancy: Randomized controlled trial. *Lancet*, **1**, 188–90.

Trudinger, B. J., Stewart, G. J., Cook, C. M., Connelly, A., and Exner, T. (1988*a*). Monitoring lupus anticoagulant positive pregnancies with the umbilical artery flow velocity waveforms. *Obstetrics and Gynecology*, **72,** 215–18.

Trudinger, B. J., Cook, C. M., Thompson, R. S., Giles, W. B., and Connelly, A. (1988*b*). Low-dose aspirin therapy improves fetal weight in umbilical placental insufficiency. *American Journal of Obstetrics and Gynecology*, **159,** 681–5.

Trudinger, B. J., Connelly, A. J., Giles, W. B., and Wilcox, G. R. (1989). The effects of prostacyclin and thromboxane analogue (U46619) on the fetal circulation and umbilical flow velocity waveforms. *Journal of Developmental Physiology*, **11,** 179–84.

Tyrrell, S., Obaid, A. H., and Lilford, R. J. (1989). Umbilical artery Doppler velocimetry as a predictor of fetal hypoxia and acidosis at birth. *Obstetrics and Gynecology*, **74,** 332–7.

Tyrrell, S. N., Lilford, R. J., MacDonald, H. N., Nelson, E. J., Porter, J., and Gupta, J. K. (1991). Randomised trial of Doppler ultrasound and biophysical scoring in high risk pregnancy. *British Journal of Obstetrics and Gynaecology*, **97,** 909–12.

Wilcox, G. R., Trudinger, B. J., Cook, C. M., and Wilcox, W. R. (1989). Reduced platelet counts in pregnancies with abnormal Doppler umbilical flow waveforms. *Obstetrics and Gynecology*, **73,** 639–43.

8. The application of uteroplacental waveforms to complicated pregnancies

Malcolm Pearce

INTRODUCTION

Doppler waveforms from the uteroplacental circulation were first described by Campbell *et al.* (1983). Using pulsed wave Doppler ultrasound they recognized small vessels running in the myometrium of the uterus which demonstrated typical waveforms. Since that time the uteroplacental circulation has not been subject to as much scrutiny as the umbilical artery, but several authors have realized that signals from the uteroplacental circulation can readily be obtained by continuous wave Doppler ultrasound (see Chapter 3).

The value of uteroplacental waveforms as a screening test is discussed in Chapter 6. This chapter looks at the use of uteroplacental waveforms, either alone or in combination with umbilical artery waveforms in complicated pregnancy.

HYPERTENSIVE DISORDERS OF PREGNANCY

Uteroplacental waveforms
Campbell *et al.* (1983) reported on 31 patients who developed hypertension in pregnancy. The patients were classified according to whether their uteroplacental waveforms were normal (Fig. 8.1) (group 1) or abnormal (Fig. 8.2) (group 2). These patients were then compared with a group of control patients. Table 8.1 illustrates the results.

Since then, other authors have reported the association between high-resistance uteroplacental waveforms and the more severe forms of pregnancy-induced hypertension. Trudinger *et al.* (1985a) reported that 75 per cent (9/12) patients with severe hypertension had abnormal uteroplacental artery waveforms, acquired from the subplacental area. Fleischer *et al.* (1986) studied 71 women who developed hypertension in pregnancy.

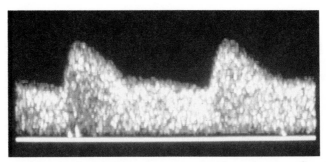

Fig. 8.1 Uteroplacental waveform from a normal pregnancy after 24 weeks' gestation.

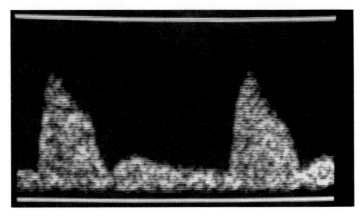

Fig. 8.2 Uteroplacental waveform from a pregnancy complicated by pre-eclampsia. Note the presence of the notch.

They classified the patients as follows:

1. Chronic hypertension: patients with pre-existing hypertension or a mean arterial pressure of more than 90 mmHg in the second trimester.

2. Pre-eclampsia: patients with an onset of hypertension in the third trimester together with proteinuria and oedema.

3. Superimposed pre-eclampsia: patients with chronic hypertension who experienced a significant increase in hypertension together with proteinuria and oedema.

They averaged the A/B (S/D) values obtained from the left and right side of the uterus. Patients with chronic hypertension had a mean (SD) ratio of 2.1 (0.4) compared with 4.3 (1.9) for pre-eclampsia and 4.7 (2.0) for superimposed pre-eclampsia. The sensitivity and specificity for prediction of an abnormal pregnancy outcome (delivery at less than 37 weeks or the

Table 8.1 Outcome of patients classified according to uteroplacental Doppler waveforms (from Campbell *et al.* 1983)

	Controls	Group 1	Group 2
Mean gestation (weeks)	39.1	38.4	35.4*
Caesarean section	1	3	10*
Mean 1-min Apgar score	8.1	8.4	6.6*
Mean birth-weight (kg)	3.28	2.94	2.05*

* $p < 0.05$.

birth of an infant weighing less than 2.5 kg) for an A/B ratio of more than 2.6 or the presence of a notch (Fig. 8.2) was 93 and 91 per cent, respectively.

Schulman *et al.* (1987) suggested that the difference between the left and right S/D (A/B) ratio may be useful in that some pregnancies with a normal S/D ratio but a high difference have poor outcomes. They suggested that a unilateral dominance might suggest errors in the placentation site. However, this conclusion is erroneous. The S/D (A/B) ratio is a non-linear ratio that can only have values of between zero and unity. Small increases in the diastolic component of the waveform will lead to large differences in the S/D ratio from each side of the uterus as the S/D ratio increases. By definition, the difference between the S/D ratios from each side of the uterus will be highly correlated with the absolute value of S/D. The difference between two non-linear ratios will also be non-linear and will have no physiological meaning.

The placental site, howver, has a marked difference on the resistance index. Pearce *et al.* (1988) demonstrated this difference using pulsed wave equipment (see Figs 4.9 and 4.10) and Kofinas *et al.* (1988) confirmed the difference with continuous wave equipment. Kofinas *et al.* (1988) reported a mean difference in the A/B ratio of 0.83 in normal pregnancies but a greater difference in pregnancies complicated by hypertension (1.66). The differences were greatest when real-time localization of the placenta demonstrated a unilateral placenta that did not cross the midline.

Uteroplacental and fetoplacental waveforms

In 1984, Campbell *et al.* first suggested that it is logical to study both circulations in complicated pregnancies. In this initial pilot study on 54 patients with hypertension or small-for-gestational age (SGA) fetuses, or both, they proposed the classification outlined in Figure 8.3. From observational studies on such patients, Steel and Pearce (1988) reported that patients did not move from one group to another, with the sole exception of patients with high-resistance uteroplacental arteries but normal umbilical artery waveforms, who developed loss of end-diastolic frequencies in the

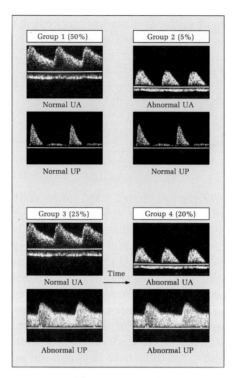

Fig. 8.3 Blood-flow groups. After presentation, patients do not appear to change groups with the exception that patients in group 3 may progress to group 4 if the pregnancy continues for long enough. UA, umbilical artery; UP, uteroplacental artery.

umbilical artery if the pregnancy was allowed to continue for long enough.

Several authors (Trudinger *et al*. 1985*b*; Al-Ghazali *et al*. 1988; Ducey *et al*. 1987; Schulman *et al*. 1989; Pearce *et al*. 1991*a, b*) have reported on the value of studying both sides of the placenta. Trudinger *et al*. (1985*b*) reported a normal outcome for small fetuses with normal umbilical and uteroplacental waveforms. Neonatal morbidity was confined to patients with abnormal umbilical artery waveforms (low or absent diastolic frequencies). The authors described two subgroups: one group of 13 cases had abnormal uteroplacental waveforms and the other group (21 cases) had normal waveforms. They felt that the former group had a primary uteroplacental lesion causing the intra-uterine growth retardation, whilst in the latter group they felt the cause was probably primarily fetal in origin.

Al-Ghazali *et al*. (1988) studied cardiac output in small fetuses; this work is discussed in detail in Chapter 13. The study confirms that normal uteroplacental and fetal waveforms are associated with a good outcome. There are too few patients with abnormal waveforms to draw conclusions. Schulman *et al.* (1989) studied both uteroplacental and umbilical artery waveforms in 250 unselected women. Unfortunately, however, the paper reported the outcomes separately for each circulation.

Ducey *et al.* (1987) proposed a system of classification of hypertensive disorders of pregnancy based on Doppler waveforms. In a study of 136 pregnant women with hypertension they classified patients into four groups as suggested by Campbell *et al.* (1984) and illustrated in Fig. 8.3. Table 8.2 illustrates the outcome. The authors concluded that prognosis was best indicated by vascular patterns than by other clinical means.

Pearce *et al.* (1992*a,b*) reported the outcome of 156 patients with the complication of hypertension and/or a small-for-gestational age fetus. These authors produced the following classification:

N   Normal uteroplacental waveforms, i.e. both placental and non-placental sides had a resistance index of less than 0.58.

A   Abnormal uteroplacental waveforms, i.e. both placental and non-placental sides had a resistance index of greater than 0.58.

M   Mixed pattern, where the placental waveform was normal but the waveform on the non-placental side was abnormal.

n   Normal umbilical artery waveforms, i.e. an A/B ratio within the data reference range.

a   Abnormal umbilical artery waveforms.

Figure 8.4 illustrates the maximum systolic and diastolic blood pressure for each of the blood flow classes, while Fig. 8.5 illustrates the incidence of hypertension and associated proteinuria. Blood pressure is significantly worse when the uteroplacental waveforms are abnormal, which occurs in at least 75 per cent of the groups. Proteinuric hypertension, for each class of uteroplacental waveform, is more likely to be associated with abnormal umbilical artery waveforms. In this study the authors did not report the

Table 8.2 Clinical outcome of patients classified according to Figure 8.3 (from Ducey *et al.* 1987)

	Group 1	Group 2	Group 3	Group 4
Proteinuria (%)	24	71	75	86
Birth-weight (kg)	3.3	2.1	2.5	1.6
< 10th centile (%)	2	29	17	51
Caesarean section for distress (%)	8	39	8	62
Neonatal intensive care unit (%)	12	68	50	89

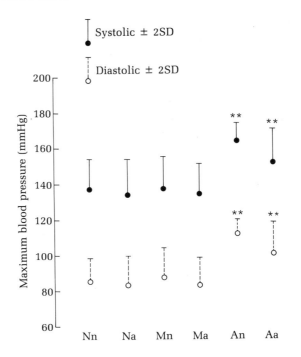

Fig. 8.4 Maximum blood pressure recorded for each blood-flow class. Utero-placental waveform patterns are: N, normal; M, mixed; A, abnormal. Umbilical artery patterns are: n, normal, a, abnormal. **p < 0.01 (From Pearce *et al.* 1991*a, b.*)

pregnancy outcome for patients with hypertension. The outcome of the pregnancies based upon the state of the uteroplacental waveforms is illustrated in Table 8.3.

SMALL-FOR-GESTATIONAL AGE FETUSES

Uteroplacental waveforms

McCowan *et al.* (1988) obtained uteroplacental waveforms on 12 women who were carrying a severely growth-retarded fetus. Six of the seven women with pre-eclampsia had abnormal uteroplacental waveforms, but waveforms were normal in four out of the remaining five women. The authors suggest that uteroplacental waveforms may indicate growth retardation associated with uteroplacental insufficiency.

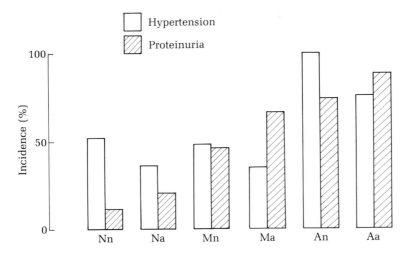

Fig. 8.5 Incidence of hypertension and associated proteinuria according to blood-flow class. Uteroplacental waveform patterns are: N, normal; M, mixed; A, abnormal. Umbilical artery patterns are: n, normal; a, abnormal. (From Pearce *et al.* 1991*a, b.*)

Uteroplacental and fetoplacental waveforms

Ducey *et al.* (1987) demonstrated that the incidence of SGA fetuses (birth-weight less than the 10th centile) was related to the state of both circulations (see Table 8.1). This was confirmed in the study by Pearce *et al.* (1992*b*) and is illustrated in Fig. 8.6. For a given pattern of uteroplacental waveforms, the birth-weight was always significantly lower in the group with abnormal umbilical artery waveforms. There is a general trend towards lower birth-weights across the blood flow classes, the exception being the Mn class in which the mean birth-weight is very similar to the normal (Nn) group. The incidence of elective deliveries is illustrated in Fig. 8.7. Deaths occurred only in babies who demonstrated abnormal umbilical artery waveforms (Fig. 8.8).

Randomized, controlled trial of uteroplacental and fetal waveforms in complicated pregnancies

Chapter 7 discusses the two randomized, controlled trials of umbilical artery waveforms that have been reported to date. Pearce *et al.* (1991*a*) reported a randomized, controlled trial of waveforms from both sides of the circulation. Blood-flow classes were as detailed above and are summarized in Table 8.4.

Table 8.3 Pregnancy outcome based on Doppler waveforms from the uteroplacental circulation in 89 pregnant women with hypertension (from Pearce and McParland 1991)

	Uteroplacental waveforms		
Outcome measure	Normal	Mixed	Abnormal
No. of patients	43	19	27
Mean maximum blood pressure (mmHg)			
Systolic	145.6	156.2	168.8
Diastolic	94.8	98.3	107.2
Proteinuria (%)	5 (12)	10 (50)	22 (82)
Gestation (mean, weeks)			
At admission	35.6	33.0	31.2
At delivery	38.5	37.7	32.3
Mean birth-weight (kg)	3.2	2.6	1.7
Fulminating hypertension (%)	0	2 (11)	19 (71)
Delivery by lower-segment caesarean section for hypertension (%)	0	3 (16)	19 (71)

The study was designed in order to stand an 80 per cent chance of reducing the death rate amongst fetuses with loss of end-diastolic frequencies from 25 to 5 per cent. A secondary aim was to reduce the length of the antenatal stay in patients who had normal waveforms. Patients admitted with hypertension and/or a fetus that had been shown to be small on real-time ultrasonography were randomized to have their Doppler results concealed (concealed group) or revealed (revealed group) to the clinicians. By the time the study was conducted all the clinicians were familiar with the interpretation of the waveforms and their possible meaning. Some 509 patients were successfully randomized and their details are shown in Table 8.5.

Table 8.6 details the gestation at admission and the length of the antenatal stay, broken down by blood flow classes. The revealed and concealed groups appear well matched but the length of the antenatal stay was significantly less in patients in the first four groups. Overall there was a reduction in the median length of stay from 25 days in the concealed group to 10 days in the revealed group ($p < 0.001$).

Overall there was no difference in caesarean section rates between the two groups (33 versus 31 per cent in the revealed group), but there were significantly more inductions in the concealed group (29 versus 19 per cent $p < 0.02$). Operative delivery for fetal distress was significantly more likely to occur in the concealed group (18 versus 7 per cent), and this was thought

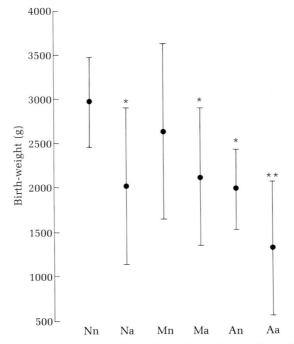

Fig. 8.6 Birth-weight in each blood-flow class. Uteroplacental waveform patterns are: N, normal; M, mixed; A, abnormal. Umbilical artery patterns are: n, normal; a, abnormal. *Indicates a significant difference ($p < 0.01$) in comparison with the Nn and Mn classes; **indicates a significant difference ($p < 0.01$) from all other classes. (From Pearce *et al.* 1991*a, b*.)

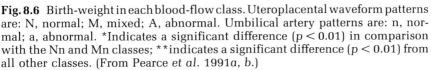

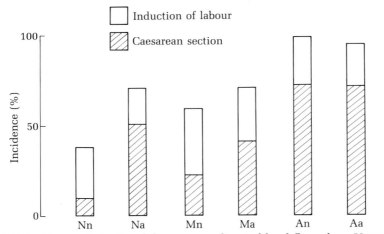

Fig. 8.7 Incidence of elective delivery according to blood-flow class. Uteroplacental waveform patterns are: N, normal; M, mixed; A, abnormal. Umbilical artery patterns are: n, normal; a, abnormal. (From Pearce *et al.* 1991*a, b*.)

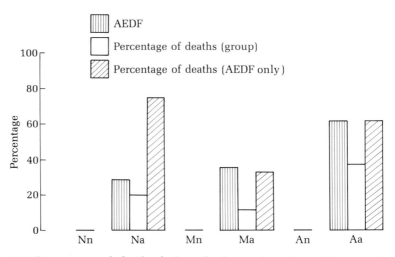

Fig. 8.8 Percentage of deaths before discharge from hospital according to blood-flow class. Uteroplacental waveform patterns are; N, normal; M, mixed; A, abnormal. Umbilical artery patterns are: n, normal; a, abnormal. AEDF, absent end-diastolic frequencies. (From Pearce *et al.* 1991*a, b.*)

to be because at-risk fetuses were delivered electively by caesarean section and not subjected to labour.

The neonatal details are illustrated in Table 8.7 and demonstrate only one clear difference between the groups. In the blood-flow class in which waveforms from both circulations were normal, birth-weights were heavier in the revealed group. This is the result of fewer elective deliveries in this group, which therefore had a longer median gestation (40.1 versus 39.2 weeks, $p < 0.05$).

Table 8.8 details the deaths before discharge from hospital. Deaths occurred only in babies with absent end-diastolic frequencies (AEDF) and these were significantly reduced in the revealed group. Overall 56 per cent of the fetuses in the concealed group with AEDF died. This figure is higher

Table 8.4 Blood-flow classes

	Fetal circulation	
Uteroplacental circulation	Normal (n)	Abnormal (a)
Normal (N)	Nn	Na
Mixed (M)	Mn	Ma
Abnormal (A)	An	Aa

Table 8.5 Randomized controlled trial of the value of the knowledge of Doppler waveforms in complicated pregnancy: patient characteristics (from Pearce *et al.* 1991*b*)

Characteristic	Concealed group	Revealed group
No. of patients	255 (50)	254 (50)
Blood flow classes		
NN	108 (42)	115 (45)
NA	14 (6)	12 (5)
MN	42 (16)	34 (13)
MA	38 (15)	46 (18)
AN	23 (9)	18 (7)
AA	30 (12)	29 (11)
Age (SD) (years)	26.2 (4.7)	225.6 (5.6)
Primips	148 (58)	153 (60)
Smokers	81 (32)	85 (33)
Race		
White	207 (82)	198 (78)
Black	38 (15)	43 (17)
Asians	10 (3)	13 (5)
Intra-uterine growth retardation		
Symmetrical	46 (18)	51 (20)
Asymmetrical	135 (53)	131 (52)
Hypertension	137 (54)	132 (52)
Proteinuria	38 (15)	41 (16)
Need for hypertensive therapy		
Oral only	28 (11)	31 (12)
Oral ± intravenous	56 (22)	53 (21)

Values in parenthesis are percentages, unless stated otherwise. N, normal; M, mixed; A, abnormal; SD, standard deviation.

than predicted from previous work (Pearce *et al.* 1992*b*) but is in keeping with recent reports (McParland *et al.* 1990). The causes of death (Table 8.8) known to be associated with reduced flow to the corpus (see also Chapter 13) were more common in the concealed group.

Table 8.9 details the number of deliveries that occurred because of an abnormal antenatal cardiotocograph. Overall, 62 per cent (18/29) of the pregnancies complicated by an abnormal antenatal cardiotocograph resulted in a perinatal or neonatal death, and all these patients had AEDF in the umbilical arteries. In the revealed group only three pregnancies were complicated by an abnormal cardiotocograph and all these babies had a normal umbilical artery circulation; none died. The authors suggest that this reduction in the number of abnormal cardiotocographs in the revealed

Table 8.6 Randomized controlled trial of the value of the knowledge of Doppler waveforms in complicated pregnancy: gestation on admission and length of antenatal stay (from Pearce 1991*b*)

Characteristic	Concealed group	Revealed group	p
No. of patients	255 (50%)	254 (50%)	NS
Gestation on admission (weeks)			
NN	35.5 (28–40)	35.0 (28–41)	NS
NA	32.5 (23–39)	34.1 (24–39)	NS
MN	33.6 (27–39)	34.0 (27–39)	NS
MA	33.3 (25–38)	32.7 (24–38)	NS
AN	33.0 (23–37)	32.2 (23–37)	NS
AA	30.3 (22–38)	29.9 (23–37)	NS
Length of antenatal stay (days)			
NN	22.6 (4–79)	3.9 (3–73)	< 0.001
NA	23.0 (8–65)	14.8 (3–29)	< 0.001
MN	24.0 (2–57)	5.4 (2–15)	< 0.001
MA	29.3 (3–85)	23.0 (3–44)	< 0.001
AN	5.0 (2–23)	5.0 (2–15)	NS
AA	8.3 (2–37)	6.0 (2–35)	NS

Values are medians and ranges, unless stated otherwise. N, normal; M, mixed; A, abnormal; NS, not significant.

group is because of elective delivery of fetuses with AEDF. The combination of these two abnormalities appears to be fatal.

Summary   Knowing that the uteroplacental and fetal circulations are normal in the face of a pregnancy complicated by hypertension or a small baby allows conservative management. Such management appears justified in that no baby appears to have suffered and such infants are heavier at birth, the result of fewer inductions of labour. Delivery of infants based upon AEDF appears to save babies' lives, in that they are less likely to succumb to the results of prolonged underperfusion. They do not appear to be more likely to die from prematurity.

OTHER CONDITIONS

Multiple pregnancy
There are no reports in the literature on the role of uteroplacental waveforms in monitoring multiple pregnancy. However, in a series of 91 sets of twins, Pearce (personal communication) reports no examples of high-

Table 8.7 Randomized controlled trial of the value of the knowledge of Doppler waveforms in complicated pregnancy: Neonatal details (from Pearce *et al.* 1991*b*)

Characteristic	Concealed group	Revealed group	*p*
Males	119 (47%)	125 (49%)	NS
Birth-weight (SD) (g)			
NN	2983.3 (467.2)	3125.0 (401.3)	0.01
NA	2020.1 (838.3)	2189.4 (927.3)	NS
MN	2611.2 (999.7)	2817.8 (606.5)	NS
MA	2100.2 (637.3)	1998.8 (675.7)	NS
AN	1979.6 (402.1)	1928.3 (493.7)	NS
AA	1308.3 (689.3)	1257.2 (711.3)	NS
Overall	2449.9 (576.6)	2517.7 (495.1)	NS
Birth-weight < 5th centile			
	81 (32%)	84 (33%)	NS
Apgar scores < 5 (SD)			
At 1 min	46 (18)	37 (15)	NS
At 5 min	11 (4)	5 (2)	NS

N, normal; M, mixed; A, Abnormal; NS, not significant.

resistance waveforms even in the 11 cases that developed proteinuric hypertension.

Anticardiolipin syndromes

Pearce (1992) reported a series of 13 women, all of whom had systemic lupus erythematosus (SLE), the lupus inhibitor, or anticardiolipin anti-bodies. In three cases, congenital fetal heart block occurred and was readily detected from Doppler surveillance. Two babies are alive and well, but the third child died from subendocardial fibro-elastosis. All pregnancies were uncomplicated by hypertension or small babies, and all three had normal uteroplacental waveforms.

Of the remaining 10 women, all but one had previous pregnancy losses; the remaining patients had SLE. There are seven live children, one of which was born pre-term (at 32 weeks) following a placental abruption. Two further patients suffered placental abruptions and lost their babies. In all three cases, there was a prior prolongation of the clotting times which had not been brought under control by the introduction of steroids. All paients were on low-dose aspirin. In none of these cases was any warning given from weekly Doppler examinations of the uteroplacental and umbilical circulation.

Table 8.8 Randomized controlled trial of the value of the knowledge of Doppler waveforms in complicated pregnancy: deaths before discharge from hospital (from Pearce *et al.* 1992*b*)

Cause	Concealed group	Revealed group
Respiratory distress syndrome	3	2
Necrotizing enterocolitis	6	3
Intraventricular haemorrhage	3	1
Pulmonary haemorrhage	1	0
Renal failure	2	0
Feeding difficulty	1	0
Still birth	4	1
Total (%)	20 (8)*	7 (2)

* $p < 0.05$.

Table 8.9 Elective delivery for an abnormal antenatal cardiotocograph

Blood-flow class	Concealed group	Revealed group
NN	2	2
NA	3	0
MN	4	1
MA	12	0
AN	0	0
AA	8	0
Total (%)	29 (11)	3 (1)

N, normal; M, mixed; A, abnormal.

Three patients suffered from proteinuric hypertension, one of whom lost her baby weighing 400 g from preterm delivery at 26 weeks. In all three cases, uteroplacental waveforms were normal at 22 weeks' gestation but demonstrated high-resistance patterns at least 7 days before the hypertension was clinically apparent. The two surviving infants were delivered as soon as they demonstrated AEDF, and both survive (1204 g at 34 weeks, 1450 g at 36 weeks).

Interestingly, the authors state that they have not observed deterioration of uteroplacental waveforms from completely normal patterns at 22–24 weeks to a very high-resistance pattern in any other situation. This suggests that the uteroplacental vessels are undergoing narrowing, possibly as the result of abnormal clotting (despite the longer clotting times).

Further work is needed, perhaps from collaborative studies, before the role of Doppler ultrasound in the management of these highly variable syndromes is understood.

Raised maternal serum alpha-fetoprotein

Recently, Aristidou *et al.* (1990) described the value of uteroplacental waveforms in 98 women with raised maternal alpha-fetoprotein (MSAFP). A notch (see Fig. 8.2) was present in 18 patients, 13 of whom suffered either a perinatal death or gave birth to a very small infant. Figure 8.9 is taken from Pearce and Robson (1992*a*), and illustrates the findings in 392 women with a raised MSAFP. Table 8.10 illustrates the outcome in those women who had a structurally normal fetus and who could be traced. Women with normal uteroplacental waveforms had a normal perinatal mortality (PNM) rate, whereas mixed and abnormal waveform patterns were associated with a very high PNM rate. A surprising finding was the 7 per cent incidence of placental abruption in this study, but this is similar to that reported by Purdie *et al.* (1983).

The same authors (Pearce and Robson 1992*b*) then carried out a randomized, controlled trial of aspirin and placebo in women with a raised MSAFP and mixed or abnormal uteroplacental waveforms. The aim was to determine whether low-dose aspirin could reduce the PNM rate in this group to the background rate. Figure 8.10 shows that the trial failed in that, although low-dose aspirin significantly reduced the incidence of deliveries before 34 weeks and of babies with birth-weights of less than the fifth centile, the reduction in the PNM rate did not achieve significance. Figure 8.11 may suggest the reason for this. Although the incidence of placental abruption did not differ between the groups (Fig. 8.11), the

Table 8.10 Pregnancy outcome in women with raised serum alpha-fetoprotein

	Doppler waveforms		
	Normal	Mixed	Abnormal
No. of patients	209	97	13
< 10th centile birthweight for gestational age	27 (13)	59 (61)	9 (69)
< 5th centile birthweight for gestational age	4 (2)	18 (19)	9 (69)
< 37 weeks gestation	23 (11)	37 (38)	13 (100)
< 34 weeks gestation	3 (1)	11 (11)	13 (100)
Abruptions	13 (6)	6 (6)	4 (31)
Deaths	0	2	4
Perinatal mortality rate (%)	9.6	268	846

Values in parentheses are percentages.

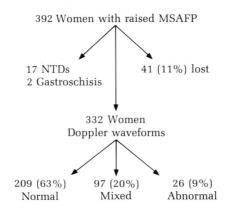

Fig. 8.9 Outcome in 392 women with raised maternal serum alphafetoprotein (MSAFP). The Doppler waveform pattern from women with a structurally normal fetus is shown on the bottom line. NTDs, neural tube defects. (From Pearce and Robson 1992*a*.)

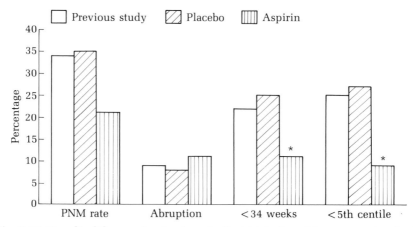

Fig. 8.10 Result of the randomized controlled trial of aspirin versus placebo in women with raised maternal serum α-fetoprotein and abnormal uteroplacental Doppler waveforms.

deaths from abruption were higher in the aspirin group and this dilutes the reduction of deaths amongst the small and pre-term babies. Although the figures are small, it appears that women who suffer a placental abruption whilst on aspirin may be more likely to lose their baby.

Oligohydramnios

The value of studying both the uteroplacental and fetal circulation is considered in Chapter 13.

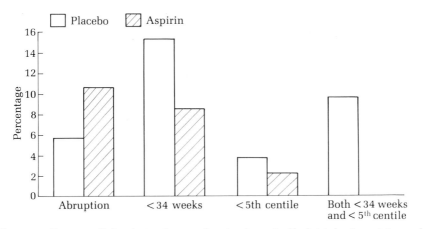

Fig. 8.11 Causes of death in the randomized controlled trial of aspirin and placebo in women with raised maternal serum α-fetoprotein and abnormal uteroplacental Doppler waveforms.

Recent developments

Transvaginal colour flow Doppler ultrasonography has recently allowed the assessment of the uteroplacental circulation from 4 to 18 weeks' gestation (Jurkovic *et al*. 1991). The colour mapping allows the pulsed Doppler signals to be obtained from both the uterine artery and from individual radial and spiral arteries. The value of this technique is at present unknown but it may be a useful tool for the study of early miscarriage.

SUMMARY

Uteroplacental waveforms appear to be of value in the classification of hypertensive disease in such a way as to allow prediction of the subsequent clinical course. The combination of waveforms from both the uteroplacental and fetal circulations appears to be useful in determining which pregnancies complicated by hypertension and/or a small baby are truly disadvantaged. These clinical findings, together with the pathophysiological findings detailed in Chapter 11, would strongly support the view that hypertensive disorders of pregnancy should be classified according to the vascular patterns from the uteroplacental circulation.

   A randomized, controlled trial has demonstrated that knowledge that both waveforms are normal allows less interference in the pregnancy, resulting in heavier babies. Acting on abnormal umbilical artery waveforms appears to save babies' lives, because it reduces deaths from causes associated with prolonged underperfusion of the fetal trunk.

REFERENCES

Al-Ghazali, W., Chapman, M. G., and Allan, L. D. (1988). Doppler assessment of the cardiac and uteroplacental circulations in normal and complicated pregnancies. *British Journal of Obstetrics and Gynaecology*, **95**, 575–80.

Aristidou, A., van den Hof, M. C., Campbell, S., and Nicolaides, K. (1990). Uterine artery Doppler in the investigation of pregnancies with raised maternal serum alphafetoprotein. *British Journal of Obstetrics and Gynaecology*, **97**, 431–5.

Campbell, S., Griffin, D. R., Pearce, J. M. F., Diaz-Recasens, J., Cohen-Overbeek, T. E., and Willson, K. (1983). New Doppler technique for assessing uteroplacental bloodflow. *Lancet*, **i**, 675–7.

Campbell, S., Hernandez, C. J., Cohen-Overbeek, T. A., and Pearce, J. M. F. (1984). Assessment of fetoplacental and uteroplacental blood flow using duplex pulsed Doppler ultrasound in complicated pregnancies. *Journal of Perinatal Medicine*, **12**, 261–5.

Ducey, J., Schulman, H., Farmakides, G., *et al.* (1987). A classification of hypertension in pregnancy based on Doppler velocimetry. *American Journal of Obstetrics and Gynecology*, **157**, 680–5.

Jurkovic, D., Jauniaux, E., Kurjak, A., Hustin, J., Campbell, S., and Nicolaides, K. (1991). Transvaginal color Doppler assessment of the uteroplacental circulation in early pregnancy. *Obstetrics and Gynecology*, **77**, 365–9.

Fleischer, A., Schulman, H., Farmakides, G., *et al.* (1986). Uterine artery Doppler velocimetry in pregnant women with hypertension. *American Journal of Obstetrics and Gynecology*, **154**, 806–13.

Kofinas, A. D., Penry, M., Greiss, F. C., Meis, P. J., and Nelson, L. H. (1988). The effect of placental localisation on uterine artery flow velocity waveforms. *American Journal of Obstetrics and Gynecology*, **159**, 1504–8.

McCowan, L. M., Ritchie, K. M. B., Mo, L., Bascom, P. A., and Sherrett, H. (1988). Uterine artery flow velocity waveforms in normal and growth-retarded pregnancies. *American Journal of Obstetrics and Gynecology*, **158**, 499–504.

McParland, P., Pearce, J. M. F., and Chamberlain, G. V. P. C. (1990). The clinical implications of absent or reversed end-diastolic frequencies in umbilical artery flow velocity waveforms. *European Journal of Obstetrics and Gynaecology*, **37**, 15–23.

Pearce, J. M. F. (1992). Doppler ultrasound in the management of the anticardiolipin syndromes. *Journal of the International Society for the Study of Ultrasound in Obsterics and Gynaecology*, (in Press).

Pearce, J. M. F. and Robson, M. (1992*a*). Doppler ultrasound in the evaluation of women with raised maternal serum alphafetoprotein. *Journal of the International Society for the Study of Ultrasound in Obstetrics and Gynaecology*, (in Press).

Pearce, J. M. F. and Robson, M. (1992*b*). A randomised controlled trial of low dose aspirin in women with raised maternal serum alphafetoprotein. *Journal of the Internationl Society for the Study of Ultrasound in Obstetrics and Gynaecology*, (in Press).

Pearce, J. M. F., Campbell, S., Cohen-Overbeek, T., Hackett, G., Hernandez, J., and Royston, J. P. (1988). Reference ranges and sources of variation for indices of pulsed Doppler flow velocity waveforms from the uteroplacental and fetal circulation. *British Journal of Obstetrics and Gynaecology*, **95**, 248–56.

Pearce, J. M. F., Campbell, S., Smith, P., and Gamsu, H. (1992*a*). A randomised controlled trial of Doppler waveforms from the uteroplacental and fetoplacental circulations. *British Journal of Obstetrics and Gynaecology*, (in Press).

Pearce, J. M. F., Campbell, S., Hernandez, J., Meizner, I., and Cohen-Overbeek, T. A. (1992*b*). The development of a blood flow classification system for waveforms from the uteroplacental and fetoplacental circulations. *British Journal of Obstetrics and Gynaecology*, (in press).

Purdie, D. W., Young, J. L., Guthrie, K. A., and Picton, C. E. (1983). Fetal growth achievement and elevated serum alphafetoprotein. *British Journal of Obstetrics and Gynaecology*, **90**, 433–6.

Schulman, H., Ducey, J., Farmakides, G., *et al.* (1987). Uterine artery Doppler velocimetry: the significance of divergent systolic/diastolic ratios. *American Journal of Obstetrics and Gynecology*, **157**, 1539–42.

Schulman, H., Winter, D., Farmakides, G., *et al.* (1989). Pregnancy surveillance with Doppler velocimetry of uterine and umbilical arteries. *American Journal of Obstetrics and Gynecology*, **160**, 192–6.

Steel, S. A. and Pearce, J. M. F. (1988). Use of Doppler ultrasound to investigate the uteroplacental and fetal circulations. *Hospital Update*, **14**, 1094–108.

Trudinger, B. J., Giles, W. B., and Cook, C. M. (1985*a*). Uteroplacental blood flow velocity waveforms in normal and complicated pregnancy. *British Journal of Obstetrics and Gynaecology*, **92**, 39–45.

Trudinger, B. J., Giles, W. B., and Cook, C. M. (1985*b*). Flow velocity waveforms in the maternal uteroplacental and fetal placental circulations. *American Journal of Obstetrics and Gynecology*, **152**, 155–63.

9. Use of Doppler ultrasound in the management of diabetic pregnancy

Frank Johnstone and J. M. Steel

INTRODUCTION

What role is Doppler flow velocity waveform (FVW) likely to play in the management of diabetic pregnancy? In non-diabetic pregnancy, Doppler ultrasonography may be establishing a place in two areas. The less well-accepted area is the use of uteroplacental blood-flow measurement in early pregnancy as a screening test (see Chapter 6) which may allow early prophylaxis (McParland *et al.* 1990*a*). The other area, with much more supportive data, is the use of umbilical artery measurement as a discriminator in suspected growth retardation or hypertensive states (see Chapter 7). In these conditions, umbilical artery Doppler ultrasonography may segregate pregnancies at very high risk (Johnstone *et al.* 1988; McParland *et al.* 1990*b*) from those at minimal risk where intensive antenatal fetal monitoring may not be required (Haddad *et al.* 1988*b*; Burke *et al.* 1990). Both of these approaches are theoretically attractive in diabetic pregnancy, where superimposed pregnancy-induced hypertension is common, and where intensive monitoring is often carried out—at least in retrospect—unnecessarily.

This chapter reviews the particular fetal monitoring problems posed by diabetic pregnancy, assesses the limited data available, and speculates further about the likely place of Doppler ultrasonography as a clinical tool.

FETAL MONITORING IN DIABETIC PREGNANCY

Historically, intra-uterine fetal death was common in diabetic pregnancy. This occurred in association with maternal keto-acidosis, when about 75 per cent of fetuses died *in utero* (White 1949), but also occurred unexpectedly in late, non-keto-acidotic, pregnancy. Even in recent times, population-based studies have shown that there is still an increased risk of fetal death in diabetic pregnancy. Thus, Connelly *et al.* (1985) found that fetal death in diabetic pregnancy was 8.7 times more common than in the total population. Lang and Kunzel (1989), in a population study from Hesse, Germany, reported a sixfold increased risk of fetal death in diabetic pregnancy, and diabetes was the most powerful single predictive factor of fetal mortality. In Kuwait, where diabetes was not always well controlled, established diabetes was associated with an 18-fold increased risk of unexplained late pregnancy still birth (Johnstone *et al.* 1991*a*).

Tight metabolic control is generally recognized as the major factor in prevention of these deaths, but even in apparently well-controlled diabetes, late fetal death still occasionally occurs. Because of this, routine fetal monitoring has become established practice. Sheldon (1989) advised the initiation of antepartum testing at 26 weeks for patients with vascular disease and by 34 weeks for all diabetic pregnancies. Miller and Horger (1985) reported several fetal deaths 4–7 days after fetal monitoring, and suggested that monitoring should be performed at least twice weekly in diabetic pregnancy, a frequency also recommended from the experience of Golde and Platt (1985). Therefore, quite intensive fetal monitoring—for many weeks—is common, sometimes often involving hospital admission. This has important, and well-recognised, economic and social consequences (Thomas and Snodgrass 1986). Many studies have reported very low fetal loss rates often using different techniques of fetal monitoring (see review by Golde and Platt 1985; Johnson *et al.* 1988). How much fetal monitoring itself contributed to these results is impossible to assess. The fact remains that only a small proportion of pregnancies result in abnormal tests, and a technique to select out these problem pregnancies would be of great clinical value.

EFFECT OF DIABETES ON BLOOD FLOW AND FLOW VELOCITY WAVEFORM

Quantitative measurements of maternal placental blood flow have been made using radio-isotope methods (Kaar *et al.* 1980; Nylund *et al.* 1982). These studies suggested that placental blood flow is decreased by about 40 per cent in diabetic pregnancy, and Nylund *et al.* (1982) suggested that the decrease might be proportional to level of diabetic control. The only studies of volume flow on the fetal side of the placenta in diabetic pregnancy appear to be the Doppler studies of Kirkinen and Jouppila (1983) and Oloffson *et al.* (1987). The former authors found low flow rates in women with severe vascular complications and with intra-uterine growth retardation. Oloffson *et al.* (1987), also using pulsed Doppler techniques, found a high volume of blood flow in diabetic pregnancy in fetal thoracic descending aorta abdominal aorta and umbilical vein. The distribution of blood flow from thoracic descending aorta to placenta, viscera, and lower extremities was similar in diabetic and reference groups. There were no differences in any flow variable in those pregnancies complicated by hypertension or non-optimally regulated diabetic control. However, there were significant increases in volume flow in the thoracic descending aorta in the cases developing fetal distress in labour ($p < 0.01$) and in those with a low cord blood pH ($p < 0.05$). The authors suggested that this unexpected finding might reflect increased cardiac output as an early compensatory mechanism for increased placental vascular resistance.

As far as qualitative measurements of blood flow are concerned, three studies have examined the relationship of umbilical artery Doppler FVWs with gestational age, and have compared values with a control group. Oloffson *et al.* (1987) studied 40 consecutive diabetic pregnancies and found the pulsatility index in the umbilical artery to be higher in the diabetic group than in the reference group at term, although not at two points earlier in the third trimester. However, this difference was entirely accounted for by the higher pulsatility index in the eight fetuses that developed fetal distress during labour. Landon *et al.* (1989) made serial measurements in 35 insulin-dependent women. They found a normal decline in mean umbilical systolic/diastolic (A/B) ratio with advancing gestation, and no statistically significant difference when compared with data from a non-diabetic population. We have studied Doppler waveforms serially in 113 diabetic women (Johnstone *et al.* 1991*b*) in order to examine the effect of uncomplicated insulin-dependent diabetes. We excluded women with hypertensive disease, pregnancy-induced hypertension, nephropathy, evidence of antenatal or early labour fetal compromise, pre-term delivery, and gestational diabetes. This left 59 pregnancies, from which 342 umbilical artery Doppler measurements were available. These measurements were indistinguishable from our normal series from pregnancies uncomplicated by diabetes mellitus.

Information about uterine artery measurements in diabetic pregnancy is sparse. In our population we studied uteroplacental waveforms, taking the average of placental and non-placental sides. The mean value for the whole of the third trimester, in all diabetic pregnancies, was 0.40 ± 0.06 and in uncomplicated diabetic pregnancy it was similarly 0.40 ± 0.06 (unpublished observations). These values do not seem greatly different from those published for non-diabetic pregnancy, using pulsed Doppler (Pearce *et al.* 1988).

It must be stressed that both established vascular disease and hypertensive complications are common in diabetic pregnancy (20 per cent of our patients have significant hypertension and proteinuria). These conditions are likely to be associated with abnormality of qualitative blood flow, as has been found by Landon *et al.* (1989). Therefore, overall, diabetic populations are likely to have waveforms indicating higher uterine and umbilical resistance. Whether entirely uncomplicated diabetic pregnancy is associated with Doppler values similar to those of non-diabetic pregnancy is uncertain, but from our own work such differences are unlikely to be large. It therefore seems appropriate at present to use reference ranges derived from a non-diabetic population.

Metabolic control

Despite the above conclusion, there is evidence that Doppler FVWs may be influenced by the degree of metabolic control. Metabolic control has invariably been assessed from blood glucose control only, either directly or by use of glycosylated haemoglobin. Bracero *et al.* (1986) studied average glucose values in '3 or 4 daily random blood samples during the 2 weeks before delivery', in 43 women, only 25 of whom were insulin dependent. They found a significant association with umbilical artery FVW ($r = 0.52$, $p < 0.001$). In a further study (Bracero *et al.* 1989), they added data from 33 well-controlled diabetic women to the data from their first report. In nine pregnancies diabetic control was judged to be poor. Umbilical artery FVWs were significantly higher in these pregnancies. Methodologically, these two studies are not ideal. Measurement of diabetic control is not defined clearly enough, and it is not obvious what allowance was made for gestation in calculating the indices from the Doppler mean FVW. No attempt was made to exclude related variables such as gestation, hypertension, growth retardation, and nephropathy which could be associated with both poor control and higher placenta resistance. Finally, if a hypothesis is generated from one set of data, it is not acceptable statistically to provide confirmatory evidence by adding to the same data.

There is, however, support for Bracero's work in a study by Kofinas *et al.* (1990). These authors studied 34 women with insulin-dependent diabetes and 31 with gestational diabetes, and found a weak positive linear correlation between maternal haemoglobin $A1_c$ and indices that represent the umbilical artery FVW ($r = 0.30$, $p < 0.02$). However, no relationship with blood glucose control was found by Landon *et al.* (1989). Similarly, in our larger study (Johnstone *et al.* 1991*b*), no relationship was found between changes in the umbilical artery FVW and glycosylated haemoglobin.

Thus, although an association between umbilical artery FVWs and blood glucose control has been reported, the evidence is not conclusive, with the association varying from study to study. It is possible that what, at most, is a weak relationship may be explained by other associated variables, or that it is seen only where diabetic control is very poor. If a relationship with diabetic control can be shown to persist on multi-variate analysis it will be important to establish the time in pregnancy when control exerts the greatest effect.

Only one study has examined uterine artery FVWs (Johnstone *et al.* 1991*b*). We found a relationship with metabolic control as judged by glycosylated haemoglobin ($r = 0.36$, $p < 0.001$). Because this was unexpected, the finding does need to be confirmed by others in a similarly large study. However, if true, it suggests that poor diabetic control not only results in increased fetal growth and a tendency to fetal hypoxaemia (see below) but also may affect placental function detrimentally. The interplay between these factors could lead eventually to asphyxia and intra-uterine fetal death.

VASCULAR COMPLICATIONS AND PREGNANCY-INDUCED HYPERTENSION

Patients with nephropathy or established hypertension are at higher risk of both superimposed pre-eclampsia and intra-uterine growth retardation, and the combination of diabetes, hypertension, and growth retardation is serious.

From what is known about the relationship between placental bed and Doppler umbilical artery FVWs it would be expected that higher resistance FVWs would be found in women with nephropathy, established hypertension, and pregnancy-induced hypertension; this has been confirmed (Landon *et al.* 1989; Kofinas *et al.* 1990; Johnstone *et al.* 1991*b*). However, such cases are already clinically identified as at higher risk, and to be of value Doppler ultrasonography should provide additional information. This could be, for example, the prediction of pregnancy-induced hypertension some time before clinical onset, or the prediction of those cases at particularly high risk of fetal compromise. There is currently no evidence that Doppler waveforms can achieve either function in diabetic pregnancies.

PREDICTION OF FETAL COMPROMISE

Potentially the most useful role for Doppler ultrasonography in diabetic pregnancy would be the long-term prediction of fetal compromise. This might allow the recognition of pregnancies at minimal risk where the woman could be spared intensive fetal monitoring.

Bracero *et al.* (1989) reported two still births. One baby was macrosomic and had congenital anomalies; the other had post-mortem findings consistent with intra-uterine anoxia. Umbilical artery recordings were abnormal in both pregnancies. Oloffson *et al.* (1987) had no cases of antenatal fetal compromise but described a significantly higher umbilical artery pulsatility index in the fetuses that subsequently developed fetal distress in labour. Individual FVW measurements were not given. Landon *et al.* (1989) delivered one fetus because of evidence of antenatal compromise diagnosed by standard means, and in this case umbilical artery FVWs showed absence of end-diastolic frequencies (AEDF). Fairlie *et al*. (1990) reported a small series of apparently unselected cases with an unusually higher mortality rate. Out of 19 women there were five perinatal losses and another three babies with serious congenital anomalies. One anatomically normal fetus with AEDF was still born. Another died from growth retardation, but Doppler results are not given.

The series from Edinburgh University of more than 120 diabetic women had only one neonatal death from congenital cardiac anomaly and no other pregnancy loss. There was evidence of antenatal fetal compromise in seven women and all were delivered promptly by Caesarean section. However, in only three of these pregnancies had Doppler been persistently abnormal (Johnstone *et al*. 1991*b*).

Thus, it seems that most, but not all, cases of antenatal fetal compromise in diabetic pregnancies can be predicted by umbilical artery FVW. The fact that, in some cases, an abnormal biophysical profile or cardiotocograph was associated with normal Doppler results is, however, unlike the situation in uncomplicated intra-uterine growth retardation or hypertension, where normal umbilical artery Doppler waveform appears highly predictive of normal antepartum fetal monitoring (Haddad *et al*. 1988*a, b*; Gudmundsson and Marsal 1988; Burke *et al*. 1990 and Chapter 7). There are two possible explanations. The first is that, in these diabetic pregnancies, abnormal antenatal monitoring does not reflect fetal compromise. Biophysical tests are influenced by maternal blood glucose levels (Ammala and Kariniemi 1983; Kariniemi *et al*. 1983; Teramo *et al*. 1983), and fetal compromise is more difficult to define in diabetic pregnancy. The second reason may be that compromise in diabetic pregnancy is not entirely due to uteroplacental insufficiency leading to chronically developing asphyxia, but may have an important metabolic component. Final deterioration in a marginally compromised situation may occur rapidly.

It is probable that Doppler ultrasonography will predict compromise in diabetic pregnancy where the mechanism is utero-placental deficiency with intra-uterine growth retardation or hypertensive disease. Whether it will do so in other situations when the baby is normal sized or large is uncertain. There have already been two reports of unexplained intra-uterine death in diabetic pregnancy preceded by normal umbilical artery FVW 3 days before hand (Bradley *et al*. 1988; Tyrrel 1988).

THE NATURE OF FETAL COMPROMISE IN DIABETIC PREGNANCY

Having examined the limited information available for examining the role of the prediction of antenatal compromise in diabetic pregnancy, we should now explore the theoretical basis for expecting a strong relationship. Although the precise mechanism of fetal death in diabetic pregnancy is uncertain, the combination of factors leading to demise is well recognised. The central factor is that the fetus of the diabetic mother tends to be hypoxaemic. This was suggested by the early work showing greatly increased extramedulary haemopoiesis in post-mortem specimens (Naeye 1965), together with the tendency of the fetus to be polycythaemic (Foley *et al.* 1981) and the finding of increased levels of erythropoietin in cord blood at delivery (Widness *et al.* 1981). Hypoxaemia has recently been demonstrated directly by measuring P_{O_2} in cord blood obtained by cordocentesis (Bradley *et al.* 1988).

The reasons for the chronic fetal hypoxaemia are excellently reviewed by Madsen (1986). There is reduced maternal placental blood flow (Kaar *et al.* 1980; Nylund *et al.* 1982), decreased villous surface area with increased placental diffusion distance (Fox 1969; Bjork and Persson 1982, 1984), and perhaps slightly decreased maternal red cell oxygen release (Ditzel 1980; Madsen 1986). However, although there is an important uteroplacental component, the placental changes found are different from those reported in association with abnormal umbilical FVWs.

The placenta in diabetic pregnancy shows a wide range of morphological change (Singer 1984). Placental infarcts are more common, and there is a tendency to villous oedema with thickening of the basement membranes of both the syncitiotrophoblast and the fetal capillaries (Fox 1969; Bjork and Persson 1984). Bjork and Persson (1984) reported an increase in syncytial knots, thinned out syncitium, and vasculosyncitial membranes approximating the fetal capillaries and maternal blood. These changes are thought to represent part of a compensatory process in response to poor placental perfusion. The abnormality reported in association with abnormal umbilical FVWs is reduction or obliteration of tertiary stem villi arterioles (see Chapter 11) and may represent an earlier failure of placentation.

In addition there is another important factor. Fetal hyperinsulinaemia stimulates fetal growth, so that the oxygen requirement of the fetus is increased (Philipps *et al.* 1981) at the same time as the oxygen supply is reduced. This imbalance may result in a baby that is hypoxaemic, but just coping within its limits of tolerance, so that no abnormality on antenatal testing is found. However, final deterioration in this setting could occur quickly. It is known that fetal hyperinsulinism is associated with hypoxaemia in lambs (Carson *et al.* 1980; Milley *et al.* 1984), and a period of maternal hyperglycaemia may be enough to precipitate that baby into a critical state. Shelley *et al.* (1974) showed in sheep that hyperglycaemia caused a rapid onset of acidosis in the mildly hypoxic fetus, and that the fetus did not recover if plasma pH fell below 7.1. This additional, acute, metabolic component, superimposed on a background of chronic hypoxaemia, may explain the failure to detect some cases of intra-uterine death in diabetic pregnancy with standard antenatal fetal monitoring. This is particularly so when diabetes has been poorly controlled (Barrett *et al.* 1981; Golde and Platt 1985; Miller and Horger 1985). Well-documented fetal compromise has been reported within a few days of a reactive cardiotocograph (non-stress test) (Schmidt *et al.* 1980; Teramo *et al.* 1983). In addition, Doppler ultrasonography could not be expected to give long-term prediction in the rare case of fetal death associated with maternal ketoacidosis. Metabolic acidosis is known to cause a marked, acute reduction in uterine blood flow (Blechner *et al.* 1975).

Thus, on theoretical grounds, it might be expected that umbilical artery Doppler FVWs would be of value where increased placental resistance is a major component, but the technique is less likely to predict cases with an acute metabolic component, particularly those associated with poor diabetic control.

CONCLUSION

Doppler uterine and umbilical artery recordings are of great research interest in diabetic pregnancy, and may help to clarify remaining uncertainties. There is currently no information about the value of uteroplacental FVWs as a screening test in diabetes. The reference ranges for indices from umbilical artery FVWs appear to be appropriate for diabetic pregnancies. There may be relationships between umbilical Doppler FVWs and the degree of metabolic control, but this is not entirely clear. Vascular complications and pregnancy-induced hypertension are common in diabetic pregnancy and in these cases umbilical artery Doppler FVWs may give useful predictive information. However, it is uncertain at present whether Doppler ultrasonography will give long-term prediction of fetal compromise in diabetic pregnancy. Although Doppler will probably have a role as a specific test of placental vasculature in diabetic pregnancy, it would be unwise to place too much reliance on normal Doppler studies until the situation becomes clearer.

REFERENCES

Ammalo, P. and Kariniemi, V. (1983). Short term variability of fetal heart rate during insulin-dependent diabetic pregnancies. *Journal of Perinatal Medicine,* **11,** 97–102.

Barrett, J. M., Salyer, S. L., and Boehm, F. H. (1981). The non-stress test: an evaluation of 1,000 patients. *American Journal of Obstetrics and Gynecology,* **141,** 153–7.

Bjork, O. and Persson, B. (1982). Placental changes in relation to the degree of metabolic control in diabetes mellitus. *Placenta,* **3**, 367–78.

Bjork, O. and Persson, B. (1984). Villous structure in different parts of the cotyledon in placentas of insulin-dependent diabetic women. A morphometric study. *Acta Obstetrica Gynaecologica Scandinavia,* **63**, 37–43.

Blechner, J. N., Stenger, V. G., and Prystowsky, H. (1975). Blood flow to the human uterus during metabolic acidosis. *American Journal of Obstetrics and Gynecology,* **121**, 789–94.

Bracero, L. A., Schulman, M., Fleischer, A., Farmakides, G., and Rochelson, B. (1986). Umbilical artery velocimetry in diabetes and pregnancy. *Obstetrics and Gynecology,* **68**, 654–8.

Bracero, L. A., Jovanovic, L., Rochelson, B., Schulman, M., Fleischer, A., and Schulman, M. (1989). Significance of umbilical and uterine artery velocimetry in the well-controlled pregnant diabetic. *Journal of Perinatal Medicine,* **34**, 273–6.

Bradley, R. J., Nicolaides, K. H., Brudenell, J. M., and Campbell, S. (1988). Early diagnosis of chronic fetal hypoxia in a diabetic pregnancy. *British Medical Journal,* **296**, 94–5.

Burke, G., Stuart, B., Crowley, P., Scanaill, S. N., and Drumm, J. (1990). Is intrauterine growth retardation with normal umbilical artery blood flow a benign condition? *British Medical Journal,* **300**, 1044–5.

Carson, B. S., Phillips, A. F., and Simmons, M. A. (1980). Effects of a sustained infusion upon glucose uptake and oxygenation of the ovine fetus. *Pediatric Reserve,* **14**, 152–5.

Connelly, F. A., Vademein, C., and Emanuel, I. (1985). Diabetes in pregnancy: a population-based study of incidence, referral for care and perinatal mortality. *American Journal of Obstetrics and Gynecology,* **151**, 598–603.

Ditzel, J. (1980). Affinity hypoxia as a pathogenetic factor of microangiopathy with particular reference to diabetic retinopathy. *Acta Endocrinologica,* **283** (Supplement), 39–53.

Fairlie, F. M., Morette, M., and Sibai, B. M. (1990). Umbilical artery velocimetry in diabetic pregnancies. *Society of Perinatal Obstetricians,* 10th Annual Meeting, Abstract no. 461, p. 478.

Foley, M. E., Collins, R., Stronge, J. M., Drury, M. I., and MacDonald, D. (1981). Blood viscosity in umbilical cord blood from babies of diabetic mothers. *British Journal of Obstetrics and Gynaecology,* **2**, 93–6.

Fox, H. (1969). Pathology of the placenta in maternal diabetes mellitus. *Obstetrics and Gynecology,* **34**, 792–8.

Golde, S. and Platt, L. (1985). Antepartum testing in diabetes. *Clinical Obstetrics and Gynecology,* **28**, 516–27.

Gudmundsson, S. and Marsal, K. (1988). Umbilical and uteroplacental blood flow velocity waveforms in pregnancies with fetal growth retardation. *European Journal of Obstetrics, Gynecology, and Reproductive Biology,* **27**, 187–96.

Haddad, G., Johnstone, F. D., Chambers, S. E., Hoskins, P. R., and McDicken, W. N. (1988a). Umbilical flow velocity waveform analysis and the outcome of hypertensive pregnancies. *British Journal of Obstetrics and Gynaecology,* **9**, 9–13.

Haddad, G., Johnstone, F. D., Chambers, S. E., and McDicken, W. N. (1988b). Umbilical artery Doppler waveforms in pregnancies with uncomplicated intrauterine growth retardation. *Gynaecological and Obstetric Investigation,* **26**, 206–10.

Johnson, J. M., Lange, I. R., Harman, C. R., Torchia, M. G., and Manning, F. A.

(1988). Biophysical profile scoring in the management of the diabetic pregnancy. *Obstetrics and Gynecology*, **72**, 841–6.

Johnstone, F. D., Haddad, N. G., Hoskins, P., McDicken, W., Chambers, S., and Muir, B. B. (1988). Umbilical artery Doppler flow velocity waveforms: the outcome of pregnancies with absent and diastolic flow. *European Journal of Obstetrics, Gynecology, and Reproductive Biology*, **28**, 171–8.

Johnstone, F. D., Nasrat, A., and Prescott, R. J. (1991*a*). The effect of established and gestational diabetes and pregnancy outcome. *British Journal of Obstetrics and Gynaecology*, (in press).

Johnstone, F. D., Steel, J. M., Haddad, N. G., McDicken, W., and Chambers, S. (1991*b*). Doppler umbilical and uterine artery velocity waveforms in diabetic pregnancy. *British Journal of Obstetrics and Gynaecology*, (in press).

Kaar, K., Jouppila, P., Kuikka, J., Koivula, A., and Jouppila, R. (1980). Intervillous blood flow in normal and complicated late pregnancy measured by means of an intravenous ^{133}Xe method. *Acta Obstetricia et Gynaecologica Scandinavica*, **59**, 7–10.

Kariniemi, V., Forss, M., Sieberg, R., and Ammala, P. (1983). Reduced short-term variability of fetal heart rate in association with maternal hyperglycaemia during pregnancy in insulin-dependent diabetic women. *American Journal of Obstetrics and Gynecology*, **147**, 793–4.

Kirkinen, P. and Jouppila, P. (1983). Ultrasonic measurements of human umbilical circulation in various pregnancy complications. In *Ultrasound annual* (ed. R. C. Sanders and M. Hill), pp. 153–5. Raven Press, New York.

Kofinas, A. D., Penry, M., and Swain, M. (1990). Uteroplacental Doppler flow velocity waveforms analysis correlates poorly with glycaemic control in diabetic pregnancy women. *Society of Perinatal Obstetricians*, 10th Annual Meeting. Abstract no. 410, p. 427.

Landon, M. B., Gabbe, S. G., Bruner, J. P., and Ludmir, J. (1989). Doppler umbilical artery velocimetry in pregnancy complicated by insulin-dependent diabetes mellitus. *Obstetrics and Gynecology*, **73**, 961–5.

Lang, V. and Kunzel, W. (1989). Diabetes mellitus in pregnancy. Management and outcome of diabetic pregnancies in the state of Hesse, F.R.G.: a five year survey. *European Journal of Obstetrics, Gynecology, and Reproductive Biology*, **33**, 115–29.

Madsen, H. (1986). Fetal oxygenation in diabetic pregnancy. *Danish Medical Bulletin*, **33**, 64–7.

McParland, P., Pearce, J. M., and Chamberlain, G. V. P. (1990*a*). Doppler ultrasound and aspirin in the recognition and prevention of pregnancy-induced hypertension. *Lancet*, **i**, 1552–5.

McParland, P., Steel, S. A., and Pearce, J. M. (1990*b*). The clinical implications of absent or reversed end-diastolic frequencies in umbilical artery flow velocity waveforms. *European Journal of Obstetrics, Gynecology, and Reproductive Biology*, **37**, 15–23.

Miller, J. M. and Horger, E. D. (1985). Antepartum heart rate testing in diabetic pregnancy. *Journal of Perinatal Medicine*, **30**, 515–18.

Milley, J. R., Rosenberg, A. A., Philipps, A. F., Molteni, R. A., Jones, M. D. Jr., and Simmons, M. A. (1984). The effects of insulin on ovine fetal oxygen extraction. *American Journal of Obstetrics and Gynecology*, **149**, 673–8.

Naeye, R. L. (1965). Infants of diabetic mothers: a quantitative morphologic study. *Pediatrics*, **35**, 980–8.

Nylund, L., Lunell, N.-O., Lewander, R., and Sarby, B. (1982). Uteroplacental blood flow in diabetic pregnancy: measurements with indium 113m and a computer-linked gamma camera. *American Journal of Obstetrics and Gynecology*, **144**, 298–302.

Oloffson, P., Lingman, G., Marsal, K., and Sjoberg, N.-O. (1987). Fetal blood flow in diabetic pregnancy. *Journal of Perinatal Medicine, 15*, 545–53.

Pearce, J. M., Campbell, S., Cohen-Overbeek, T., Hackett, G., Hernandez, J., and Royston, J. P. (1988). Reference ranges and sources of variation for indices of pulsed Doppler flow velocity waveforms from the uteroplacental and fetal circulations. *British Journal of Obstetrics and Gynecology*, **95**, 248–56.

Philipps, A. A., Dubin, J. W., and Raye, J. R. (1981). Fetal metabolic response to endogenous insulin release. *American Journal of Obstetrics and Gynecology*, **139**, 441–5.

Schmidt, P. L., Thorneycroft, I. H., and Goebelsmann, U. (1980). Fetal distress following a reactive nonstress test. *American Journal of Obstetrics and Gynecology*, **136**, 960–2.

Sheldon, G. W. (1989). Diabetes and pregnancy. *Obstetric and Gynecology Clinics of North America, 15*, 379–90.

Shelley, M. J., Bassett, J. M., and Milner, R. D. G. (1974). Control of carbohydrate metabolism in the fetus and newborn. *British Medical Bulletin*, **31**, 37–43.

Singer, D. B. (1984). The placenta in pregnancies complicated by diabetes. *Perspectives in Pediatric Pathology, 8*, 199–212.

Teramo, K., Ammala, P., Ylinen, K., and Raivio, K. O. (1983). Pathologic fetal heart rate associated with poor metabolic control in diabetic pregnancies. *Obstetrics and Gynecology*, **61**, 559–65.

Thomas, E. J. and Snodgrass, C. A. (1986). Social consequences of admission to the antenatal ward. *American Journal of Obstetrics and Gynecology*, **152**, 155–63.

Tyrrel, S. N. (1988). Doppler studies in diabetic pregnancy. *British Medical Journal*, **296**, 428.

White, P. (1949). Pregnancy complicating diabetes. *American Journal of Medicine, 7*, 609–16.

Widness, J. A., Susa, J. B., Garcia, J. F., *et al.* (1981). Increased erythropoiesis and elevated erythropoietin in infants born to diabetic mother and hyperinsulinaemic Rhesus fetuses. *Journal of Clinical Investigation*, **67**, 637–442.

10.   The use of Doppler ultrasound in a district general hospital

Simon Tyrrell

INTRODUCTION

The decision as to when to introduce a new technology into routine clinical practice is difficult. Currently, there is a large body of favourable evidence for a role for Doppler waveforms from the umbilical artery. They have been shown to distinguish the truly compromised fetus from the fetus that is constitutionally small (see Chapter 7). The place of umbilical artery Doppler waveforms is now being established by randomized, controlled trials.

There now seems to be an argument for the routine use of Doppler waveforms in well-defined clinical situations. After its introduction, it is likely that Doppler equipment will be used and interpreted by a range of professional staff, many of whom will not have either the understanding of the limitations of the technique nor the enthusiasm of research staff. Apart from providing adequate training, staff should have easy and rapid access to a team leader to resolve problems of recording, reporting, and interpreting waveforms.

With these thoughts in mind, the current uses of Doppler ultrasound will be reviewed to determine their suitability for use in a district general hospital.

CURRENT INDICATIONS

Use as a screening test

Umbilical artery waveforms   Chapter 5 discusses this situation in detail and comes to the firm conclusion that at the present time umbilical artery waveforms have no role as a screening test for the small-for-gestational age fetus. Therefore, screening of the low-risk pregnant population that attends most district general hospitals is not indicated.

Uteroplacental waveforms   Results of available studies are reviewed in Chapter 6, but may be summarized by saying that there is so much variation in the waveforms that they cannot be recommended for screening the entire low-risk population. They may, however, have a role to play in subgroups that are at somewhat higher risk, such as primigravidae (Steel *et al.* 1990) or Afro-Caribbeans (see Chapter 6).

On a practical note, however, the implementation of routine antenatal screening at 18–20 weeks, and perhaps again at 24 weeks, may not be feasible in a district general hospital. Although the two large studies of screening (Steel *et al.* 1990; see Chapter 6) combined the Doppler examination with the 18–20 week, real-time, ultrasound examination with little extra expense or time, not all hospitals scan women at this time. Many hospitals provide ultrasound examination only at the time of the booking visit, so that it would be necessary for the women to return for special visits.

There is only one randomized, controlled trial of the value of uteroplacental waveforms (McParland *et al.* 1990). The results of this study are detailed in Chapter 6, and reference to Table 6.5 suggests that potential cost savings may be made in terms of hospitalization. Some 17 per cent of women with abnormal uteroplacental waveforms developed hypertension before 37 weeks' gestation, and all of these patients were hospitalized for a minimum of 3 days (J. M. F. Pearce, personal communication, 1991). No patients in the aspirin-treated group developed early hypertension and the usual response to late-onset hypertension was induction of labour, rather than admission. In the absence of a statistical difference in perinatal mortality rates, we need a cost–benefit study before justifying the routine use of screening with uteroplacental waveforms.

Use in high-risk situations

Umbilical artery waveforms   Evidence to support the hypothesis that abnormal umbilical artery flow velocity waveforms can identify the fetus at risk of asphyxia is reviewed in Chapter 6, but is most directly obvious from the studies of Nicolaides *et al.* (1988) and Tyrrell *et al.* (1989). Tyrrell *et al.* (1989) also demonstrated a progressive increase in the risk of hypoxia and acidosis with increasingly abnormal umbilical artery waveforms. This suggests that in an obstetric population at high risk of fetal asphyxia, umbilical artery waveforms should be a useful adjunct to current methods of fetal surveillance (see also suggested scheme in Chapter 6).

Three prospective, randomized, controlled trials investigating the use of Doppler ultrasound in high-risk pregnancies have now been reported (Trudinger *et al.* 1987; Pearce *et al.* 1992; Tyrrell *et al.* 1991). All showed a reduction in the perinatal morbidity rate in the group where Doppler waveforms were used as an adjunct to standard clinical management, without a concomitant increase in obstetric intervention or iatrogenic prematurity. One trial (Pearce *et al.* 1991) demonstrated a clear reduction in the rate of perinatal and early infant deaths (see Chapter 8). These trials are sufficient evidence for the use of Doppler ultrasound in high-risk pregnancies.

Practically, all high-risk pregnancies are scanned serially for fetal biometric growth studies and for estimation of amniotic fluid columns. If fetal growth is abnormal and the Doppler equipment is located in the ultrasound department, there is virtually no extra administration and minimal additional time is required (usually less than 5 min) to obtain Doppler waveforms from the umbilical artery.

Practically speaking, evidence is accumulating that in the absence of an acute event, such as an abruption, umbilical artery waveforms rarely go from being completely normal to the loss of end-diastolic frequencies (AEDF) within 1 week (see also Chapter 8). The evidence that changes in Doppler umbilical artery waveforms pre-date changes in standard means of fetal surveillance is now clear (see Chapter 6). Thus, the following seems to be a logical management of a fetus that has an abnormal growth pattern on real-time ultrasonography:

1. Derive the A/B (S/D) ratio from three to five umbilical artery waveforms. If the value lies within normal limits on the data reference range (see Chapter 4) then:
    (i)   Repeat the Doppler scan weekly;
    (ii) Repeat the fetal biometric measurement fortnightly;
    (iii) Further fetal surveillance and/or delivery is not required while there are recordable frequencies in end-diastole and growth continues.

2. If AEDF are found in the umbilical artery, then arrange detailed methods of fetal surveillance (see Chapter 6) or delivery. The decision as to when to deliver is difficult, but should be actively considered over 28 weeks' gestation. There is increasing evidence that the combination of an abnormal cardiotocograph and AEDF has a very high mortality rate (Pearce *et al.* 1991; see Chapters 6 and 8).

3. AEDF in a symmetrically small fetus (particularly if there are also normal uteroplacental waveforms) should lead to a search for maternal infection and structural abnormalities. Karyotyping should also be considered if there are markers suggestive of chromosome abnormality.

Uteroplacental waveforms   The role of uteroplacental waveforms is less clear (see Chapter 8). There is only one randomized, controlled trial that has examined the value of such waveforms (Pearce *et al.* 1991). This trial studied waveforms from both the uteroplacental and the umbilical circulations (see Chapter 8). Broadly speaking, uteroplacental waveforms seem to predict the more severe forms of hypertensive disorder but, when considered alone, are not predictive of fetal compromise. This trial appears to support the work of Ducey *et al.* (1987) which suggests that an adverse fetal outcome (other than that inflicted by iatrogenic pre-term delivery because of worsening hypertension) occurs only in the presence of abnormal umbilical artery waveforms. The only additional reason for acquiring utero-placental waveforms may be that the finding of AEDF in the umbilical artery in the presence of completely normal uteroplacental waveforms should raise the question of a fetal abnormality or infection (see Chapter 8). Such patients should have detailed real-time ultrasound studies, searching for structural abnormalities and markers of chromosome anomalies.

SPECIAL SITUATIONS

Having defined a firm role for umbilical artery waveforms in the fetus found to be small on real-time ultrasonography, and a possible role for uteroplacental waveforms in the hypertensive patient, there appears to be no place for Doppler waveforms in a district general hospital in the following subgroups.

Maternal diabetes mellitus   The current evidence for the present role of Doppler waveforms from the umbilical artery and uteroplacental circulation is reviewed in Chapter 9. Although umbilical artery waveforms may be of use in those pregnancies complicated by increased umbilical placental resistance, and uteroplacental waveforms may be predictive of pregnancy-induced hypertension, Doppler waveforms in diabetic pregnancies are currently firmly in the area of research. Of great concern is the false reassurance that may be gained from normal umbilical artery waveforms, because there has been at least one case of a still birth not associated with abnormal umbilical artery waveforms (Tyrrell 1988).

Rhesus disease   Simple continuous wave Doppler ultrasonography has no role in the management of Rhesus disease. Although there is an increase in velocity in response to fetal anaemia, this reverses as the fetus decompensates. Chapter 12 details the value of pulsed Doppler in managing Rhesus disease. It is probably that both the pulsed Doppler equipment and the Rhesus patient should be at a regional centre under the care of specialist in fetal–maternal medicine.

Post-maturity   This is reviewed in Chapter 6. The evidence is conflicting but, at present Doppler ultrasonography cannot be recommended as part of fetal surveillance for post-dates pregnancy. Even though the large study suggests that it is more sensitive than amniotic fluid column measurement or cardiotocography (non-stress testing) (Pearce and McParland 1991), this has not been evaluated by means of a randomized, controlled trial.

CHOICE OF MACHINE

This is largely limited by two factors:

1. At present, the only justifiable use of Doppler equipment in the district general hospital is that of umbilical waveforms in fetuses shown to be small on real-time ultrasonography.
2. Financial constraints: Simple, portable continuous wave equipment costs £7000–10 000, which is approximately the price of an antenatal fetal heart rate monitor. These machines can often be acquired by appeals to charities, benevolent individuals, or the friends of the hospital.

Pulsed Doppler equipment is expensive and may be 'stand alone' or an 'add on' to current real-time equipment. Pulsed Doppler machines make identification of the umbilical cord easier, especially in twin pregnancies. They are essential if the district general hospital has a sub-specialist in fetal–maternal medicine who wishes to back up the continuous wave findings with recordings from individual fetal vessels. Failing such equipment patients with AEDF in the umbilical artery who are not to be delivered should be referred to a regional centre and colour flow and pulsed Doppler ultrasonography at the DGH can then not be justified.

WHO SHOULD PERFORM DOPPLER STUDIES?

It is unrealistic to expect to take on new staff purely to perform Doppler studies. In addition, Doppler ultrasound equipment should be located close to facilities used for real-time ultrasound investigation of fetal growth, normality, and biophysical parameters. This means one of two sites:

1. In the obstetric ultrasound department.
2. In the fetal welfare laboratory. This is usually a site in which women with high-risk pregnancies can be assessed as day cases.

In either case, the most appropriate people to carry out Doppler studies are those who use the real-time apparatus, be they ultrasonographers, midwives, or doctors. The ability to acquire Doppler waveforms is readily learnt, but unless there is regular feedback from clinicians to workers on the value of the waveforms in individual cases, recording waveforms can become very boring.

Finally, it is better to have a formal protocol for planning who should have Doppler examinations, when, and how often. Guide-lines are best agreed between the consultant obstetric staff, led by the specialist or sub-specialist in fetal–maternal medicine, together with the ultrasound staff. This makes for less argument and also reduces unnecessary referrals.

Reporting Doppler waveforms

This is a contentious area, but for use in most district general hospitals the information given in Chapter 3 is appropriate and maybe summarized as follows:

1. Record the A/B (S/D) ratio from the umbilical artery and plot it on the chosen reference range. Report the waveform in words, that the umbilical artery waveform is normal. There are, currently, no studies to suggest that a fetus that demonstrates a gradually worsening wave-form but never loses end-diastolic frequencies does any worse than the fetus whose waveform remains within normal limits. When there are absent or reversed frequencies in the umbilical artery waveforms, report this in words.

2. Report uteroplacental waveforms according to the pattern obtained from both sides of the uterus, namely:
   (i) low resistance: waveforms from both sides with a resistance index within normal limits;
   (ii) high resistance: waveforms from both sides with a resistance index outside normal limits;
   (iii) mixed resistance: one waveform within normal limits and one waveform outside normal limits.

CONCLUSIONS

There is now evidence to justify the purchase of simple continuous wave Doppler equipment for every district general hospital. Its use should be limited to determining which fetuses found to be small on real-time ultra-sonography are truly disadvantages. Another possible use may be the recording of uteroplacental waveforms in women with hypertensive disease of pregnancy.

The equipment should be used by those individuals who carry out real-time ultrasonography, either in the obstetric ultrasound clinic or the fetal welfare laboratory. Protocols for its use should be agreed and there should be regular feedback on the outcome of clinical cases to the Doppler ultrasound operators.

REFERENCES

Ducey, J., Schulman, H., Farmakides, G., *et al.* (1987). A classification of hypertension in pregnancy based on Doppler velocimetry. *American Journal of Obstetrics and Gynecology,* **157,** 680–5.

McParland, P., Pearce, J. M. F., and Chamberlain, G. V. P. (1991). Doppler ultrasound and aspirin in recognition and prevention of pregnancy-induced hypertension. *Lancet,* **335,** 1552–5.

Nicolaides, K. H., Bilardo, C. M., Soothill, P. W., and Campbell, S. (1988). Absence of end-diastolic frequencies in the umbilical artery: a sign of fetal hypoxia and acidosis. *British Medical Journal,* **297,** 1026–7,

Pearce, J. M. and McParland, P. (1991). A comparison of Doppler flow velocity waveforms, amniotic fluid columns and non-stress tests as a means of monitoring post-dates pregnancy. *Obstetrics and Gynecology,* **77,** 204–8.

Pearce, J. M. F., Campbell, S., Smith, P., and Gamsu, H. (1992). A randomised, controlled trial of Doppler waveforms from the uteroplacental and feteroplacental circulation. *British Journal of Obstetrics and Gynaecology,* (in press).

Steel, S. A., Pearce, J. M., McParland, P., and Chamberlain, G. V. P. (1990). Early Doppler ultrasound screening in the prediction of hypertensive disorders of pregnancy. *Lancet,* **335,** 1548–51.

Trudinger, B. J., Cook, C. M., Giles, W. B., Connelly, A., and Thompson, R. S. (1987). Umbilical artery flow velocity waveforms in high risk-pregnancy. *Lancet,* **i,** 188–90.

Tyrrell, S. N. (1988). Doppler waveforms in diabetes mellitus. *British Medical Journal,* **296,** 428.

Tyrrell, S. N., Lilford, R. J., and Obaid, A. H. (1989). Umbilical artery Doppler velocimetry as a predictor of fetal hypoxia and acidosis at birth. *Obstetrics and Gynecology,* **74,** 332–7.

Tyrrell, S. N., Lilford, R. J., MacDonald, H. N., Nelson, E. J., Porter, J., and Gupta, J. K. (1991). Randomised trial of Doppler ultrasound and biophysical scoring in high risk pregnancy. *British Journal of Obstetrics and Gynecology,* **97,** 909–16.

11. The pathophysiological basis of abnormal flow velocity waveforms

Robert Morrow, Lee Adamson, Knox Ritchie, and Malcolm Pearce

INTRODUCTION

Flow velocity waveforms (FVWs) in any vessel may be influenced by many factors such as cardiac contractility, the characteristics of the vessel wall, blood viscosity, and the vascular arrangement downstream from the vessel (Burns 1987). Difficulties with investigations in the human fetus have led to the study of appropriate animal models, particularly to elucidate the changes observed in the umbilical artery. Changes in the uteroplacental circulation have been largely related to work from placental bed biopsies.

THE UMBILICAL CIRCULATION

Placental vascular resistance

Clinical studies   Analogy with other vascular beds suggests that the velocity information contained in waveforms is influenced by downstream vascular resistance (Skidmore *et al.* 1980). This suggests that the micro-vasculature of the fetal placental bed is the logical starting point to examine the changes that are observed in the umbilical artery waveforms. Microscopy of the placental vasculature reveals no obvious difference in structure but a difference in the number of small-calibre placental resistance vessels.

Giles *et al.* (1985) examined the placentas from three groups of women: those with normal pregnancies and a normal S/D (A/B) ratio from the umbilical artery; those with an at-risk pregnancy but a normal S/D ratio; and those with an at-risk pregnancy but an abnormal S/D ratio. The demonstrated that the number of tertiary stem arterioles was reduced in women with abnormal S/D ratios. Tertiary stem arterioles are the level at which there is a maximum fall in blood pressure, i.e. they are fetal placental resistance vessels. This work has been confirmed by McCowan *et al.*

(1989), who also demonstrated a linear inverse relationship between the S/D ratio and the numbers of small arterioles.

There are two possible explanations for these findings: either there is a deficiency in the formation of these small arterioles or they are subsequently obliterated. Obliteration could arise because of reduced uteroplacental perfusion leading to hypoxic ischaemia of the intervillous space and vaso-constriction of the fetal placental vessels (Rankin and McLaughlin 1979). Alternatively, changes in the constituency of fetal blood may encourage coagulation and thrombosis. In any event reduction in the number of patent small arterioles leads to an increase in peripheral resistance which is reflected in the abnormal umbilical FVWs.

Animal studies   The major problem with clinical studies of physiological mechanisms is that it is difficult to establish cause and effect. Thus, even though abnormal placental vascular counts have been demonstrated in cases of abnormal umbilical waveforms, they may not be the cause. Morrow *et al.* (1990*a*, *b*) have used an animal model in an attempt to dissect out this problem. A Doppler probe was directly implanted into the umbilical artery of a fetal sheep (Fig. 11.1) allowing observation of the FVWs over prolonged periods with the sheep in an undisturbed state. In addition, the lamb was also instrumented to allow direct measurement of its blood pressure and placental vascular resistance; access to the fetal circulation was also available for the infusion of drugs or blood gas meas-urements. Such a model was used to test hypotheses generated from clinical observations.

In order to determine the effect of a reduction in the number of fetal

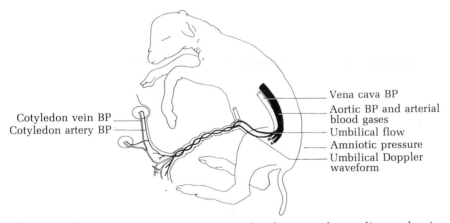

Cotyledon vein BP
Cotyledon artery BP

Vena cava BP
Aortic BP and arterial blood gases
Umbilical flow
Amniotic pressure
Umbilical Doppler waveform

Fig. 11.1 Diagram to show the placement of catheters and recording probes in the fetal sheep. The Doppler crystal is placed in a cuff around one of the umbilical arteries.

placental resistance vessels these were occluded by means of plastic emboli of 50 μm in diameter (Morrow *et al.* 1989). These emboli were introduced through the distal abdominal aorta so that they were carried into the umbilical circulation and eventually became lodged in the fetal side of the placenta (Fig. 11.2). With increasing embolization, a gradual change was observed in the FVW. The diastolic component was progressively reduced until it became absent and eventually reversed (Fig. 11.3). These changes were directly related to an increase in placental vascular resistance. It is apparent from these studies that occlusion of the fetal placental vascular bed can produced abnormal FVWs, similar to those observed in growth-retarded fetuses (see Figs 7.1 and 7.2).

In order to determine whether the site of raised placental vascular resistance affects the waveforms, the same animal model was infused with angiotensin II. Angiotensin II causes a substantial but transient elevation of the placental vascular resistance (Adamson *et al.* 1990) but, unlike embolization, it causes vasoconstriction of the umbilical artery and its major branches but not of the distal vasculature. Angiotensin II causes a rise in placental resistance of up to 10-fold and a decrease in umbilical blood flow of about one-third of control values, but the umbilical artery waveform S/D ratio is not significantly altered (Fig. 11.4). Thus, it can be

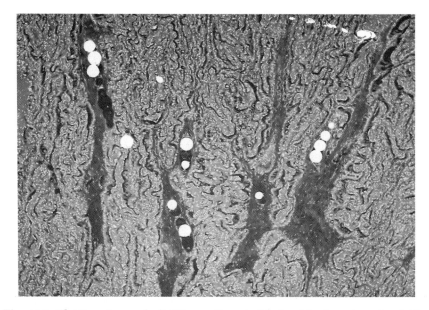

Fig. 11.2 Plastic microemboli (50 μm diameter) lodged in the microcirculation of the placenta of the fetal sheep. The emboli appear to be different sizes as they are sectioned in different planes.

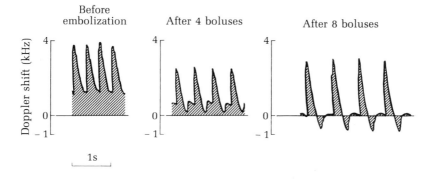

Fig. 11.3 Umbilical artery waveform changes in the fetal sheep in response to progressive embolization of the placenta: before embolization; after 4 boluses; and after 8 boluses. (Reproduced by permission of the *American Journal of Obstetrics and Gynecology*.)

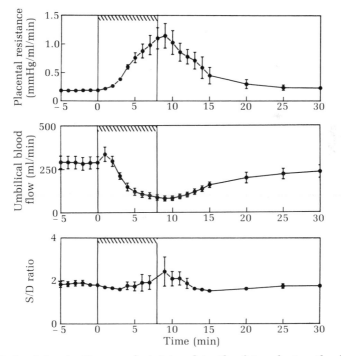

Fig. 11.4 Angiotensin II was administered to the fetus during the hatched period. There was a rise in placental vascular resistance (top) but the S/D ratio (A/B ratio) was not significantly altered (bottom).

concluded that changes in the small resistance vessels on the fetal side of the placenta are responsible for the changes observed in the umbilical artery waveform.

Giles *et al.* (1989) conducted a series of experiments of sheep involving carunculectomy. Before pregnancy, the sheep uterus is lined with caruncles, and removal of some of these results in a small placenta which has normal anatomy with normal perfusion per weight of placenta and normal placental resistance. Carunculectomy results in an overall reduction in blood flow to the placenta in growth-retarded fetal lambs but normal umbilical artery waveforms.

It is apparent, therefore, that not only is the overall resistance in the fetal, placental circulation important, but the actual site of elevated resistance within the vascular tree is crucial to the waveform shape. Changes in the small placental resistance vessels result in changes in the umbilical artery waveform, but narrowing umbilical artery (or its major branches) from poor development or from vasoconstriction has no effect of the waveform.

Fetal asphyxial changes

There is a known association in human pregnancies between abnormal umbilical artery waveforms and fetal hypoxaemia and acidaemia as established by cordocentesis (Nicolaides *et al.* 1987). This suggests that abnormal umbilical artery waveforms may be useful indicators of hypoxaemia since it is known that hypoxaemia leads to a redistribution of fetal blood flow with preferential flow to the fetal brain, heart, and adrenal glands (Cohn *et al.* 1974).

Morrow *et al.* (1990*a*) induced hypoxaemia in fetal lambs in order to assess the effect on the umbilical artery waveforms. Figure 11.5 demonstrates that despite a significant fall in the fetal arterial P_{O_2} the waveforms remained normal. This does not exclude the possibility that chronic hypoxia might ultimately induce that placental changes that result in abnormal waveforms, but it clearly demonstrates that a normal waveform does not guarantee normal blood gases nor does hypoxaemia necessarily result in an abnormal waveform. In a further series of experiments Morrow *et al.* (1990*b*) exposed fetal lambs to prolonged hypoxia such that acidaemia resulted. Figure 11.6 demonstrates that even when the fetal pH was reduced to 6.8 the umbilical artery waveform remained normal in many animals. This confirms that profound hypoxia and acidaemia are not the cause of the umbilical artery changes.

Other asphyxial changes

Theoretically, it may be expected that a rise in blood viscosity may cause abnormal waveforms. Poiseuille's law, which governs flow of fluids through rigid tubes, suggests that increased blood viscosity would give rise to an increase in vascular resistance and hence decreased blood flow. Growth-

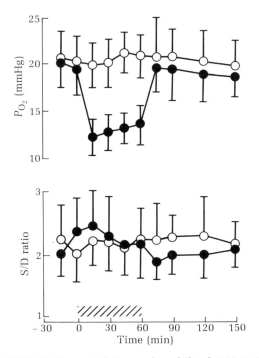

Fig. 11.5 Mean (SEM) fetal arterial P_{O_2} and umbilical S/D (A/B) ratio during control experiments (open circles) and hypoxaemia experiments (closed circles). The 60 min. period of gas infusion into the ewe (air or nitrogen) is indicated by the stripped bar above the axis. (Reproduced from *Obstetrics and Gynecology* by permission of the American College of Obstetrics and Gynecology.)

retarded fetuses become polycythaemic and blood viscosity increases (Makanson and Oh 1980). Because increased viscosity reduces blood flow, it has been suggested that hyperviscosity may cause waveform abnormalities. This has not been confirmed over the range of viscosities observed in clinical practice (Giles and Trudinger 1986; Steel *et al.* 1989).

Morrow *et al.* (1990*b*) doubled the viscosity of the blood in fetal sheep and observed no significant change in the umbilical artery waveform (Fig. 11.7). The infusion of packed cells that resulted in the increased viscosity also increased directly measured placental resistance by 50 per cent, again demonstrating that the umbilical artery waveform does not necessarily change in response to placental resistance under all circumstances.

Maternal hypertensive disease of pregnancy is often associated with abnormal umbilical artery waveforms (see Chapter 7). This led Morrow *et al.* (1990*b*) to investigate the effects of blood pressure of the umbilical

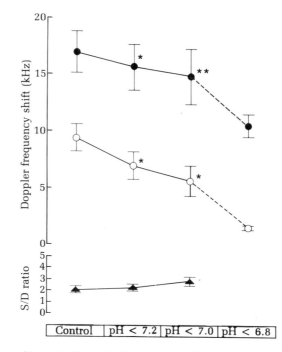

Fig. 11.6 Systolic and diastolic frequency shift (proportional to blood flow) and S/D (A/B) ratio are shown for both control and progressive acidaemia. Only four of the seven fetuses survived to pH less than 6.8 so the data points are joined by dashed lines and not subjected to statistical analysis. (*p < 0.025 compared with controls, **p = 0.002 compared with controls.) (Reproduced with permission from the *American Journal of Obstetrics and Gynaecology*.)

waveforms. Large rises in blood pressure (more than 50 mmHg) in the pregnant sheep had no observed effect on the umbilical artery waveform. In contrast, however, fetal hypotension led to abnormal umbilical artery waveforms as myocardial activity failed following profound ischaemia.

Conclusions

Results from animal studies show that occlusion of the small vessels of the fetal, placental vasculature is the most effective way of causing abnormal umbilical artery Doppler waveforms. The clinical and experimental evidence to date strongly suggest that abnormal umbilical artery waveforms are primarily a reflection of occlusion of small placental vessels. Normal waveforms may be observed even when the fetus is hypoxic, acidotic, hyperviscous, or has reduced placental blood flow. Clinical studies should be interpreted in the light of these findings.

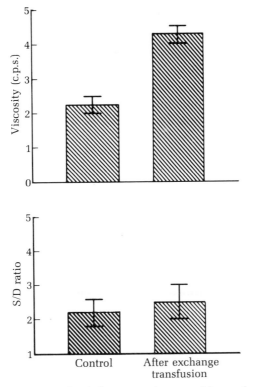

Fig. 11.7 Blood viscosity in fetal sheep was increased by exchange transfusion of packed cells but there was no significant change in umbilical artery waveform shape.

THE UTEROPLACENTAL CIRCULATION

Development of the maternal placental bed

The maternal placental bed develops from the original implantation site (Gruenwald 1972) and, at term, maternal blood enters the intervillous space through 100 to 200 spiral arteries (Brosens and Dixon 1966). The pressure of the blood entering the intervillous space is about 25 mmHg which is higher than the pressure within the space (15–20 mmHg), so the blood is directed towards the roof of the space (the chorionic plate). Flow is dampened such that the blood then flows slowly over the fetal villi, so allowing time for gaseous and metabolic exchange. Maternal blood then drains to the floor of the intervillous space and on into the endometrial veins (Ramsey and Donner 1980). The intervillous space of the mature placenta contains about 150 ml of blood which is replaced three to four times a minute (Aherne and Dunnill 1966). Uteroplacental blood flow increases from about 50 ml/min at 10 weeks' gestation to about 600 ml/min at term (Martin 1968). In order to achieve this vast increase, the spiral arteries of the non-pregnant uterus are modified into the uteroplacental arteries of pregnancy.

Trophoblast can be found in the maternal spiral arteries from the first time that these arteries communicate with the intervillous space (Hamilton and Boyd 1966; Harris and Ramsey 1966). The trophoblast disrupts the wall of the spiral artery, destroying its muscle and elastic coats and replacing them with fibrinoid tissue (Brosens *et al.* 1967; de Wolf *et al.* Dixon 1973). Invasion of the spiral arteries occurs in two separate waves (Robertson *et al.* 1975). The first wave occurs at the time of implantation and lasts until about 10 weeks' gestation; it is limited in depth to the decidual parts of the spiral arteries. The second wave starts at 14–16 weeks' gestation and lasts for 4–6 weeks. This wave invades as far as the radial artery (Fig. 11.8).

This second wave of invasion allows progressive distension of the arteries such that they become uteroplacental vessels and can thus accommodate the increased uteroplacental blood flow. In addition, the lack of a muscular wall renders them insensitive to circulating pressor agents.

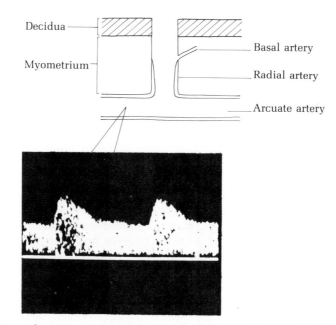

Fig. 11.8 Schematic representation of the state of the spiral arteries in a normal pregnancy after 24 weeks gestation. The trophoblast has stripped the muscle coat down to the level of the radial artery, resulting in a waveform from the arcuate arteries demonstrating a low resistance index and pulsatility.

Pathology of the placental bed

From the pioneering work of Robertson *et al.* (1967) and Brosens *et al.* (1972) on Caesarean hysterectomy specimens, it was discovered that patients with severe pre-eclampsia had a universal failure of the second wave of invasion (Robertson *et al.* 1967). Thus, only the decidual portion of each spiral artery was converted to a uteroplacental vessel (Fig. 11.9). This has the following effects: (1) decreased perfusion of the intervillous space; and (2) maternal systemic hypertension. The retention of about 1 cm of muscle coat on each of some 200 spiral arteries prevents the mid-trimester fall in peripheral resistance. In addition, these uninvaded portions are sensitive to circulating pressor agents and are subject to acute atherosis (de Wolf *et al.* 1975; Khong and Pearce 1987). This is an acute necrotizing arteriopathy similar to that observed in malignant hypertension. It further narrows the spiral arteries.

In pregnancies complicated by intra-uterine growth retardation but not by hypertension, about 50 per cent of such women demonstrate inadequate invasion of the spiral arteries based on placental bed biopsy results (Sheppard and Bonnar 1976; Robertson *et al.* 1981). Because not all causes of

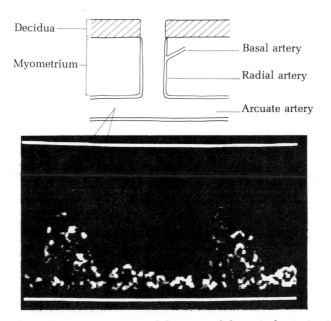

Fig. 11.9 Schematic representation of the state of the spiral arteries in a pregnancy complicated by pre-eclampsia. Invasion of the trophoblast is limited to the decidual portion of the spiral arteries resulting in an arcuate artery waveform with increased pulsatility and resistance index.

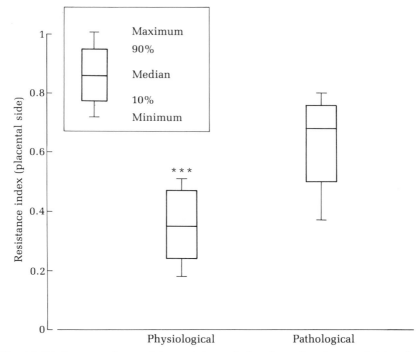

Fig. 11.10 A comparison of the resistance index from the placental side of the uterus with the depth of invasion of the trophoblast. This was determined from placental bed biopsies taken at the time of caesarean section (***p < 0.001).

smallness are related to inadequate placental perfusion, and because both studies used a statistical cut-off point for defining intra-uterine growth retardation (less than the 10th centile), it is not surprising that this was not a universal finding.

Clinical studies

The observation that the resistance index (RI) from the uteroplacental circulation fell until about 22–24 weeks' gestation (see Chapter 4, Figs 4.9 and 4.10) but then appeared unchanged led to the suggestion that utero-placental waveforms may be the result of trophoblastic invasion. Despite the problems in defining the precise site from which the waveforms arose, Khong and Pearce (1987) demonstrated a significant difference in the RI obtained from the placental side of the uterus in cases of pathological and physiological invasion.

This work has been extended and the results are illustrated in Figs 11.10 and 11.11. There is a highly significant difference in both the median RI and its distribution in patients demonstrating physiological invasion and in

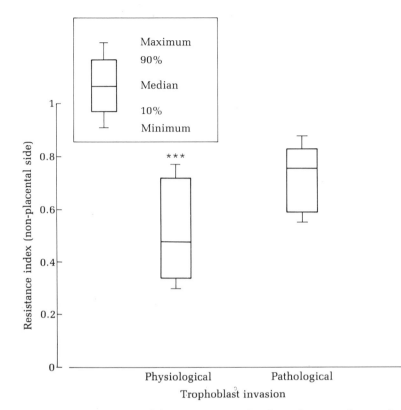

Fig. 11.11 A comparison of the resistance index from the non-placental side of the uterus with the depth of invasion of the trophoblast. This was determined from placental bed biopsies taken at the time of Caesarean section (***$p < 0.001$).

those demonstrating pathological invasion. This difference is most marked in the RI obtained from the placental side of the uterus. This suggests that the uteroplacental waveform truly reflects the depth of trophoblastic invasion.

Figure 11.12 demonstrates the resistance index for the clinical classification of the patients. Patients requiring Caesarean section for hypertensive disease of pregnancy have a significantly higher RI than controls. The number of patients with small-for-gestational age (SGA) infants without hypertension is small, but the range of RI is large, reflecting the diverse reasons for SGA babies.

Such studies provide insight into the pathophysiology of disease and go some way towards explaining the Doppler waveform changes. Care must be taken, however, because placental bed biopsies often contain only one spiral artery and may therefore not reflect the general state of invasion of

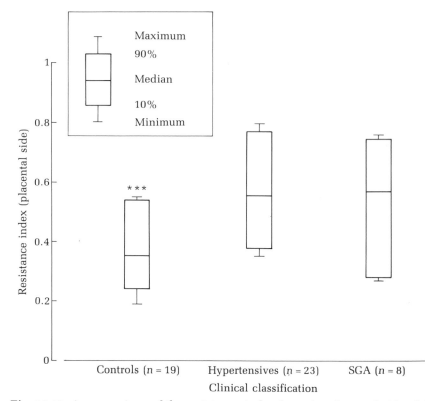

Fig. 11.12 A comparison of the resistance index from the placental side of the uterus with the clinical classification of patients undergoing caesarean section (***p < 0.001 for controls versus hypertensive patients).

the spiral arteries. In addition, women requiring Caesarean section for hypertension and/or SGA fetuses represent the most severe examples of the disease process. It can only be truly concluded, therefore, that at the extremes of the disease the RI represents the depth of trophoblastic invasion.

Figure 11.13 demonstrates the correlation between the birth-weight (expressed as birth-weight centile after correction for gestational age and sex) and the RI. The depth of trophoblastic invasion, as expressed by the RI, explains only about 40 per cent of the variation in birthweight. Figure 11.14 demonstrates that, although there is a highly statistically significant difference in the median birth-weight centiles of the two groups, there is considerable overlap in the range.

Eclampsia is rare in the UK, and there is little or no information on such cases from Doppler ultrasonography or placental bed biopsies. Table 11.1 illustrates the clinical, histopathological, and Doppler details on six cases.

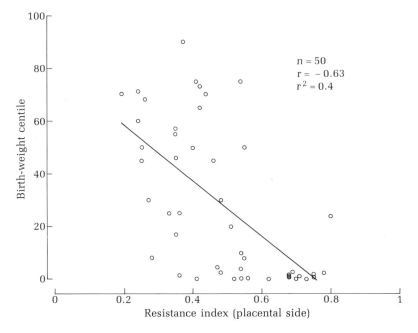

Fig. 11.13 The correlation between the birth-weight centile and the resistance index from the placental side of the uterus. Only about 40 per cent of the variability in birthweight is explained by the depth of trophoblastic invasion.

In all six, physiological invasion of the uteroplacental arteries appeared complete and all had normal Doppler waveforms from the uteroplacental circulation. Although there are small numbers, this strongly suggests that the eclampsia oberved in UK obstetric practice is not the end-result of pre-eclampsia.

Biochemical changes in pregnancy

Figure 11.15 illustrates the changes in the haemodynamic state during normal pregnancy. Normal trophoblastic invasion increases the circulating capacity and leads to an increase in the ratio of prostacyclin to thromboxane. This, in turn, leads to a resistance in the vasoconstrictor action of angiotensin II (for a review of evidence, see McParland and Pearce 1991). The resultant hypotension activates the renin–angiotensin system and causes an increase in the secretion of aldosterone and atrial naturetic peptide (ANP). This maintains homoeostasis, although blood pressure is usually slightly lower than in the non-pregnant state.

There is much dispute over the classification of hypertensive disorders in pregnancy. This makes the interpretation of any biochemical changes difficult and the literature is beset with differing results. Slater *et al.* (1992)

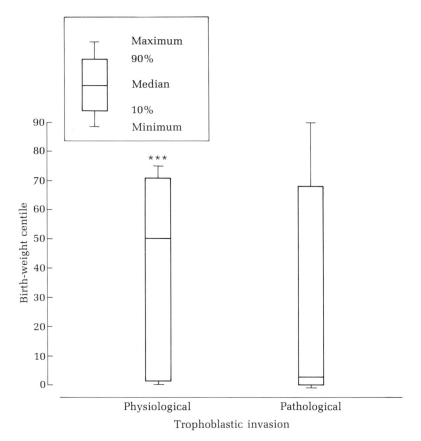

Fig. 11.14 A comparison of birthweight centiles with the depth of trophoblastic invasion (***p < 0.001).

classify hypertensive disorders of pregnancy based upon the Doppler waveforms from the uteroplacental circulation:

1. Pre-eclampsia was considerd to exist when uteroplacental waveforms demonstrated a high-resistance pattern, with an RI of more 0.58 in the presence of hypertension.

2. Pregnancy-induced hypertension was considered to exist if the uteroplacental waveforms demonstrated a low-resistance pattern in the presence of hypertension.

Figures 11.16–11.24 illustrate the findings. Figure 11.16 is a schema representing the suggested changes observed in hypertension of pregnancy but in the presence of normal uteroplacental waveforms. Activation of the renin–angiotensin system and increased aldosterone production occur as in

Table 11.1 Clinical, Doppler and pathological features of six eclamptic women

Uteroplacental waveforms	Trophoblast invasion	Clinical comment
NN	Physiological	Post-natal fit × 2 Normotensive antenatally
NN	Physiological	Post-natal fit × 5 Blood pressure 140/90 in labour No proteinuria
NN	Physiological	Post-natal fit × 2 Proteinuric hypertension developed in labour
NN	Physiological	Intrapartum fit Normotensive antenatally
NN	Physiological	Antepartum fit × 3 Hypertensive from 38 weeks No proteinuria
NN	Physiological	Antepartum fit × 1 Hypertensive from 34 weeks Proteinuria

NN, Doppler waveforms normal from both sides of the uterus.

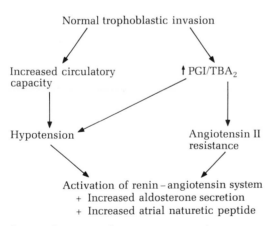

Fig. 11.15 The haemodynamic changes in normal pregnancy (PGI, prostacyclin; TBA$_2$, thromboxane A$_2$).

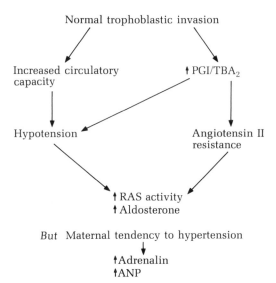

Fig. 11.16 The haemodynamic changes in hypertensive disease of pregnancy but in the presence of normal uteroplacental Doppler waveforms (PGI, prostacyclin; TBA₂, thromboxane A₂; ANP, atrial naturetic peptide; RAS, renin–angiotensin II system).

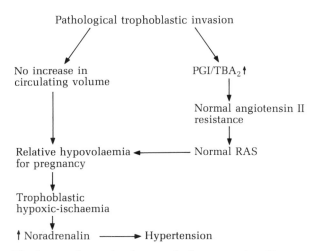

Fig. 11.17 The haemodynamic changes in hypertensive disease of pregnancy but in the presence of abnormal uteroplacental Doppler waveforms—pre-eclampsia (PGI, prostacyclin; TBA₂, thromboxane A₂; ANP, atrial naturetic peptide; RAS, renin–angiotensin II system).

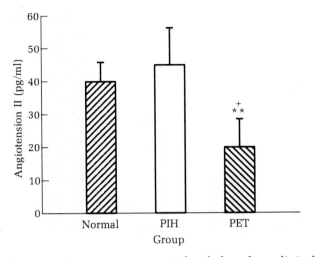

Fig. 11.18 Maternal plasma angiotensin II levels based on clinical classification. Normal, not hypertensive and normal uteroplacental Doppler waveforms; PIH, pregnancy induced hypertension that is hypertension but with normal uteroplacental Doppler waveforms; PET, pre-eclampsia, which is hypertension with abnormal waveforms. (**$p < 0.01$ PET *vs.* normal, +$p < 0.01$ PET *vs.* PIH)

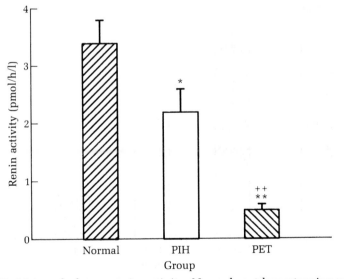

Fig. 11.19 Maternal plasma renin activity. Normal, not hypertensive and normal uteroplacental Doppler waveforms; PIH, pregnancy induced hypertension that is hypertension but with normal uteroplacental Doppler waveforms; PET, pre-eclampsia, which is hypertension with abnormal Doppler waveforms. (**$p < 0.01$ PET *vs.* normal, ††$p < 0.01$ PET *vs.* PIH, *$p < 0.05$ PIH *vs.* normal)

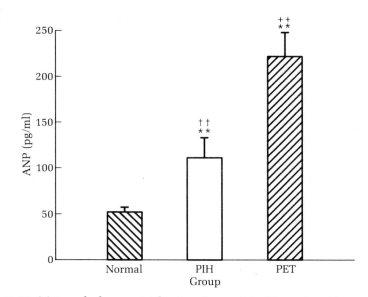

Fig. 11.20 Maternal plasma atrial naturetic peptide. Normal, not hypertensive and normal uteroplacental Doppler waveforms; PIH, pregnancy induced hypertension that is hypertension but with normal uteroplacental Doppler waveforms; PET, pre-eclampsia, which is hypertension with abnormal Doppler waveforms. (**$p < 0.01$ PET *vs.* normal, $^{++}p < 0.01$ PET *vs.* PIH, ††$p < 0.01$ PIH *vs.* normal)

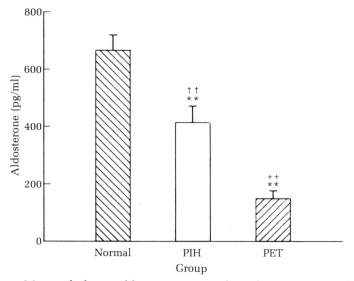

Fig. 11.21 Maternal plasma aldosterone. Normal, not hypertensive and normal uteroplacental Doppler waveforms; PIH, pregnancy induced hypertension that is hypertension but with normal uteroplacental Doppler waveforms; PET, pre-eclampsia, which is hypertension with abnormal Doppler waveforms. (**$p < 0.01$ PET *vs.* normal, $^{++}p < 0.01$ PET *vs* PIH, ††$p < 0.01$ PIH *vs.* normal)

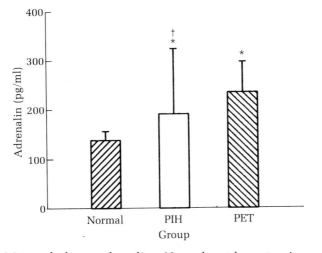

Fig. 11.22 Maternal plasma adrenaline. Normal, not hypertensive and normal uteroplacental Doppler waveforms; PIH, pregnancy induced hypertension that is hypertension but with normal uteroplacental Doppler waveforms; PET, pre-eclampsia, which is hypertension with abnormal Doppler waveforms. (*$p < 0.05$ PET *vs.* normal, †$p < 0.05$ PIH *vs.* normal)

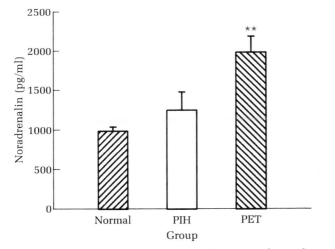

Fig. 11.23 Maternal plasma nor-adrenaline levels. Normal, not hypertensive and normal uteroplacental Doppler waveforms; PIH, pregnancy induced hypertension that is hypertension but with normal uteroplacental Doppler waveforms; PET, pre-eclampsia, which is hypertension with abnormal Doppler waveforms. (**$p < 0.01$ PET *vs.* normal)

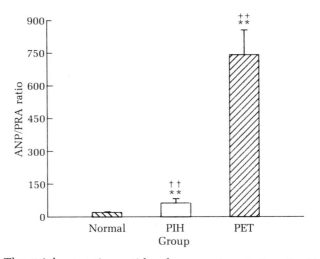

Fig. 11.24 The atrial naturetic peptide: plasma renin activity ratio. Normal, not hypertensive and normal uteroplacental Doppler waveforms; PIH, pregnancy induced hypertension that is hypertension but with normal uteroplacental Doppler waveforms; PET, pre-eclampsia, which is hypertension with abnormal Doppler waveforms. (**$p < 0.01$ PET *vs.* normal, $^{++}p < 0.01$ PET *vs.* PIH, ††$p < 0.01$ PIH *vs.* normal)

normal pregnancy (see Fig. 11.15), but the underlying maternal tendency to hypertension is accompanied by an increase in the circulating levels of adrenalin. There is also a rise in the levels of ANP but, because the renin–angiotensin system is normal, the ratio of ANP to plasma renin activity is only moderately changed (Fig. 11.24).

In pre-eclampsia, failure of trophoblastic invasion (as demonstrated by high-resistance uteroplacental waveforms) results in failure to activate the renin–angiotensin system and in normal aldosterone levels. However, this results in underperfusion of the trophoblast, which responds by increasing noradrenalin production, and hence the blood pressure rises. This rise in blood pressure stimulates the release of ANP but as the plasma renin activity is normal, the ANP to plasma renin activity ratio increases massively (Fig. 11.24).

Summary

Histopathological studies on placental bed biopsies suggest that the RI of the uteroplacental waveforms reflects the depth of trophoblastic invasion. Biochemical studies demonstrate that classifying hypertension in pregnancy on the basis of Doppler waveforms is justified. This further backs up the clinical evidence that such a classification is superior to current means of classifying hypertensive disorders in pregnancy (see Chapter 8).

REFERENCES

Adamson, S. L., Morrow, R. J., Langille, B. L., Bull, S. B., and Ritchie, J. W. K. (1990). Site dependent effects of increases in placental vascular resistance on the umbilical arterial velocity waveform in sheep. *Ultrasound in Medicine and Biology,* **16,** 19–27.
Aherne, W. and Dunnill, M. S. (1966). Quantitative aspects of placental structure. *Journal of Pathology and Bacteriology,* **91,** 123–39.
Brosens, I. and Dixon, H. G. (1966). Anatomy of the maternal side of the placenta. *Journal of Obstetrics and Gynaecology of the British Commonwealth,* **73,** 357–63.
Brosens, I., Robertson, W. B., and Dixon, H. G. (1967). The physiological response of the vessels of the placental bed to normal pregnancy. *Journal of Pathology and Bacteriology,* **93,** 569–79.
Brosens, I., Robertson, W. B., and Dixon, H. G. (1972). The role of the spiral arteries in the pathogenesis of pre-eclampsia. *Obstetric and Gynaecological Annual,* **1,** 177–91.
Burns, P. N. (1987). Doppler flow estimations in the fetal and maternal circulations: principles, techniques and some limitations. In: *Doppler ultrasound measurements of maternal fetal haemodynamics* (ed. D. Maulik and D. H. McNellis), pp. 43–76. Perinatology Press, Ithaca, New York.
Cohn, M. E., Sacks, E. J., Heyman, M. A., and Rudolph, A. M. (1974). Cardiovascular responses to hypoxaemia and acidosis in fetal lambs. *American Journal of Obstetrics and Gynecology,* **120,** 817–24.
de Wolf, F., de Wolf-Peeters, C., and Brosens, I. (1973). Ultrastructure of the spiral arteries in the human placental bed at the end of normal pregnancy. *American Journal of Obstetrics and Gynecology,* **117,** 833–48.
de Wolf, F., Robertson, W. B., and Brosens, I. (1975). The ultrastructure of acute atherosis in hypertensive pregnancy. *American Journal of Obstetrics and Gynecology,* **123,** 164–74.
Giles, W. B. and Trudinger, B. J. (1986). Umbilical cord whole blood viscosity and the umbilical artery flow velocity waveform: a correlation. *British Journal of Obstetrics and Gynaecology,* **93,** 466–70.
Giles, W. B., Trudinger, B. J., and Baird, P. J. (1985). Fetal umbilical artery flow velocity waveforms and placental resistance: a pathological correlation. *British Journal of Obstetrics and Gynecology,* **92,** 31–8.
Giles, W. B., Trudinger, B. J., Stevens, D., Alexander, G., and Bradley, L. (1989). Umbilical artery flow velocity waveforms in normal ovine pregnancy and after carunculectomy. *Journal of Developmental Physiology,* **11,** 135–8.
Gruenwald, P. (1972). Expansion of the placental site and maternal blood supply in the primate placenta. *Anatomy Records,* **173,** 189–204.
Hamilton, W. J. and Boyd, J. D. (1966). Trophoblast in human uteroplacental arteries. *Nature,* **212,** 906–8.
Harris, J. W. S. and Ramsey, E. H. (1966). The morphology of the human uteroplacental vasculature. *Contributions to Embryology,* **38,** 43–58.
Khong, Y. T. and Pearce, J. M. F. (1987). Development and investigation of the placenta and its blood supply. In *The human placenta* (ed. J. P. Lavery), pp. 25–46. Aspen, Rockville, Maryland.
McCowan, L. M., Mullen, B. M., and Ritchie, J. W. K. (1989). Umbilical artery flow velocity waveforms and the placental vascular bed. *American Journal of Obstetrics and Gynecology,* **157,** 900–2.

McParland, P. and Pearce, J. M. F. (1991). Prostaglandins, aspirin and pre-eclampsia. In *Progress in obstetrics and gynaecology* (ed. J. W. W. Studd), Vol. 9, pp. 55–82. Churchill Livingstone, Edinburgh.

Makanson, D. O., and Oh, W. (1980). Hyperviscosity in the small for gestational age infants. *Biology of the Neonate*, **37**, 109–12.

Martin C. B. (1968). The anatomy and circulation of the placenta. In Barns, A. C. (ed. *Intrauterine development* A. C. Barns) pp. 35–67. Lea and Febiger, Philadelphia.

Morrow, R. J., Adamson, S. L., Bull, S. B., and Ritchie, J. W. K. (1989). The effect of placental embolization on the umbilical artery waveform in sheep. *American Journal of Obstetrics and Gynecology*, **161**, 1055–60.

Morrow, R. J., Adamson, S. L., Bull, S. B., and Ritchie, J. W. K. (1990*a*). Acute hypoxaemia does not affect umbilical artery waveforms in sheep. *Obstetrics and Gynecology*, **75**, 590–3.

Morrow, R. J., Adamson, S. L., Bull, S. B., and Ritchie, J. W. K. (1990*b*). Hypoxic acidaemia, hyperviscosity and maternal hypertension do not affect the umbilical artery velocity waveform in fetal sheep. *American Journal of Obstetrics and Gynecology*, **163**, 1313–20.

Nicolaides, K. M., Billardo, C. M., Soothill, P. W., and Campbell, S. (1987). Absence of end-diastolic frequencies in the umbilical artery: a sign of fetal hypoxia and acidosis. *British Medical Journal*, **297**, 1026–7.

Ramsey, E. M. and Donner, M. W. (1980). *Placental vasculature and circulation.* Saunders, Philadelphia.

Rankin, J. H. G. and McLaughlin, M. K. (1979). The regulation of placental blood flow. *Journal of Developmental Physiology*, **1**, 3–30.

Robertson, W. B., Brosens, I., and Dixon, H. G. (1967). The pathological response of the vessels of the placental bed to hypertensive pregnancy. *Journal of Pathology and Bacteriology*, **93**, 581–92.

Robertson, W. B., Brosens, I., and Dixon, H. G. (1975). Uteroplacental vascular pathology. *European Journal of Obstetrics, Gynecology, and Reproductive Biology*, **5**, 47–65.

Robertson, W. B., Brosens, I., and Dixon, H. G. (1981). Maternal blood supply in fetal growth retardation. In *Fetal growth retardation* (ed. F. A. van Assche and W. B. Robertson), pp. 126–38. Churchill Livingstone, Edinburgh.

Sheppard, B. L. and Bonnard, J. (1976). The ultrastructure of the arterial supply of the human placenta in pregnancy complicated by fetal growth retardation. *British Journal of Obstetrics and Gynecology*, **83**, 948–59.

Skidmore, R., Woodcock, J. P., and Wells, P. N. T. (1980). Physiological interpretation of Doppler shift waveforms. III. *Ultrasound in Medicine and Biology*, **6**, 227–31.

Slater, D., Pearce, J. M. F., Wilson, K., Hole, D., and Chamberlain, G. V. P. (1992). Vasoactive substance in pregnancy: a study based on a Doppler waveform classification of hypertension (in press).

Steel, S. A., Pearce, J. M. F., Nash, G., Christopher, B., Dromandy, J., and Bland, J. M. (1989). Correlation between Doppler flow velocity waveforms and cord blood viscosity. *British Journal of Obstetrics and Gynecology*, **96**, 1168–72.

III Pulsed wave and colour flow Doppler ultrasound

12. Pulsed Doppler examination of the normal human fetus

Sanjay Vyas

INTRODUCTION

Duplex systems are an improvement on simple, continuous wave Doppler systems in that they provide concurrent imaging so that the angle of vessel insonation can be determined, thus allowing velocity calculations to be made (see Chapter 1). Despite this ability, many authors have continued to use the indices that are derived from the maximum frequency outline, especially the pulsatility index (PI). The introduction of colour flow Doppler ultrasound has allowed the easier recognition of vessels that may be below the resolution of real-time ultrasound.

DESCENDING THORACIC AORTA

This is a relatively straight blood vessel which, owing to its size, is easily accessible for duplex studies.

Method

A longitudinal view of the fetal aorta with a good length of thoracic aorta is visualized (Fig. 12.1). The range gate is then placed cephalad to the diaphragm, avoiding obstruction by the fetal limbs or spine and also interference from fetal heart pulsations (Griffin *et al.* 1984). Figure 12.2 illustrates a flow velocity waveform (FVW) from a normal fetus. Signals for analysis should be acquired in the absence of gross body movements, because these make accurate placement of the range gate difficult, and during fetal apnoea. Fetal breathing movements have a marked effect of the waveform (Marsal *et al.* 1984, 1987).

The range gate is adjusted so that it is just slightly bigger than the vessel, thus ensuring that all Doppler frequencies are recorded. This is essential for mean velocity and volume flow calculations, but for derivation of the PI a small range gate placed in the centre of the vessel has been used by some authors. The angle of insonation should ideally be kept below 45° to optimize the height of the returning signal, thus avoiding artefactual loss of

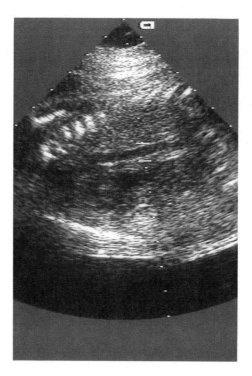

Fig. 12.1 Longitudinal view of the fetus demonstrating the thoracic aorta with the line of the Doppler beam (dotted line) and the range gate (horizontal lines) superimposed on the real-time image.

end-diastolic frequencies and subsequent errors in velocity calculations (Griffin *et al*. 1983).

Factors affecting the aortic FVW

There have been no studies on the effect of fetal heart rate on velocity calculations or on the fetal descending aorta *per se*. Extrapolating from the studies on the umbilical artery (see Chapter 3), it seems unlikely that the variations in fetal heart rate observed in clinical practice will affect the PI or the velocity calculations.

Fetal behavioural states are detailed in Chapter 3. Van Eyck *et al*. (1985) demonstrated higher end-diastolic frequencies in the descending aorta with a lower PI in fetuses in the active state, 2F, compared with the quiescent state, 1F. The reduction in the PI was felt by the authors to be due to increased perfusion of the fetal limbs to meet the oxygen demands of exercising muscles. In practice, it is difficult to control for behavioural states when recording waveforms from the descending aorta. As growth-

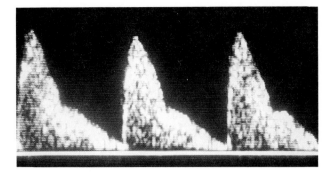

Fig. 12.2 Descending thoracic aorta flow velocity waveform from a normal fetus at 26 weeks' gestation.

retarded fetuses show no differences in waveforms between states 1F and 2F it is unlikely that behavioural states will affect clinical interpretation of waveforms as long as gross body movements are avoided.

Data references ranges

Bilardo *et al.* (1988) examined 70 fetuses at 17–42 weeks' gestation and reported their data reference range for aortic PI and mean blood velocity. There was forward movement throughout the cardiac cycle and the PI remained constant with increasing gestation. Figure 12.3 demonstrates an increase in mean velocity up to 32 weeks' gestation; thereafter it remains constant until term, when there is a small decrease. Similar results have been reported by Lingman and Marsal (1986) and Griffin *et al.* (1984). Pearce *et al.* (1988), however, reported a slight but significant rise in the PI from the fetal aorta in their longitudinal study of 40 normal pregnancies.

There is a marked fall in impedance to flow in the umbilical circulation with increasing gestation (see Chapter 3). Both Bilardo *et al.* (1988) and Pearce *et al.* (1988) argued that in order for there to be no or minimal change in the PI from the descending aorta with increasing gestation, there must be an increase in the impedance to flow in the other branches of the aorta, particularly the renal and mesenteric arteries.

Griffin *et al.* (1983) measured the time-averaged mean velocity in 75 normal fetuses from 28–40 weeks' gestation and found that the increase in mean velocity occurred concurrently with an increase in aortic diameter; thus, aortic flow also increased with gestation. Although the methodological errors in measurement of the aortic diameter (see Chapter 2) preclude comment on normal physiological values, these findings suggest that cardiac output increases with gestation to fulfil the needs of the growing fetus (see also Chapter 15). When aortic volume flow was corrected for estimated fetal weight, the values remained constant from 28 to 38 weeks'

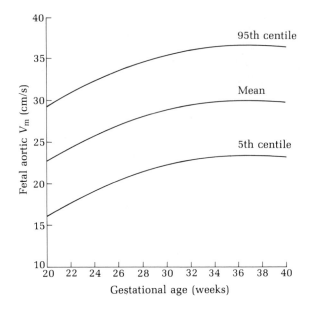

Fig. 12.3 Data reference range of intensity-weighted, time-averaged mean aortic velocity (V_m) with gestation.

gestation (246 ml/kg/min) and fell slightly thereafter. These findings imply that the fetal demand for oxygenated blood is relatively constant in the third trimester, although the fall at term is inexplicable.

FETAL CEREBRAL CIRCULATION

Studies on the fetal circulation have included examinations of the common carotid artery, the intracranial portion of the internal carotid artery, and branches of the circle of Willis, notably the middle cerebral artery.

Method

Flow velocity waveforms from the common carotid artery are usually easy to obtain because this is a relatively straight vessel, so the range gate can be placed on its proximal portion before it branches into the internal and external carotid arteries (Fig. 12.4). Waveforms from the internal carotid artery are more difficult to obtain. The fetal head must be in a occipito-transverse position so that the section on which the biparietal diameter is measured can be obtained. The transducer is then moved towards the base of the skull until the cerebral peduncles are visible. The pulsations of the

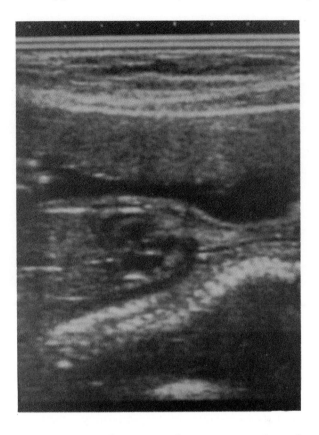

Fig. 12.4 The common carotid artery can be seen arising from the arch of the aorta and in its passage through the neck.

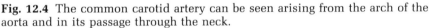

internal carotid artery are then seen just anterior to the peduncles (Wladimiroff *et al.* 1986).

Pulsations running laterally from the internal carotid artery are thought to represent the middle cerebral artery (Fig. 12.5), while the posterior cerebral artery may be seen pulsating lateral to the cerebral peduncles. The anterior cerebral artery is usually visualized just anterior to the peduncles (Fig. 12.5). Van der Wijngaard *et al.* (1989*a*) reported successful examinations of these vessels in third trimester fetuses as follows: internal carotid artery, 89 per cent; middle cerebral artery, 91 per cent; posterior cerebral artery, 58 per cent; and anterior cerebral artery, 64 per cent. End-diastolic frequencies were present in all vessels examined, indicating flow to a low-impedance circulation.

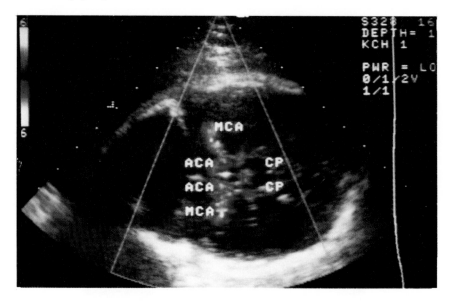

Fig. 12.5 Transverse section of the fetal brain demonstrating the anterior communicating artery (ACA) and the middle cerebral artery (MCA) by colour flow imaging. The cerebral peduncles (CP) are clearly seen.

Problems

Fetal head compression   Vyas *et al.* (1990*a*) demonstrated that application of pressure on the ultrasound transducer during the Doppler examination may result in an increase in impedance to flow in the cerebral circulation. Thus, the PI from the internal carotid and middle cerebral arteries was observed to fall and there was also a decrease in the mean velocity measurements from the middle cerebral artery. These changes were independent of changes in fetal heart rate and were directly proportional to the pressure applied. Similar changes were not observed in the descending fetal aorta (Fig. 12.6 and Table 12.1).

The fetal brain is readily compressible but is contained within a confined space. External pressure may, therefore, be expected to result in an increase in intracranial pressure and a rise in impedance to flow within the cerebral circulation. Since most of the pressures recorded by Vyas *et al.* (1990*a*) were observed during normal imaging of the fetal head, it is impossible to say over what pressure range such an effect is absent.

Increased intracranial pressure may also be the underlying cause of the reported alterations seen in Doppler waveforms from the intracranial vessels in some fetuses with hydrocephaly (Kirkinen *et al.* 1987). In

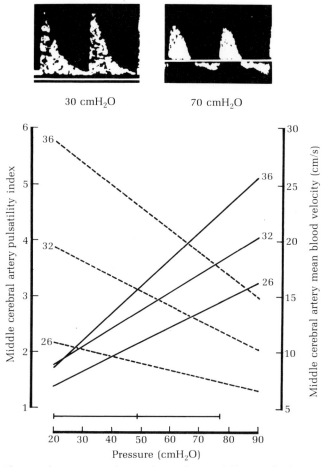

Fig. 12.6 Flow velocity waveforms from the middle cerebral artery during minimal head compression (left), demonstrating the presence of end-diastolic frequencies. As more pressure is applied there is reversal of end-diastolic frequencies (right). The regression lines demonstrate the increase in pulsatility index (———) together with a decrease in mean velocity (– – – – –) with increasing degrees of pressure at 26, 32, and 36 weeks' gestation. The horizontal bar represents the mean (± 2SD) pressure exerted during a routine measurement of the fetal biparietal diameter. (From Vyas *et al.* (1990*a*), with permission.)

contrast, fetal thoracic compression is not associated with alteration in waveforms from the descending thoracic aorta, presumably because the intrathoracic pressure is not raised. With advancing gestation, transducer pressure has less effect on the waveforms from intracranial vessels, possibly owing to increased rigidity of the fetal brain and skull; but as the fetal

Table 12.1 Correlation coefficients of the relationships of pressure applied to the maternal abdomen (cmH$_2$O) and fetal heart rate (beats/min), pulsatility index, and mean blood velocity (cm/s) in the respective vessels examined

Gestational age (weeks)	Vessel	Pressure Mean	Pressure SD	Correlation with pressure (r) FHR	Correlation with pressure (r) PI	Correlation with pressure (r) V_m
26	MCA	52.05	19.43	−0.148	0.640**	−0.480*
26	ICA	50.83	18.19	0.078	0.740**	—
26	AOR	44.78	13.57	−0.157	0.455	—
32	MCA	61.19	19.07	−0.150	0.650**	−0.524*
32	ICA	55.93	18.94	−0.304	0.750**	—
32	AOR	48.97	16.57	−0.053	−0.113	—
36	MCA	58.13	20.61	−0.236	0.620*	−0.755**
36	ICA	60.67	17.47	−0.282	0.381	—
36	AOR	47.37	14.41	0.091	0.008	—

MCA, middle cerebral artery; ICA, internal carotid artery; AOR, descending thoracic aorta; FHR, fetal heart rate (beats/min); PI, pulsatility index; V_m, mean blood velocity (cm/s); * $p < 0.05$; ** $p < 0.01$.

skull diameter increases, there is also an increase in the distance of the intracranial vessels from the origin of the pressure.

During Doppler examination of the intracranial vessels, care should be taken to minimize compression of the fetal skull. Indeed, it has been suggested that compression of the fetal head may cause the high impedance to flow that is observed in the internal carotid artery of fetuses with renal agenesis and anhydramnios (van der Wijngaard *et al.* 1989*b*).

Fetal head position   Intracranial flow cannot be investigated with the fetal head in the occipito-posterior or anterior position, or once the fetal head has engaged. In these circumstances it is often possible to continue to record waveforms from the common carotid artery.

Fetal behavioural state   Van Eyck *et al.* (1987) demonstrated a reduction in the PI from the internal carotid artery in state 2F as opposed to 1F, again suggesting that Doppler waveforms from the fetal circulation should not be recorded at times of gross body movements. The change in PI is independent of the fetal heart rate and is believed to indicate increased fetal cerebral perfusion in state 2F.

Data reference ranges

Bilardo *et al.* (1988) examined common carotid artery blood flow in the 70 fetuses described above. End-diastolic frequencies are commonly absent until 32 weeks' gestation, but progressively increase thereafter (Fig. 12.7). Mean velocity in the common carotid artery increases linearly with advancing gestation (Fig. 12.8), whereas the PI remains constant until 32 weeks' gestation and then falls steeply thereafter (Fig. 12.9).

(a)   (b)

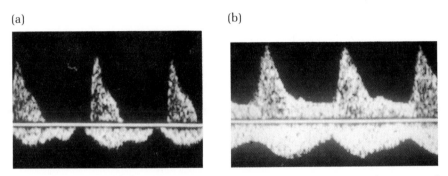

Fig. 12.7 Flow velocity waveforms from the fetal common carotid artery and internal jugular vein. (a) was recorded at 26 weeks' gestation, while (b) was at 34 weeks' gestation and shows recordable end-diastolic frequencies.

Bilardo *et al.* (1988) expressed both the PI and the mean velocity from the common carotid artery as a ratio of the aortic PI and mean velocity. There was a linear increase in the common carotid/aortic mean velocity ratio with increasing gestation, whilst the common carotid/aortic PI ratio remained constant until 32 weeks' gestation, whereafter it fell steeply. Thus, both curves are principally influenced by the changes in the common carotid artery that occur with advancing gestation (Figs 12.8 and 12.9). The authors postulate that a progressively increasing fraction of cardiac output is directed to the fetal brain and further suggest that this redistribution is in response to the fall that is known to occur in umbilical venous P_{O_2} with advancing gestation (Soothill *et al.* 1986; Nicolaides *et al.* 1989).

Van der Wijngaard *et al.* (1989*a*) used duplex Doppler ultrasound to examine the intracranial circulation of 55 normal pregnancies at 25–41 weeks' gestation and reported that end-diastolic frequencies were present in all vessels examined. Kirkinen *et al.* (1987) reported on 83 normal

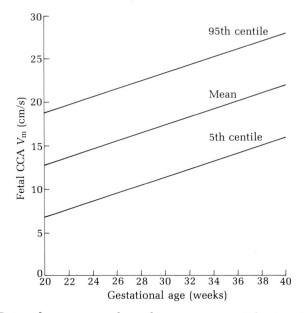

Fig. 12.8 Data reference range from the common carotid artery for intensity-weighted, time-averaged mean blood velocity (CCA V_m) with gestation.

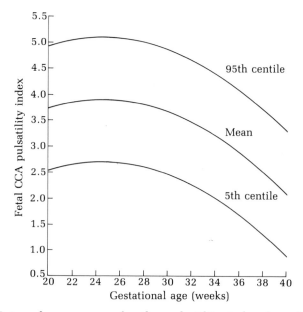

Fig. 12.9 Data reference range for the pulsatility index from the common carotid artery (CCA) with gestation.

pregnancies at 25–42 weeks' gestation. Although they were unsure of the exact origin of the signals, they argued that they most probably arose from the intracranial portion of the internal carotid artery, the middle cerebral artery, or a mixture of both. They noted forward flow in all waveforms recorded. Woo *et al.* (1987) used the same methodology in a longitudinal study of 15 normal pregnancies and reported that absence of end-diastolic frequencies was observed at 24–26 weeks' gestation, but did not state in how many of the fetuses.

The discrepancy in the above studies are not due to differing high-pass filters (all used 100 Hz) but may be due to recordings from different intracranial vessels. The introduction of colour flow imaging has largely overcome this problem. As colour flow mapping recognizes red-cell movement rather than relying upon real-time imaging of the vessel walls, FVWs can be obtained from small vessels that are below the resolution of real-time images. Figure 12.5 illustrates colour flow imaging of part of the circle of Willis.

Vyas *et al.* (1990*b*) used colour flow imaging to identify the middle cerebral artery for subsequent pulse Doppler examination and obtained satisfactory waveforms in 90 per cent (154/172) of cases. Failure to obtain waveforms was due to deep engagement of the fetal head or persistent occipito-posterior or anterior position rather than to ambiguity over the intracranial anatomy. Intra-observer variation was not significant (5.3 per cent). End-diastolic frequencies were recorded above the 125Hz vessel wall filter in about 75 per cent of fetuses at 18–33 weeks' gestation and in all 66 fetuses after 34 weeks' gestation (Fig. 12.10). Figure 12.11 illustrates the change in the PI from the middle cerebral artery with increasing gestation.

Vyas *et al.* (1990*b*) also measured the intensity-weighted, mean velocity in 106 of 154 fetuses. The data were not normally distributed so the data reference range illustrated in Fig. 12.12 was derived after a logarithmic transformation.

There is a similarity in the pattern of reduction of impedance to flow in the cerebral vasculature which mirrors the changes observed in the common carotid artery with increasing gestation. This suggests that the fall in the PI observed in the common carotid artery is predominantly due to a reduction in impedance to flow in the cerebral vasculature. Furthermore, the inverse relationship found between middle cerebral artery blood flow and PI (Fig. 12.13) suggests that the increase in flow in the middle cerebral artery is significantly associated with a decrease in impedance to flow with increasing gestation. Mean blood flow in intracranial vasculature has not been previously reported because of the difficulties in imaging the vessel with B-mode ultrasound, and therefore an inability to measure the angle of insonation accurately.

(a)   (b)

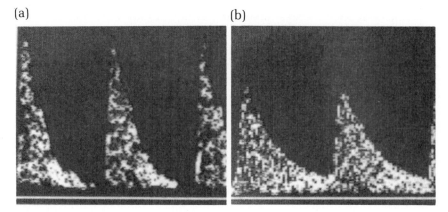

Fig. 12.10 Flow velocity waveforms from the middle cerebral artery at 24 weeks' (a) and 38 weeks' gestation (b).

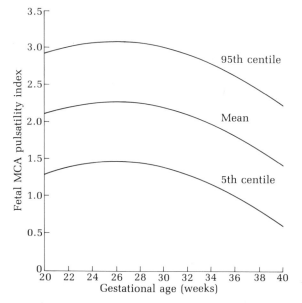

Fig. 12.11 Data reference range for the pulsatility index from the middle cerebral artery (MCA) with gestation.

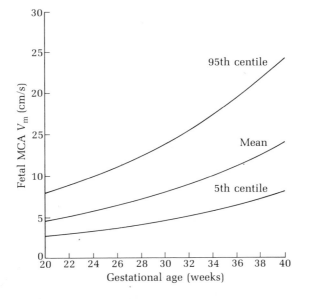

Fig. 12.12 Data reference range for intensity-weighted, mean velocity from the middle cerebral artery (MCA V_m) with gestation.

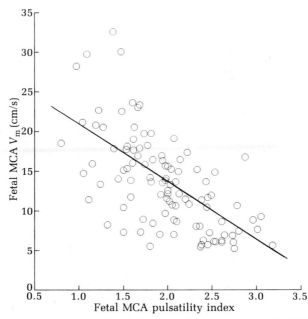

Fig. 12.13 Relationship between the middle cerebral artery (MCA) flow and pulsatility index in appropriate-for-gestational age fetuses.

THE FETAL RENAL ARTERY

Animal studies have demonstrated that in fetal hypoxia there is a redistribution of blood flow favouring the fetal brain, heart, and adrenal glands at the expense of the viscera (Cohn *et al.* 1974; Peeters *et al.* 1979). Colour flow imaging has now allowed studies on the fetal visceral circulation, and the first to be reported was the fetal renal artery (Vyas *et al.* 1989).

Method

A longitudinal view of the fetal kidneys and aorta is obtained by real-time ultrasonography. The colour flow imaging is then switched on and the renal artery is imaged running directly towards the transducer from its origin on the aorta towards the hilus of the kidney (Fig. 12.14). In this orientation the beam to vessel angle for the renal artery is close to $0°$ while that from the aorta is almost $90°$. This ensures that the signal from the renal artery is maximal whilst little or no Doppler-shifted signal is obtained from the aorta (cosine $90° = 0$). The pulsed Doppler range gate is then placed over the renal artery, rather than one of its branches. In practice, the length of blood vessel visualized is insufficient for accurate measurement of the angle of insonation, so the PI is reported.

To date, satisfactory recordings have been obtained from 91 per cent

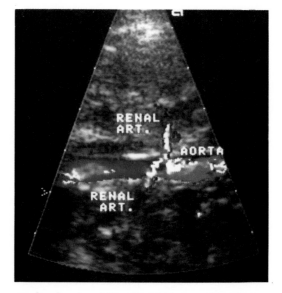

Fig. 12.14 Longitudinal axis of the fetal kidney with renal arteries and aorta demonstrated by colour flow imaging.

(a) (b)

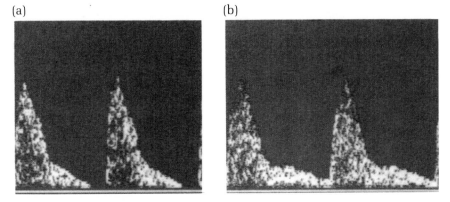

Fig. 12.15 Flow velocity waveforms from the renal artery at 26 weeks' (a) and 38 weeks' gestation (b).

(192/212) cases. The waveforms became more pulsatile and end-diastolic frequencies were more common with increasing gestation. Thus, end-diastolic frequencies were recorded in 19/113 (22 per cent) cases at 18–34 weeks' gestation but in 90 per cent of cases at 35–43 weeks' gestation (Fig. 12.15). This is also reflected in the PI, which fell steeply from 32 weeks' gestation (Fig. 12.16).

During renal angiogenesis there is lengthening of the developing nephrons and branching of the arterioles. This process begins in the early second trimester and is completed by the late third trimester (Hudlicka and Tyler 1986). Thus, the observed reduction in impedance to flow with increasing gestation is likely to be the result of a maturation process representing an increase in the total arteriolar cross-sectional area.

If it is assumed that fetal blood pressure remains constant with increasing gestation, then renal perfusion must increase. This may offer an explanation for the increase in fetal urine production rates that are observed with increasing gestation (Rabinowitz *et al.* 1989). This is in agreement with studies on chronically catheterized fetal lambs where the total renal blood flow and filtration rate are significantly higher near term than in the early third trimester (Robillard *et al.* 1981).

Pearce *et al.* (1988) reported a slight but significant increase in the PI for the descending fetal aorta, whilst Bilardo *et al.* (1988) demonstrated that it remains constant. Since approximately 40 per cent of the cardiac output is distributed to the umbilical circulation (Rudolph and Heymann 1967), where the impedance to flow falls with gestation (see Chapter 4), Pearce *et al.* (1988) suggested that impedance to flow in the other major branches of the aorta must increase in order to produce a minimal net effect on the impedance to flow in the aorta. Studies on the renal artery do not support

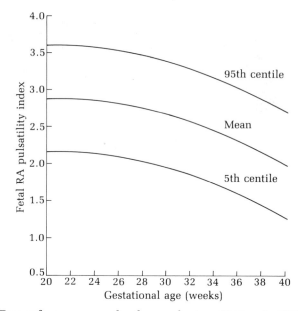

Fig. 12.16 Data reference range for the renal artery (RA) pulsatility index with gestation.

this view, but because the renal arteries receive only about 3 per cent of the cardiac output (Rudolph and Heymann 1967) changes in impedance to flow in the renal circulation may have little net effect on the impedance to flow in the aorta.

Bilardo *et al.* (1988) and van den Wijngaard *et al.* (1989*a*) suggested that the decrease in impedance to flow in the cerebral circulation during normal pregnancy represents a physiological increase in cerebral perfusion in response to falling P_{O_2} levels (Soothill *et al.* 1986; Nicolaides *et al.* 1989). If this were the case then, from studies on hypoxic sheep (Cohn *et al.* 1974; Peeters *et al.* 1979), one would expect that the PI of the renal arteries would increase with advancing gestation. However, this is not the case, and the steepest fall in the PI from both the renal and the cerebral circulations occurs at the time of maximum arteriolar proliferation (Hudlicka and Tyler 1986). This suggests that the reduction in impedance to flow in both these circulations is unrelated to alterations in blood gases.

REFERENCES

Bilardo, C. M., Campbell, S., and Nicolaides, K. H. (1988). Mean blood velocity and flow impedance in the fetal descending thoracic aorta and common carotid artery in normal pregnancy. *Early Human Development,* **18,** 213–17.

Cohn, H. E., Sacks, E. J., Heyman, M. A., and Rudolph, A. M. (1974). Cardiovascular responses to hypoxaemia and acidaemia in fetal lambs. *American Journal of Obstetrics and Gynecology,* **120,** 817–24.

Griffin, D. R., Cohen-Overbeek, T., and Campbell, S. (1983). Fetal and uteroplacental blood flow. *Clinics in Obstetrics and Gynaecology,* **10,** 565–72.

Griffin, D. R., Bilardo, K., Diaz-Recasens, J., Pearce, J. M., Wilson, K., and Campbell, S. (1984). Doppler blood flow waveforms in the descending thoracic aorta of the human fetus. *British Journal of Obstetrics and Gynaecology,* **91,** 997–1002.

Hudlicka, O. and Tyler, K. R. (1986). *Angiogenesis.* Academic Press, London.

Kirkinen, P., Muller, R., Huch, R., and Huch, A. (1987). Blood flow velocity waveforms in human fetal intra-cranial arteries. *Obstetrics and Gynecology,* **70,** 617–21.

Lingman, G. and Marsal, K. (1986). Fetal central blood circulation in the third trimester of pregnancy. I. Aortic and umbilical blood flow. *Early Human Development,* **13,** 137–42.

Marsal, K., Lindblad, A., Lingman, G., and Eik-Nes, S. H. (1984). Blood flow in the descending aorta: intrinsic factors affecting fetal blood flow, i.e. fetal breathing movements and cardiac arrhythmia. *Ultrasound in Medicine and Biology,* **10,** 339–41.

Marsal, K., Laurin, J., Lindblad, A., and Lingman, G. (1987). Blood flow in the descending thoracic aortas. *Seminars in Perinatology,* **11,** 322[N]5.

Nicolaides, K. H., Economides, D. L., and Soothill, P. W. (1989). Blood gases, pH and lactate in appropriate and small for gestational age fetuses. *American Journal of Obstetrics and Gynecology,* **161,** 996–1001.

Pearce, J. M., Campbell, S., Cohen-Overbeek, T., Hackett, G., Hernandez, J., and Royston, P. (1988). Reference ranges and sources of variation for indices of pulsed Doppler flow velocity waveforms from the uteroplacental and fetal circulation. *British Journal of Obstetrics and Gynaecology,* **95,** 248–52.

Peeters, L. L. H., Sheldon, R. E., Jones, M. D., Makowski, E. L., and Meschia, G. (1979). Blood flow to fetal organs as a function of arterial content. *American Journal of Obstetrics and Gynecology,* **135,** 637–41.

Rabinowitz, R., Peters, M. T., Vyas, S., Campbell, S., and Nicolaides, K. H. (1989). Measurement of fetal urine production in normal pregnancy by real time ultrasonography. *American Journal of Obstetrics and Gynecology,* **161,** 1264–7.

Robillard, J. E., Weitzman, R. E., Burmeister, L., and Smith, F. G. (1981). Developmental aspects of the renal response to hypoxaemia in the fetal lamb. *Circulation Research,* **48,** 128–32.

Rudolph, A. M. and Heymann, M. A. (1967). The circulation of the fetus *in utero.* Methods for studying distribution of blood flow, cardiac output and organ blood flow. *Circulation Research,* **21,** 163–7.

Soothill, P. W., Nicolaides, K. H., Rodeck, C. H., and Campbell, S. (1986). Effect of gestational age on fetal and intervillous blood gas and acid–base values in human pregnancy. *Fetal Therapy,* **1,** 68–75.

van Eyck, J., Wladimirroff, J. W., Noordam, M. J., Tonge, H. M., and Prechtl, H.

F. R. (1985). The blood flow velocity waveform in the fetal descending aorta: its relationship to fetal behavioural states in normal pregnancy at 37–38 weeks. *Early Human Development,* **12,** 137–43.

van Eyck, J., Wladimiroff, J. W., van der Wijngaard, J. A. G., Noordam, M. J., and Prechtl, H. F. R. (1987). The blood flow velocity waveform in the fetal internal carotid and umbilical artery: its relationship to fetal behavioural states in normal pregnancy at 37–38 weeks. *British Journal of Obstetrics and Gynaecology,* **94,** 736–41.

van der Wijngaard, J. A. G. W., Groenenberg, I. A. L., Wladimiroff, J. W., and Hop, W. C. J. (1989*a*). Cerebral Doppler ultrasound in the human fetus. *British Journal of Obstetrics and Gynaecology,* **96,** 845–9.

van den Wijngaard, J. A. G. W., Wladimiroff, J. W., Reuss, A., and Stewart, P. A. (1989*b*). Oligohydramnios and fetal cerebral blood flow. *British Journal of Obstetrics and Gynaecology,* **95,** 1309–11.

Vyas, S., Nicolaides, S., and Campbell, S. (1989). Renal artery blood flow velocity waveforms in normal and hypoxaemic fetuses. *American Journal of Obstetrics and Gynecology,* **161,** 168–75.

Vyas, S., Campbell, S., Bower, S., and Nicolades, K. H. (1990*a*). Maternal abdominal pressure alters fetal cerebral blood flow. *British Journal of Obstetrics and Gynaecology,* **97,** 740–2.

Vyas, S., Nicolaides, K. H., Bower, S., and Campbell, S. (1990*b*). Middle cerebral artery flow velocity waveforms in fetal hypoxaemia. *British Journal of Obstetrics and Gynaecology,* **97,** 797–82.

Wladimiroff, J. W., Tonge, H. M., and Stewart, P. A. (1986). Doppler ultrasound assessment of cerebral blood flow in the human fetus. *British Journal of Obstetrics and Gynaecology,* **93,** 471–5.

Woo, J. S., Liang, S. T., Lo, R. L. S., and Chan, F. Y. (1987). Middle cerebral artery Doppler flow velocity waveforms. *Obstetrics and Gynecology,* **70,** 613–17.

13. The clinical value of waveforms from the descending aorta

Karel Marsal, Kypros Nicolaides, Petros Kaminpetros, and Gerry Hackett

FETUSES THAT ARE SMALL FOR GESTATIONAL AGE

Introduction

Initial work on the fetal descending aorta used duplex Doppler equipment to estimate volume flow (Eik-Nes *et al.* 1980). In normal fetuses, the weight-related volume flow decreases slightly during the last trimester (Griffin *et al.* 1984; Tonge *et al*; Lingman and Marsal 1986*a*). Differences in volume flow between well-grown fetuses and those that are small for gestational age show a marked overlap (Laurin *et al.* 1987). This is thought to be due to errors inherent in estimating volume flow (see Chapter 1), and so most investigators have abandoned this method in favour of analysis of the maximum blood flow velocity waveform (FVW).

The shape of the maximum FVW recorded from the descending aorta is subject to several factors: cardiac contractility, blood pressure, vessel wall compliance, blood viscosity, and peripheral resistance. The closer to the heart that the recording is made, the greater the effect of the central circulation. Recorded high in the fetal thorax, the descending aortic FVW shows high pulsatility with a low frequency in end-diastole (Fig. 13.1), while recordings made in the abdominal aorta show an increase in these frequencies (Fig. 13.2). Accordingly, in normal fetuses the pulsatility index (PI) will always be lower in the abdominal aorta (Lingman and Marsal 1986*b*) and recording should therefore be standardized; most authors have located the sample volume just above the diaphragm. Comparable measurements are obtained irrespective of whether the aorta is insonated in the upstream or downstream direction.

Waveform classification

In situations of increased peripheral resistance, for example owing to a reduction in the placental vascular bed (see Chapter 11), aortic diastolic flow diminishes and eventually disappears. The absence of end-diastolic frequencies has been associated with impaired fetal health and a poor pregnancy outcome (Jouppila and Kirkinen 1984; Lingman *et al.* 1986).

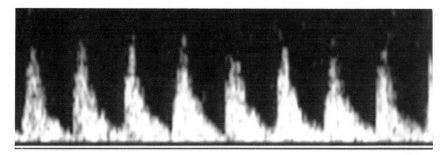

Fig. 13.1 Flow velocity waveform from the fetal descending thoracic aorta.

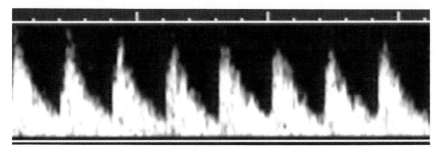

Fig. 13.2 Flow velocity waveform from the fetal abdominal aorta.

Because intra-uterine and neonatal morbidity rates appear to correlate with the pathological changes in the aortic waveform, a semi-quantitative method of assessing the waveform has been evolved, with four blood-flow classes being defined to describe the waveform, with special emphasis on the diastolic part (Fig. 13.3). The blood-flow classes (BFC) are defined as (Laurin *et al.* 1987):

1. *BFC 0 (normal)*: positive flow throughout the cardiac cycle; normal PI.
2. *BFC I*: positive flow throughout the cardiac cycle; PI outside the reference range for normal pregnancies.
3. *BFC II*: undetectable end-diastolic frequencies.
4. *BFC III*: absence of forward frequencies throughout the majority of diastole and/or reversed frequencies.

This approach has been simplified by a simple qualitative evaluation of the presence or absence of end-diastolic frequencies (AEDF) (Hacket *et al.* 1987*b*; Arabin *et al.* 1988; Marsal and Persson 1988).

Problems When evaluating end-diastolic frequencies in the aorta an arte-factual loss may be due to a high angle of insonation or a high value for the high-pass filter, or both. For example, at an angle of 75°, and with a 150Hz

(a)   (b)

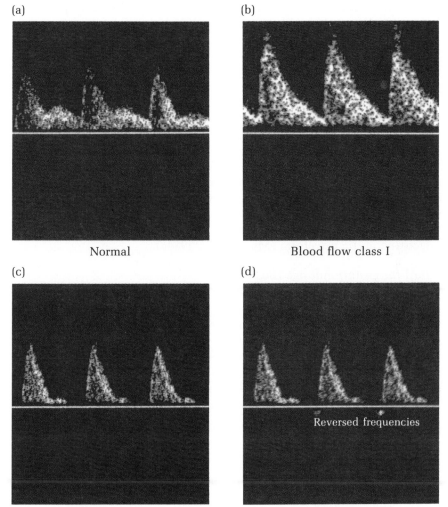

Normal   Blood flow class I

(c)   (d)

Reversed frequencies

Blood flow class II   Blood flow class III

Fig. 13.3 Blood-flow classes (see text for explanation).

high-pass filter, Doppler frequencies of less than 22 cm/s will not be detected. Thus, the recommendation of the European Association of Perinatal Medicine (1989) that the angle of insonation should be less than 55° and that the high-pass filter should be less than 100 Hz are valid not just for estimating mean velocity but also for analysing the maximum frequency outline of the waveform.

In uncomplicated late gestation, the peak velocity in the thoracic descending aorta of the fetus is reported to be 70–116 cm/s, with least diastolic velocities of 17–20 cm/s. The PI in the third trimester is thought by most authors to be stable (see Chapter 12) with values of between 1.83 and 2.49 (Griffin *et al*. 1984; Tonge *et al*. 1984; Jouppila and Kirkinen 1984; Lingman and Marsal 1986*a*, see Chapter 12). The aortic PI is dependent on the fetal heart rate (Lingman and Marsal 1986*b*) within the normal range of heart rate (r = − 0.43), and this negative correlation is even more pronounced in cases of fetal arrhythmia (Lingman and Marsal 1986*c*).

The aortic PI is affected by fetal behavioural states, at least in the last 4 weeks of gestation (van Eyck *et al*. 1985; see Chapter 12). During the active fetal state (2F) the PI was found to be lower than in the quiet state (1F), with higher frequencies being recorded in end-diastole. The authors suggested that this may be due to decreased peripheral resistance in the skeletal muscles due to enhanced perfusion to meet the increased energy needs. Measurements should therefore be made only during quiescent periods, and fetal breathing movements should also be avoided as this affects the aortic waveform (Marsal *et al*. 1984*a*).

Small-for-gestational age (SGA) fetuses
Uteroplacental blood flow is probably the single most effective determinant of fetal growth (Wootton *et al*. 1977). Restricted flow to the placental vascular bed may result in intra-uterine growth retardation with subsequent redistribution of fetal blood flow with preferential blood supply to the brain, myocardium, and adrenals (see Chapter 11). In the human fetus, this brain-sparing effect is reflected in a low PI in the common carotid artery and cerebral circulation (see Chapter 14) and a concomitant rise in the PI in the descending aorta (Marsal *et al*. 1984*a*; Wladimiroff *et al*. 1986; Arabin *et al*. 1987; Kirkinen *et al*. 1987).

Use in management of SGA fetuses   FVWs from the descending aorta of some SGA fetuses show a reduction or absence of end-diastolic frequencies with a subsequent increase in the PI (Griffin *et al*. 1984; Jouppila and Kirkinen 1984), similar to changes seen in the umbilical artery (see Chapter 7). This suggests an increase in peripheral resistance in the vascular bed. The descending aorta supplies the placenta and the lower fetal body, including the kidneys and the legs. As the aortic waveform is subject not only to resistance in the varying parts of the vascular bed but also to heart action, aortic waveforms do not yield the same type of information as umbilical artery waveforms.

Aortic waveforms from SGA fetuses that are developing signs of intra-uterine distress show loss of end-diastolic frequencies (Jouppila and Kirkinen 1984); Lingman *et al*. 1986; Laurin *et al*. 1987; Arabin *et al*. 1988; Illyes and Gati 1988) and fall into blood-flow classes II or III. These changes precede cardiotocographic changes with a median lag time of 3 days

(Laurin *et al.* 1987; Arabin *et al.* 1988), although this may be up to several weeks. A relationship has been found between the degree of fetal hypoxia, hypercapnia, acidosis, and hyperlactaemia, as diagnosed on fetal blood samples from cordocentesis, and both the mean fetal aortic velocity (Soothill *et al.* 1986) and the velocity waveform (Bilardo *et al.* 1988). However, owing to the considerable overlap between growth-retarded fetuses and the control group, it is impossible to predict the fetal metabolic status using the Doppler findings.

Laurin *et al.* (1987) demonstrated that the PI from the fetal aorta predicted 63 per cent of fetuses that developed fetal distress in labour and that this figure could be increased to 87 per cent by use of blood-flow classes (Fig. 13.3). Furthermore, Hackett *et al.* (1987*b*) have demonstrated that AEDF in the aorta predicts significant neonatal morbidity (Fig. 13.4).

Use in screening for SGA fetuses   Several studies have evaluated the ability of aortic waveforms to predict the birth of an SGA infant. Most show poor results and may be exemplified by the prospective study on 159

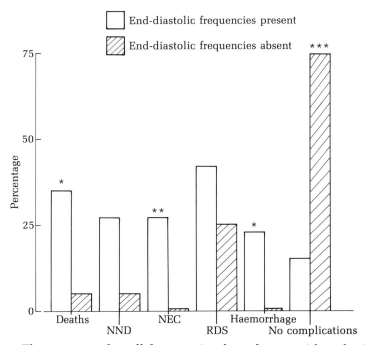

Fig. 13.4 The outcome of small for gestational age fetuses with and without end-diastolic frequencies (from Hackett *et al.* 1987*b*) (deaths = Deaths in the first year of life, NND = neonatal deaths, NEC = necrotizing enterocolitis, RDS = respiratory distress syndrome). (*$p < 0.05$, **$p < 0.01$, ***$p < 0.001$)

clinical small fetuses (Laurin *et al.* 1987). Forty-one per cent of infants with birth-weights of less than the 10th centile for gestational age were predicted by use of the PI from the aortic waveform, and this was increased to 57 per cent if blood-flow classes (see Fig. 13.3) were used.

Conclusion

The accumulated evidence suggests that fetal aortic waveform monitoring is better suited to use as a secondary test in fetuses that have been demonstrated to be small on real-time ultrasound examination (Marsal and Persson 1988), similar to the current usage of umbilical artery waveforms (see Chapter 7). Gudmundsson and Marsal (1991) have performed a direct comparison of umbilical artery and aortic waveforms in the prediction of fetal outcome in fetuses known to be small on real-time ultrasonography. The umbilical artery waveforms performed slightly better.

Waveforms from the descending fetal aorta therefore currently seem to have a place only in the monitoring of the fetus that is small and demonstrates centralization of blood flow (see Chapter 14).

RED-CELL ISO-IMMUNIZATION

This section reviews the application of Doppler ultrasonography in the study of red-cell iso-immunized pregnancies and considers its role in defining pregnancies at risk of fetal anaemia. Data from a series of 95 consecutive affected pregnancies that were examined at King's College Hospital, London, using colour flow mapping and pulsed Doppler velocimetry are also presented.

Pathophysiology of fetal haemolytic disease

In red-cell iso-immunized pregnancies, the life-span of fetal erythrocytes is reduced because antibody-coated red cells are destroyed in the fetal reticulo-endothelial system (Nicolaides *et al.* 1988*b*). In mild–moderate anaemia there is associated reticulocytosis, suggesting a compensatory increase in intramedullary erythropoiesis (Fig. 13.5) (Nicolaides *et al.* 1988*a*). With severe anaemia there is recruitment of extramedullary erythropoietic sites, resulting in macrocytosis and erythroblastaemia (Fig. 13.6) (Nicolaides *et al.* 1988*a*, 1989*b*).

The fetal blood oxygen content decreases in proportion to the degree of anaemia. Fetal blood P_{O_2}, P_{CO_2}, and pH usually remain within the normal ranges, except in extreme anaemia when hypoxia and acidosis occur (Fig. 13.7). (Nicolaides 1989; Soothill *et al.* 1988*a*). The fetal 2,3- diphosphoglycerate concentration is increased and the consequent decrease in haemoglobin oxygen affinity presumably improves delivery of oxygen to

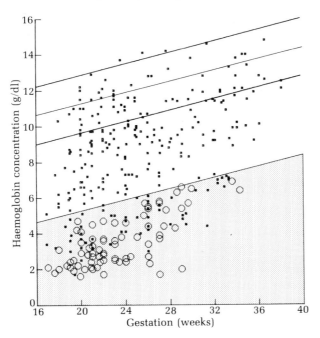

Fig. 13.5 Fetal haemoglobin concentration (■) from 231 red-cell iso-immunized pregnancies at the time of the first fetal blood sampling is plotted on the reference range (mean, 5th, and 95th centiles) for gestation. Hydrops fetalis (○) is associated with severe anaemia (shaded area). In the absence of hydrops, there are no consistent ultrasonographically detectable markers that can reliably distinguish mild from severe haemolytic disease.

the tissues (Soothill *et al.* 1987*b*). In moderate anaemia, the umbilical arterial plasma lactate concentration is increased but this is cleared by a single passage through the placenta, and normal umbilical venous levels are maintained (Soothill *et al.* 1987). In severe anaemia, when the oxygen content is less than 2 mmol/l, the placental capacity for lactate clearance is exceeded and the umbilical venous concentration increases exponentially. These data suggest that in the fetus systemic metabolic acidocis can be prevented, unless the oxygen content decreases below the critical level of 2 mmol/l(Soothill *et al.* 1987).

When the fetal haemoglobin concentration deficit exceeds 6 g/dl, hydrops fetalis develops (Nicolaides *et al.* 1988*b*). This may result from extensive infiltration of the liver by erythropoietic tissue leading to portal hypertension, parenchymal compression of portal vessels, and/or hypoproteinemia due to impaired protein synthesis (Nicolaides *et al.* 1985). Furthermore, at this haemoglobin concentration deficit, the oxygen content decreases below the critical level of 2 mmol/l.

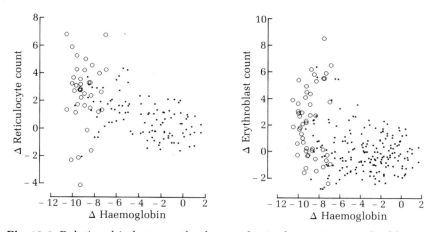

Fig. 13.6 Relationship between the degree of reticulocytosis or erythroblastosis and fetal anaemia in non-hydropic (■) and hydropic (○) fetuses from red-cell iso-immunized pregnancies. In mild–moderate anaemia there is associated reticulocytosis suggesting a compensatory increase in intramedullary erythropoiesis. With severe anaemia there is recruitment of extramedullary erythropoietic sites, resulting in erythroblastaemia. △ values represent the number of standard deviations from the appropriate normal mean for gestation.

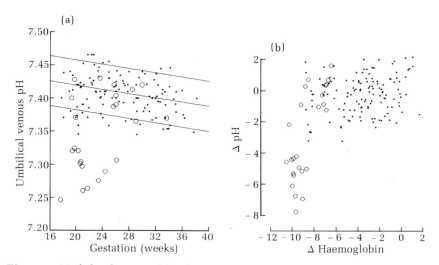

Fig. 13.7 Umbilical venous blood pH from red-cell iso-immunized pregnancies at the time of the first fetal blood sampling are plotted on the reference range (mean, 5th, and 95th centiles) for gestation. (a) Acidaemia develops only in some extremely anaemic, hydropic (○) fetuses. (b) △ values represent the number of standard deviations from the appropriate normal mean for gestation.

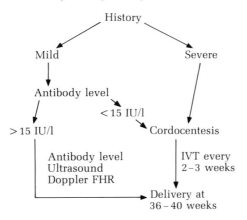

Fig. 13.8 In the management of red-cell iso-immunized pregnancies, patients with a previous severely affected pregnancy should have cordocentesis at approximately 10 weeks before the time of the earliest previous fetal or neo-natal death, fetal transfusion, or birth of a severely affected baby, but not before 16–17 weeks' gestation. In patients with mild or no previous affected pregnancy, cordocentesis should be performed: (i) when the maternal haemolytic antibody level is >15 IU/ml; (ii) if the fetus develops ascites; (iii) if the fetal heart rate (FHR) is sinusoidal or decelerative; or (iv) if Doppler studies demonstrate hyperdynamic fetal circulation. If at cordocentesis the fetus is anaemic, an intravascular fetal blood transfusion (IVT) is given and this is repeated every 2–3 weeks.

Diagnosis and treatment of fetal anaemia

The severity of fetal haemolysis can be predicted from:

(1) the history of previously affected pregnancies;

(2) the level of maternal haemolytic antibodies;

(3) the altered morphometry of fetus and placenta;

(4) the presence of pathological fetal heart rate (FHR) patterns;

(5) changes in the FVWs obtained by Doppler studies of the fetal circulation (Nicolaides 1989).

However, there is a wide scatter of values around the regression lines describing the associations between the degree of fetal anaemia and the data obtained from these indirect methods of assessment.

The only accurate method for determining the severity of the disease is blood sampling by cordocentesis and measurement of the fetal haemo-globin concentration. However, the indication for, and the timing of, fetal blood sampling in the context of this disease have not yet been fully defined. Neverthless, it could be argued that cordocentesis should be performed for all patients with a history of severe disease and those with high haemolytic antibody levels (≥ 15 IU/ml), pathological FHR patterns or abnormal FVWs (Fig. 13.8) (Nicolaides *et al.* 1989*a*, 1990; Vyas *et al.* 1990; Nicolaides and Rodeck 1991).

At cordocentesis a fetal blood sample is first obtained and the haemoglobin concentration is determined. If this is below the normal range, the tip of the needle is kept in the lumen of the umbilical cord vessel and fresh, packed, Rhesus-negative blood compatible with that of the mother is infused manually into the fetal circulation through a 10-ml syringe. At the end of the transfusion, a further fetal blood sample is aspirated for determination of the final haemoglobin concentration (Nicolaides *et al.* 1986*a,b*).

Subsequent transfusions are given at 1–3-weekly intervals until 34–36 weeks (Fig. 13.9) and their timing is based on the findings of non-invasive tests, such as Doppler studies and FHR monitoring, and the knowledge that after a fetal blood transfusion the mean rate of decrease in fetal haemoglobin is approximately 0.3 g/dl per day (Nicolaides *et al.* 1986*b*).

Doppler findings

Uteroplacental circulation   In a longitudinal series of 12 fetuses, Copel *et al.* (1988) included the uterine artery PI, together with the descending

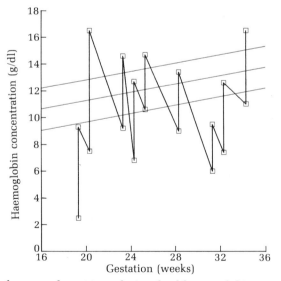

Fig. 13.9 Serial pre- and post-transfusion fetal haemoglobin concentrations in a severe case of red-cell iso-immunization plotted on the reference range (mean, 5th, and 95th centiles) for gestation.

thoracic aortic peak velocity, in a multiple regression model to predict whether the fetal haematocrit was below or above 25 per cent before the second fetal blood transfusion. The authors suggested that the significant contribution of uterine artery PI to the model could be explained by the effect of resolving placental oedema after the correction of fetal anaemia by the second transfusion. However, this is unlikely because there was no difference in uterine PI or resistance index (RI) between hydropic and non-hydropic fetuses.

In a series of 95 red-cell iso-immunized pregnancies treated at King's College Hospital, London, that had not yet received intra-uterine transfusions, the uterine artery RI was within the normal range in all cases (Fig. 13.9) and there was no significant association between uterine RI and the degree of fetal anaemia. Therefore, it is unlikely that fetal anaemia alters the uteroplacental circulation.

Fetoplacental circulation   Rightmire *et al.* (1986) found a significant inverse correlation between umbilical artery RI and fetal haematocrit measured at fetoscopy. It was suggested that increased impedance to flow in the fetoplacental microcirculation may be due to hypoxaemia-mediated capillary endothelial cell damage, or clogging of the placental capillaries by the large fetal erythroblasts.

In contrast, Warren *et al.* (1987) found that the umbilical arterial systolic to diastolic ratio was not abnormal in pregnancies with a high amniotic fluid bilirubin concentration. Similarly the King's College Hospital group measured the umbilical artery PI immediately before 95 cordocenteses for blood transfusion and found no significant association with fetal anaemia (Fig. 13.10).

Fetal cardiac Doppler studies   Meijboom *et al* (1986) measured maximal and mean temporal velocity and early passive to late active ventricular filling phase (E/A) ratio on the atrioventricular orifices in 12 fetuses immediately before fetoscopic blood transfusion. There was a non-significant increase in both maximal and mean temporal velocities. Furthermore, there was a significant reversal in the E/A ratio in the tricuspid valve FVWs. In normal fetuses these two peaks present an 'M' shape, whereas in anaemic fetuses the E peak is dominant, suggesting that in fetal anaemia there is an increased pre-load in the right atrium.

Copel *et al.* (1989) found that before intra-uterine transfusion anaemic fetuses had significantly higher stroke volumes and ventricular outputs than normal controls. The increase was shared proportionately by both ventricles. However, there was no significant relationship between fetal haematocrit and cardiac output. Nevertheless, extremely compromised fetuses demonstrated diminished cardiac function as a terminal finding. In

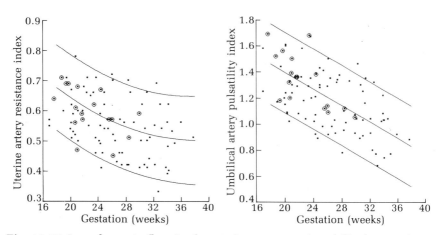

Fig. 13.10 Impedance to flow in the uterine artery and umbilical artery in 95 red-cell iso-immunized pregnancies, including 17 with fetal hydrops (○), plotted on the appropriate reference range (mean, 5th, and 95th centiles) for gestation.

contrast, Barss *et al.* (1987) reported a case of hydrops fetalis where the cardiac output measured before an intravascular transfusion was close to the normal mean for gestation.

Rizzo *et al.* (1990) measured right and left cardiac outputs (by multiplying the tricuspid or mitral mean temporal velocities, valvular area, and heart rate) in 12 anaemic fetuses before blood transfusion by cordocentesis. Both left and right cardiac outputs were significantly higher for gestation than in 187 normal controls. Furthermore the E/A ratios of both atrioventricular valves were higher than normal.

The findings of increased fetal cardiac output in anaemia are in agreement with the results of animal studies and confirm the prediction, from a mathematical model, that in fetal anaemia the cardiac output is increased to maintain an adequate oxygen delivery to the tissues (Huikeshoven *et al.* 1985). Possible mechanisms include decreased blood viscosity leading to increased venous return and cardiac pre-load, and/or peripheral vasodilatation as a result of a fall in blood oxygen content and therefore reduced cardiac after-load. The high E/A ratio is suggestive of increased cardiac pre-load. Because right to left cardiac output ratio is normal, there is no evidence of redistribution in cardiac output similar to that described in hypoxaemic growth-retarded fetuses. These findings suggest that in fetal anaemia the changes in fetal cardiac output are mainly due to low blood viscosity.

Impedance to flow in fetal vessels   Vyas *et al.* (1990) measured the PI in the middle cerebral artery (MCA) of 24 previously untransfused, non-hydropic fetuses from red-cell iso-immunized pregnancies at 18–35 weeks' gestation. Although the mean PI was significantly lower than the mean for gestation, there were no significant associations with either the degree of fetal anaemia or the degree of deficit in oxygen content measured in samples obtained by cordocentesis.

In the King's College Hospital series of 95 previously untransfused fetuses undergoing cordocentesis for Rhesus disease, the MCA PI was not significantly different from normal controls (Fig. 13.11). In this same series of fetuses undergoing cordocentesis for Rhesus disease the aortic PI was not significantly different from that of normal controls (Fig. 13.11). Furthermore, there were no significant associations between PI and either fetal anaemia or deficit in oxygen content.

The findings of MCA and aortic PI indicate that inpedance to flow is not affected by anaemic hypoxia and the alterations of blood constituents, such as hypoproteinaemia, or of red-cell morphology, such as the erythroblastaemia that accompanies severe anaemia.

Blood velocity in fetal vessels Rightmire *et al.* (1986) measured the fetal inferior vena caval time-averaged mean velocity immediately before the first intravascular fetal blood transfusion in 19 Rhesus-affected pregnancies at 18–28 weeks' gestation. Although the velocity was higher than in non-anaemic controls, there was no significant correlation with fetal hematocrit. In the same study, the intrahepatic umbilical venous velocity was not significantly different from that of non-anaemic controls.

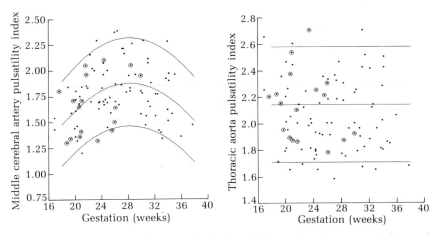

Fig. 13.11 Impedance to flow in the fetal middle cerebral artery and descending thoracic aorta in 95 red-cell iso-immunized pregnancies, including 17 with fetal hydrops (O), plotted on the appropriate reference range (mean, 5th and 95th centiles) for gestation.

In contrast, Kirkinen *et al.* (1983) examined 18 Rhesus iso-immunized pregnancies within the 4 days prior to delivery and reported that in anaemic fetuses the volume flow in the intrahepatic umbilical vein was significantly increased due to both increased blood velocity and vessel diameter. Similarly, Warren *et al.* (1987) performed serial measurements of fetal blood flow in 51 Rhesus iso-immunized pregnancies and reported that increased flow was associated with subsequent develoment of fetal hydrops or rise in amniotic fluid bilirubin concentration. It was postulated that the increased flow was the result of reduced blood viscosity due to the reduced haematocrit.

Rightmire *et al.* (1986), from their study of 21 previously untransfused iso-immunized fetuses, reported an increase in aortic time-averaged, intensity-weighted mean blood velocity (aortic V_m). Furthermore, there was a significant inverse correlation between aortic V_m and the haematocrit of umbilical cord blood samples obtained by fetoscopy. This association was independent of the significant association between aortic V_m and gestational age.

Similarly, from the examination of 68 previously untransfused fetuses at 17–37 weeks' gestation, Nicolaides *et al.* (1990) reported a significant association between aortic V_m measured immediately before cordocentesis and the degree of fetal anaemia. However, separate analysis of non-hydropic ($n = 51$) and hydropic ($n = 17$) fetuses demonstrated that in the former group there was a significant positive correlation between increased aortic V_m and fetal anaemia, whilst in the latter group there was a significant negative correlation between these two parameters.

Copel *et al.* (1988) measured the peak velocity (V_p) in 16 fetuses immediately before cordocentesis and derived a series of formulae for the prediction of whether the fetal haematocrit was above or below 25 per cent. The best prediction was achieved for the untransfused fetuses (haematocrit = $7.78 - (0.088 \times V_p) + (0.968 \times$ no. of weeks' gestation) $- (10.911$ if hydrops is present)). For subsequent transfusions, different formulae had to be used, presumably because of the different rheological properties of adult rather than fetal blood in the fetal circulation.

In the King's College Hospital series of 95 previously untransfused fetuses undergoing cordocentesis for Rhesus disease there was a significant increase in aortic V_m with the degree of fetal anaemia (Figs 13.12 and 13.13). Although in some hydropic fetuses aortic V_m was decreased, in the majority of cases the aortic V_m was elevated. In an additional series of 212 fetuses that had a transfusion 2–3 weeks previously, the relation between aortic V_m and anaemia was weaker (Fig. 13.14).

Bilardo *et al.* (1989) measured the common carotid artery, mean velocity (CCA V_m) in 12 previously untransfused anaemic fetuses immediately before cordocentesis. There was a significant correlation between the

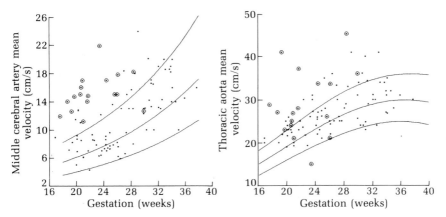

Fig. 13.12 In 95 red-cell iso-immunized pregnancies, including 17 with hydropic fetuses (○), Doppler studies demonstrate increased blood velocity in both the fetal middle cerebral artery and the descending thoracic aorta. Values are plotted on the appropriate reference range (mean, 5th, and 95th centiles) for gestation. If it is assumed that, in anaemia, the cross-sectional area of these vessels does not change, the increased velocity would reflect an increase in blood flow and cardiac output.

degree of fetal anaemia and the increase in CCA V_m. The authors speculated that this increase in CCA V_m reflected increased cardiac output associated with fetal anaemia rather than a chemoreceptor-mediated redistribution in blood flow as seen in hypoxaemic growth-retarded fetuses (Bilardo *et al.* 1990). Vyas *et al.* (1990), in a study of 24 previously untransfused, non-hydropic fetuses from red-cell iso-immunized pregnancies at 18–35 weeks' gestation, reported a significant correlation between the increase in MCA V_m and the degree of fetal anaemia measured in samples obtained by cordocentesis.

In the King's College Hospital series of 95 previously untransfused fetuses undergoing cordocentesis for Rhesus disease, there was a significant association between the increase in MCA V_m with the degree of fetal anaemia (Figs 13.11 and 13.12). In an additional series of 212 fetuses that had had a transfusion 2–3 weeks previously, the relation between MCA V_m and anaemia was weaker (Fig. 13.13).

The findings of increased aortic V_m and MCA V_m with anaemia are compatible with the data from the fetal cardiac Doppler studies. If it is assumed that in anaemia, the cross-sectional area of these fetal vessels does not change, the increased velocity would reflect an increase in both central and peripheral blood flow due to increased cardiac output.

In some hydropic fetuses the aortic V_m decreased with worsening anaemia. Therefore, in severe anaemia there is cardiac decompensation, presumably resulting from the associated hypoxia and lactic acidosis and

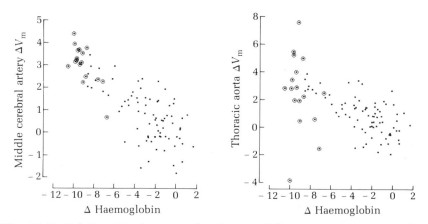

Fig. 13.13 Relationship between the degree of fetal anaemia, measured at cordocentesis, and mean blood velocity in the fetal middle cerebral artery or the descending thoracic aorta in 95 previously untransfused fetuses from red-cell iso-immunized pregnancies. △ values represent the number of standard deviations from the appropriate normal mean for gestation. In some hydropic fetuses ○, aortic velocity is decreased.

from the impaired venous return due to liver infiltration with haemopoietic tissue (Nicolaides *et al.* 1988*a*).

Haemodynamic changes following fetal blood transfusion

Intraperitoneal transfusion   Kirkinen *et al.* (1983) and Warren *et al.* (1987) found a temporary increase in umbilical venous blood flow immediately after a transfusion and subsequent gradual decrease from above to within the normal range. It was suggested that the gradual decrease in flow, coinciding with resolution of fetal ascites, was the result of absorption of the transfused blood and correction of the fetal anaemia.

Intravascular exchange transfusion   Copel *et al.* (1988) measured impedance to flow in the uterine and umbilical arteries and peak velocity in the descending thoracic aorta immediately before and 12 h after fetal blood transfusion by cordocentesis; no differences were found.

Intravascular top-up transfusion   Doppler studies of impedance to flow in the umbilical artery before and soon after intravascular transfusion have provided conflicting results. In a study of 43 cases, Bilardo *et al.* (1989) found no significant changes. In contrast, Weiner and Anderson (1989) and Hanretty *et al.* (1989) reported a significant decrease in impedance immediately after fetal blood transfusion. It was postulated that simple needling of fetal vessels stimulated a humoral vasodilator mechanism. Supportive evidence was provided by the finding that substances with vasodilatory

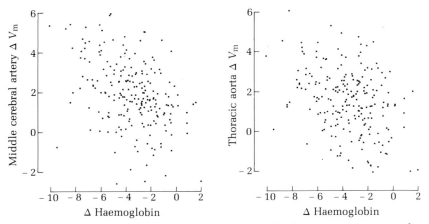

Fig. 13.14 Relationship between the degree of fetal anaemia, measured at corocentesis, and mean blood velocity in the fetal middle cerebral artery or the descending thoracic aorta in 212 fetuses from red-cell iso-immunized pregnancies that had received blood transfusions 2–3 weeks previously. Δ values represent the number of standard deviations from the appropriate normal mean for gestation.

effects, such as prostaglandins and atrial natriuretic peptide, have higher levels in the fetus after an intravascular transfusion (Panos *et al.* 1989; Weiner and Robillard 1989). However, as Welch and Rodeck (1990) pointed out, the possible changes in indices of impedance after an intra-uterine transfusion may not be simply due to vasodilatation but due to the

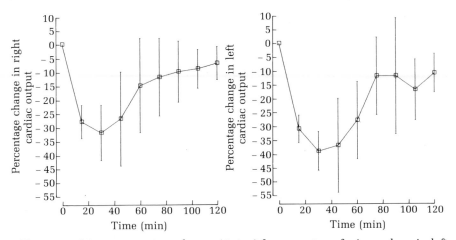

Fig. 13.15 Mean percentage change ($\pm$ 1SD) from pre-transfusion values in left and right fetal cardiac output during the 2 h following an intravascular blood transfusion in 12 red-cell iso-immunized pregnancies.

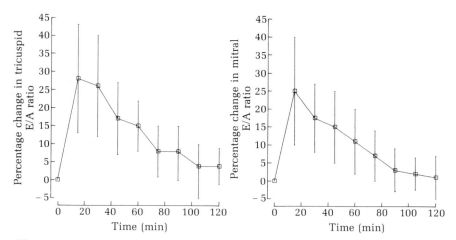

Fig. 13.16 Mean percentage change (± 1SD) from pre-transfusion values in trans-tricuspid and trans-mitral E/A ratios during the 2 h following an intravascular blood transfusion in 12 red-cell iso-immunized pregnancies.

complex influences of altered fetal whole blood viscosity, increased number of scattering particles (red cells), and vaso-active compounds.

Bilardo *et al.* (1989) performed fetal Doppler studies in 43 cases immediately before and within 30 min of an intravascular transfusion. There was a significant decrease in both aortic V_m and CCA V_m. These findings were attributed to decrease in cardiac output following the transfusion due to: (a) increased blood haemoglobin concentration and viscosity, and consequent decrease in venous return; (b) congestive heart failure due to overloading of the fetal circulation; or (c) cardio-inhibition due to increased baroreceptor activity.

Confirmatory evidence of decrease in cardiac output following the transfusion was provided by Rizzo *et al.* (1990). They measured cardiac outputs from the left and right ventricles before and at 15-min intervals for 2 h after an intravascular transfusion in 12 fetuses. After transfusion there was a significant temporary fall in both right and left cardiac outputs. Furthermore, the E/A ratios in both the tricuspid and mitral valves were increased, suggesting that cardiac pre-load was also increased. Within 2 h after transfusion both parameters were returned towards the normal range (Figs 13.15 and 13.16). The fall in cardiac output was significantly related to the amount of expansion of the fetoplacental volume due to the transfusion. The most likely explanation for these findings is that transfusion results in temporary cardiovascular overload. Animal studies have also shown that the fetal heart has very limited reserve capacity to increase its output in response to acute overload and that massive increases in fetal blood volume are associated with a decrease in cardiac output. After transfusion there is a rapid rate of fluid loss and this explains the rapid recovery in E/A ratios and cardiac output (Gillbert 1980).

The short-lived nature of the haemodynamic effects of intravascular transfusion can also explain the findings of Mari *et al.* (1990) who reported that the MCA PI, internal carotid artery PI, and umbilical artery PI before and the day after fetal transfusion were not significantly different. Similarly, Copel *et al.* (1989) in a study of cardiac output at 12 h after intravascular blood transfusion found no significant differences from the pre-transfusion levels.

Conclusion

In red-cell iso-immunized pregnancies, indices of impedance to flow in the uterine, umbilical, and fetal circulations are not altered significantly. In contrast, cardiac output and blood velocity in the fetal circulation are increased in proportion to the degree of fetal anaemia. Intravascular blood transfusion results in temporary cardiovascular overload.

FETAL ABNORMALITIES, OLIGOHYDRAMNIOS, AND POLYHYDRAMNIOS

There is, as yet, little published work describing the changes in fetal Doppler waveforms associated with fetal structural abnormality. This is understandable given that the majority of defects would not be expected to result in a disturbance of the fetal circulation. Currently, real-time imaging of fetal abnormalities is of such exceptional quality that adjunctive methods are rarely required. Exceptions to this are seen in fetuses with cardiac malformation (see Chapter 15), in small-for-gestational age fetuses with an abnormal circulation but a normal uteroplacental circulation (see Chapter 8), and in oligohydramnios when Doppler waveforms may be very informative.

Oligohydramnios

Doppler evaluation of the descending aorta may prove to be of value in severe oligohydramnios when ultrasound imaging of the fetus is impaired because of loss of the acoustic window that amniotic fluid usually provides. Oligohydramnios is best appreciated by an experienced ultrasound practitioner but is commonly reported in terms of the biggest vertical column of amniotic fluid that can be measured, 2–8 cm being considered as representative of normal pregnancy. Ahydramnios is a term reserved for situations in which there are no visible pockets of amniotic fluid.

Oligohydramnios is a particular problem when it occurs in the second trimester. In general, it has an extremely poor outlook (Campbell and Pearce 1983) but it is not universally adverse (Mercer and Brown 1986), so accurate diagnosis is important in order to give a prognosis and to determine management.

In a study of 41 cases, Hackett *et al.* (1987*a*) found Doppler waveforms from the descending fetal aorta and uteroplacental circulation to be of value in determining aetiology. Diagnosis in all cases was confirmed at subsequent post-mortem or delivery. Waveforms from the aorta were classified as abnormal if there were no frequencies recordable in end-diastole whilst waveforms from the uteroplacental circulation were considered abnormal if the RI was greater than 0.58. Four groups of patients could be defined:

1. Group 1 included fetuses with renal agenesis and dysplasia, and such pregnancies had normal waveforms from both the fetal aortic and uteroplacental circulation.

2. Group 2 fetuses had chromosome abnormalities, viral infections, or dysmorphic syndromes; no characteristic pattern was discernable as befits multiple pathologies. However, it is interesting that both fetuses with chromosomal abnormalities had abnormal aortic but normal uteroplacental circulations.

3. Group 3 fetuses were growth retarded but without evidence of structural defect, chromosomal abnormality, or viral infections, and they demonstrated uniformly abnormal waveforms. This suggests that poor uteroplacental perfusion may occasionally compromise the fetal circulation in the second trimester, usually leading to oligohydramnios and fetal death.

4. Group 4 consisted of patients who were eventually demonstrated to have pre-term, premature rupture of the membranes (PPROM). In these cases Doppler studies were normal.

Normal Doppler waveforms in the presence of oligohydramnios therefore suggest a renal defect or PPROM. Early severe intra-uterine growth retardation is usually associated with abnormal waveforms from both the uteroplacental circulation and the aorta. The presence of an abnormal fetal circulation with normal aortic waveforms should raise the possibility of a chromosome abnormality.

In oligohydramnios, the waveform from the fetal aorta is a more reliable guide than the umbilical artery as this may be compressed giving artefactual loss of end-diastolic frequencies. Instillation of saline (often used to improve real-time ultrasonic visualization of fetal organs) may result in the return of end-diastolic frequencies in the umbilical artery.

Finally, the recent introduction of colour flow mapping has aided in the diagnosis renal agenesis. This is often a difficult diagnosis to make using real-time ultrasonography because the absence of amniotic fluid makes inspection of the renal areas difficult (Campbell and Pearce 1983). One renal area tends to lie in the spinal shadow, and echoes from adrenal glands can easily be mistaken for the kidney. However, in renal agenesis the normal colour signal obtained from the renal artery (Figs 12.14 and 13.17) cannot be visualized. Recently, Pearce *et al.* (1991) have reported on 14 cases of second trimester oligohydramnios in which the renal area could not be adequately inspected. In the six cases of complete renal agenesis, no renal artery signal could be obtained (Fig. 13.18), while six out of the eight cases in which the renal artery could be visualized had normal kidneys at post mortem. One of the remaining cases had a unilateral renal signal and so was managed conservatively. An intra-uterine death occurred at 26 weeks' gestation, and postmortem demonstrated a shrunken, single kidney. In the other case postmortem demonstrated renal arteries but bilateral renal agenesis.

Polyhydramnios

There appears to be only one reported study on the value of umbilical artery waveforms in polyhydramnios (Rochelson *et al.* 1990). Of 54 cases studied in the third trimester, 11 (20 per cent) fetuses had abnormal Doppler waveforms from the umbilical artery. Six of these fetuses had abnormal karyotypes and the remaining five were SGA. Macrosomia was observed in 15 fetuses, all of whom had normal umbilical artery waveforms. The authors suggest that the finding of an abnormal waveform in the presence of polyhydramnios should raise the possibility of a chromosomal abnormality and that considerations should be given to karyotyping.

Chromosome abnormality

Tests of fetal well-being are often abnormal in the presence of a lethal abnormality and may therefore lead to inappropriate operative intervention. New techniques of assessing fetal health should therefore also investigate findings in cases of fetal abnormality. In 1985, Trudinger and Cook investigated a group of fetuses with anomalies and reported that all four fetuses with abnormal karyotypes also had abnormal umbilical artery waveforms. Hseith *et al.* (1988) reported on eight fetuses dying in association with congenital abnormalities, all of whom had abnormal umbilical artery waveforms and four of whom also had lethal chromosomal abnormalities.

There is now a wealth of data of umbilical artery waveforms in SGA

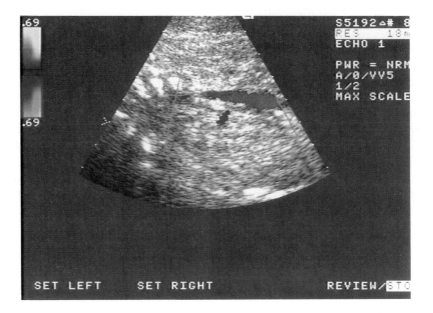

Fig. 13.17 Colour flow Doppler image demonstrating the descending aorta (red) and a renal artery (blue).

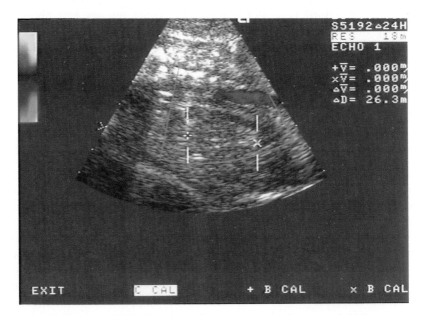

Fig. 13.18 Severe oligohydramnios but an apparently normal kidney on real time scan. There is no renal artery visible and no kidney found at postmortem.

fetuses (see Chapter 7), and up to 16 per cent of such fetuses may have a chromosomal defect (Daffos *et al.* 1985). From these data it is possible to state that fetuses with chromosomal abnormalities are consistently reported as demonstrating abnormal umbilical artery waveforms (McCowan *et al.* 1987; Reed *et al.* 1987; Rochelson *et al.* 1987). Trudinger and Cook (1985) have suggested that these findings are due to a reduced fetal stimulus for development of the placental circulation. It is well known that chromosomal aberrations are associated with abnormal placentae (Battaglia 1978), with the trisomic placenta demonstrating vascular architecture that is immature for the stage of gestation. As the umbilical A/B (S/D) ratio falls with increasing gestation (see Chapter 4), the high-resistance pattern observed in trisomic fetuses may be a reflection of the immature vasculature.

However, caution should be applied when extrapolating the results from selected groups to the general population. Absent end-diastolic frequencies may be associated with diverse maternal and fetal pathology. In a study of 450 high-risk patients, Wenstrom *er al.* (1991) reported 22 (5 per cent) pregnancies to be associated with absent or reversed end-diastolic frequencies. All had detailed real-time ultrasound examination and 18 fetuses are shown in Table 13.1.

Studies on aortic waveforms in chromosomal abnormalities are few, report small numbers of cases, and are conflicting. Hackett *et al.* (1987*a*) reported abnormal aortic waveforms in both cases of chromosomal abnormalities, while Arduini and Rizzo (1988) reported normal waveforms in their two cases. Clearly, no conclusion can be drawn from such small studies.

Structural abnormalities

Doppler waveforms have been reported in cases of fetal abnormality where structural or vascular defects have been suspected. Lindfors *et al.* (1986) reported a series of fetuses with suspected abdominal-wall defects where pulsed Doppler examination allowed differentiation of extruded bowel from umbilical cord. Doppler studies may also be of value in determining the nature of arteriovenous malformations of the cerebral circulation, both in the fetus (Rizzo *et al.* 1987) and the neonate (Vaksmann *et al.* 1989).

Both Trudinger and Cook (1985) and Meizner *et al.* (1987) reported abnormal umbilical artery waveforms in about half of fetuses with structural abnormalities. Table 13.2 summarizes the results of these two studies.

Recently, Burke *et al.* (1990) studied 179 fetuses who were SGA on the basis of real-time ultrasound measurements. Of the group with abnormal umbilical artery Doppler waveforms, 11 per cent had major congenital abnormalities compared with only 4 per cent in fetuses with normal umbilical artery Doppler waveforms.

Table 13.1 Outcome of 22 fetuses with absent end-diastolic frequencies

n	Outcome
3	Trisomy
1	Inversion, holoprosencephaly, renal agenesis, polydactyly
2	Non-immune hydrops fetalis
1	Ventriculomegaly
1	Gastroschisis
1	Body-wall defect with exencephaly
1	Complete heart block
12	Small for gestational age

In normal pregnancy, fetal growth and development is associated with parallel placental growth and a progressive decrease in umbilical placental resistance (see Chapters 4 and 11). Abnormal Doppler waveforms are associated with increased resistance in the tertiary stem arterioles, i.e. the resistance vessels within the umbilical fetal circulation (see Chapter 11). Both Trudinger and Cook (1985) and Meizner *et al.* (1987) found normal uteroplacental waveforms in most patients with fetal abnormalities and an abnormal umbilical artery waveform, suggesting that the increased placental resistance was not secondary to underperfusion of the intervillous space. Trudinger and Cook (1985) also examined the placental weights, expressing them as a ratio of placental to fetal weight. In cases were the placental to fetal weight ratio was low for gestational age, the umbilical artery waveform was normal, whereas an increase in the placental to fetal weight ratio was strongly associated with an abnormal umbilical artery waveform. This suggests that cases of fetal abnormality associated with a normal umbilical artery waveform demonstrate low growth potential, whilst in those associ-

Table 13.2 Umbilical artery waveforms in fetuses with structural abnormalities

System	Normal	Abnormal
Central nervous system	11	7
Gastro-intestinal tract	5	7
Urinary tract	7	5
Musculoskeletal system	2	2
Fetal tumour	0	2
Ascites	0	2
Total	25	25

ated with abnormal umbilical artery waveforms vascular obliteration may be triggered by the abnormal fetus rather than uteroplacental ischaemia. However, even the same abnormality may result in different umbilical artery patterns. For instance, Trudinger and Cook (1985) reported three cases of renal agenesis delivered at approximately 34 weeks' gestation; two had normal umbilical artery waveforms.

Conclusion

Umbilical artery waveforms alone cannot differentiate between intrinsic and extrinsic causes of an SGA fetus (McCowan *et al.* 1987). Nevertheless, the finding of an SGA fetus with normal amniotic fluid and with normal uteroplacental and abnormal umbilical artery Doppler waveforms should initiate a careful search for structural fetal abnormalities and markers suggestive of chromosomal abnormalities.

REFERENCES

Arabin, B., Bergmann, P. L., and Saling, E. (1987). Simultaneous assessment of blood flow velocity waveforms in uteroplacental vessels, the umbilical artery, the fetal aorta and the fetal common carotid artery. *Fetal Therapy*, **2**, 17–26.

Arabin, B., Siebert, M., Jimenez, E., and Saling, E. (1988). Obstetrical characteristics of a loss of end-diastolic velocities in the fetal aorta and/or umbilical artery using Doppler ultrasound. *Gynecological and Obstetrical Investigations*, **25**, 173–80.

Arduini, D. and Rizzo, G. (1988) Differential diagnosis of small for gestational age fetuses by Doppler ultrasound. *Fetal Therapy*, **3**, 31–6.

Barss, V. A., Doubilet, P. M., St. John-Sutton, M., Cartier, M. S., and Frigoletto, F. D. (1987). Cardiac output in a fetus with erythroblastosis fetalis: assessment using pulsed Doppler. *Obstetrics and Gynecology*, **70**, 442–4.

Battaglia, F. C. (1978). Intrauterine growth retardation: an invitational symposium. *Journal of Reproductive Medicine*, **21**, 283–6.

Bilardo, C. M., Nicolaides, K. H., and Campbell, S. (1988). The relationship of fetal blood gases and pH to Doppler investigations of the fetal circulation. In *Third International Conference on Fetal and Neonatal Physiological Measurements*, Malmo, Sweden (ed. K. Marsal), pp. 106–00.

Bilardo, C. M., Nicolaides, K. H., and Campbell, S. (1989). Doppler studies in red cell isoimmunization. *Clinics in Obstetrics and Gynecology*, **32**, 719–27.

Bilardo, C. M., Nicolaides, K. H., and Campbell, S. (1990). Doppler measurements of fetal and uteroplacental circulation: relationship with umbilical venous blood gases measured at cordocentesis. *American Journal of Obstetrics and Gynecology*, **162**, 115–20.

Burke, G., Stuart, B., Crowley, P., Scanaill, S. N., and Drumm, J. (1990). Is intrauterine growth retardation with normal umbilical artery blood flow a benign condition? *British Medical Journal*, **300**, 1044–5.

Campbell, S. and Pearce, J. M. F. (1983). The prenatal diagnosis of fetal structural abnormalities by ultrasound. *Clinics in Obstetrics and Gynecology*, **10**, 475–89.

Copel, J. A., Grannum, P. A., Belanger, K., Green, J., and Hobbins, J. C. (1988).

Pulsed Doppler flow-velocity waveforms before and after intrauterine intravascular transfusion for severe erythroblastosis fetalis. *American Journal of Obstetrics and Gynecology*, **158**, 768–74.

Copel, J. A., Grannum, P. A., Green, J. J., Hobbins, J. C., and Kleinman, C. S. (1989). Fetal cardiac output in the isoimmunized pregnancy: a pulsed Doppler echocardiographic study of patients undergoing intravascular intrauterine transfusion. *American Journal of Obstetrics and Gynecology*, **161**, 361–4.

Daffos, F., Capella-Pavlovsky, M., and Forestier, F. (1985). Fetal blood sampling during pregnancy with use of a needle guided by ultrasound: a study of 600 consecutive cases. *American Journal of Obstetrics and Gynecology*, **153**, 655–6.

Eik-Nes, S. H., Brubbakk, A. O., and Ulstien, M. (1980). Measurement of human fetal blood flow. *British Medical Journal*, **1**, 283–4.

European Association of Perinatal Medicine (1989). Regulation for the use of Doppler technology in perinatal medicine. In *Consensus of Barcelona*, pp. 22–6. Instituto Barcelona.

Gillbert, R. D. (1980). Control of fetal cardiac output during changes in blood volume. *American Journal of Physiology*, **238**, 1180–6.

Griffin, D., Bilardo, K., Masini, L., *et al.* (1984). Doppler flow velocity waveforms in the descending thoracici aorta of the human fetus. *British Journal of Obstetrics and Gynaecology*, **91**, 997–1006.

Gudmundsson, S. and Marsal. K. (1991). Blood velocity waveforms in the fetal aorta and umbilical artery as predictors of fetal outcome: a comparison. *American Journal of Perinatology*, **8**, 1–6.

Hackett, G. A., Nicolaides, K. H., and Campbell, S. (1987*a*). Doppler assessment of fetal and uteroplacental circulations in severe second trimester oligohydramnios. *British Journal of Obstetrics and Gynaecology*, **94**, 1074–7.

Hackett, G. A., Campbell, S., Gamsu, H., Cohen-Overbeek, T. A., and Pearce, J. M. F. (1987*b*). Doppler studies in the growth retarded fetus and prediction of neonatal necrotising enterocolitis, haemorrhage and neonatal morbidity. *British Medical Journal*, **294**, 13–16.

Hanretty, K. P., Whittle, M. J., Gilmore, D. H., McNay, M. B., Howie, C. A., and Rubin, P. C. (1989). The effect of intravascular transfusion for Rhesus haemolytic disease on umbilical artery Doppler flow velocity waveforms. *British Journal of Obstetrics and Gynaecology*, **96**, 960–3.

Hseith, F.-J., Chang, F.-M., and Ko, T.-M. (1988). Umbilical artery flow velocity waveforms in fetuses dying with congenital abnormalities. *British Journal of Obstetrics and Gynaecology*, **95**, 478–82.

Huikeshoven, F. J., Hope, I. D., Power, G. G., Gilbert, R. D., and Longo, L. D. (1985). A comparison of sheep and human fetal oxygen delivery systems with use of a mathematical model. *American Journal of Obstetrics and Gynecology*, **151**, 449–55.

Illyes, M. and Gati, I. (1988). Reverse flow in the human fetal descending aorta as a sign of severe fetal asphyxia preceding intrauterine death. *Journal of Clinical Ultrasound*, **16**, 403–10.

Jouppila, P. and Kirkinen, P. (1984). Increased vascular resistance in the fetal descending aorta of the human fetus in hypoxia. *British Journal of Obstetrics and Gynaecology*, **91**, 853–6.

Kirkinen, P., Jouppila, P., and Eik-Nes, S. (1983). Umbilical vein blood flow in Rhesus isoimmunization. *British Journal of Obstetrics and Gynaecology*, **90**, 719–27.

Kirkinen, P., Muller, R., Huch, R., and Huch, A. (1987). Blood flow velocity waveforms in human fetal intracranial arteries. *Obstetrics and Gynecology*, **70**, 617–21.

Laurin, J., Lingman, G., Marsal, K., and Perrson, P. H. (1987). Fetal blood flow in pregnancies complicated by intrauterine growth retardation. *Obstetrics and Gynecology*, **69**, 895–902.

Lindfors, K. K., McGahan, J. P., and Walter, J. P. (1986). Fetal omphalocele and gastroschisis: pitfalls in sonographic diagnosis. *American Journal of Roentgenology*, **147**, 797–800.

Lingman, G. and Marsal, K. (1986*a*). Fetal central blood circulation in the third trimester of normal pregnancy. I. Aortic and umbilical blood flow. *Early Human Development*, **13**, 137–50.

Lingman, G. and Marsal, K. (1986*b*). Fetal central blood circulation in the third trimester of normal pregnancy. II. Aortic blood velocity waveforms. *Early Human Development*, **13**, 151–9.

Lingman, G. and Marsal, K. (1986*c*). Circulatory effects of fetal heart arrhythmias. *Journal of Pediatric Cardiology*, **7**, 67–74.

Lingman, G., Laurin, J., and Marsal, K. (1986). Circulatory changes in fetuses with imminent asphyxia. *Biology of the Neonate*, **49**, 66–73.

McCowan, L. M., Erskine, L. A., and Ritchie, K. (1987). Umbilical artery Doppler blood flow studies in the preterm, small for gestational age fetus. *American Journal of Obstetrics and Gynecology*, **156**, 655–9.

Mari, G., Moise, K. J., Russell, L. D., Kirshon, B., Stefos, T., and Carpenter, R. J. (1990). Flow velocity waveforms of the vascular system in the anemic fetus before and after intravascular transfusion for severe red cell allimmization. *American Journal of Obstetrics and Gynecology*, **162**, 1060–4.

Marsal, K. and Perrson, P. H. (1988). Ultrasonic measurement of fetal blood velocity waveform as a secondary diagnostic test in screening for intrauterine growth retardation. *Journal of Clinical Ultrasound*, **16**, 239–44.

Marsal, K., Lingman, G., and Giles, W. (1984*a*). Evaluation of the carotid, aortic and umbilical blood velocity waveforms in the human fetus. *Society for the Study of Fetal Physiology, XI Annual Conference*, Oxford, p. C33. The Nuffield Institute, Oxford.

Marsal, K., Lindblad, A., Lingman, G., and Eik-Nes, S. H. (1984*b*). Blood flow in the fetal descending aorta: intrinsic factors affecting fetal blood flow, i.e. fetal breathing movements and fetal cardiac arrhythmia. *Ultrasound in Medicine and Biology*, **10**, 339–48.

Meijboom, E. J., de Smedt, M. C. H., Visser, G. H. A., Jager, W., and Nicolaides, K. H. (1986). Fetal cardiac output measurements by Doppler echocardiography. *Proceedings of the Sixth Annual Meeting of the Society of Perinatal Obstetricians*. San Antonio, Texas. Abstract 17.

Meizner, I., Katz, M., Lunenfeld, E., and Insler V. (1987). Umbilical and uterine flow velocity waveforms in pregnancies complicated by major fetal abnormalities. *Prenatal Diagnosis*, **7**, 491–6.

Mercer, L. J. and Brown, L. G. (1986). Fetal outcome with oligohydramnios in the second trimester. *Obstetrics and Gynecology*, **156**, 840–2.

Nicolaides, K. H. (1989). Studies on fetal physiology and pathophysiology in Rhesus disease. *Seminars in Perinatology*, **13**, 28–37.

Nicolaides, K. H. and Rodeck, C. H. (1991). Maternal serum anti-D concentration in the assessment of Rhesus isoimmunisation. *British Medical Journal*, (in press).

Nicolaides, K. H., Bilardo, C. M., and Campbell, S. (1990). Prediction of fetal anaemia by measurement of mean blood velocity in the fetal aorta. *American Journal of Obstetrics and Gynecology*, **162**, 209–12.

Nicolaides, K. H., Warenski, J. C., and Rodeck, C. H. (1985). The relationship of fetal protein concentration and haemoglobin level to the development of hydrops in Rhesus isoimmunization. *American Journal of Obstetrics and Gynecology*, **152**, 341–4.

Nicolaides, K. H., Soothill, P. W., Rodeck, C. H., and Campbell, S. (1986*a*). Ultrasound guided sampling of umbilical cord and placental blood to assess fetal wellbeing. *Lancet*, **i**, 1065–7.

Nicolaides, K. H., Soothill, P. W., Rodeck, C. H., and Clewell, W. (1986*b*) Rh disease: intravascular fetal blood transfusion by cordocentesis. *Fetal Therapy*, **1**, 185–92.

Nicolaides, K. H., Thilaganathan, B., Rodeck, C. H., and Mibashan, R. S. (1988*a*).
Erythroblastosis and reticulocytosis in anemic fetuses. *American Journal of Obstetrics and Gynecology*, **159**, 1063–5.

Nicolaides, K. H., Soothill, P. W., Clewell, C. H., Mibashan, R., and Campbell, S. (1988*b*). Fetal haemoglobin measurement in the assessment of red cell isoimmunization. *Lancet*, **i**, 1073–6.

Nicolaides, K. H., Sadovsky, G., and Cetin, E. (1989*a*). Fetal heart rate patterns in red cell isoimmunized pregnancies. *American Journal of Obstetrics and Gynecology*, **161**, 351–6.

Nicolaides, K. H., Snijders, R. J. M., Thorpe-Beeston, J. G., van den Hof, M. C., Gosden, C. M., and Bellingham, A. J. (1989*b*). Mean red cell volume in normal, small and anemic fetuses. *Fetal Therapy*, **4**, 1–13.

Panos, M. Z., Nicolaides, K. H., Anderson, J. V., Economides, D. L., Rees, L., and Williams, R. (1989). Plasma atrial natriuretic peptide: response to intravascular blood transfusion. *American Journal of Obstetrics and Gynecology*, **161**, 357–61.

Pearce, J. M. F., Leach, G., and Jeffries, I. (1992). The value of colour flow Doppler in second trimester oligohydramnios. *Prenatal Diagnosis*, (in press).

Reed, K., Anderson, C. F., and Shenker, L. (1987). Changes in intracardiac Doppler blood flow velocities in fetuses with absent umbilical artery diastolic flow. *American Journal of Obstetrics and Gynecology*, **157**, 774–9.

Rightmire, D. A., Nicolaides, K. H., Rodeck, C. H., and Campbell, S. (1986). Fetal blood velocities in Rh isoimmunization: relationship to gestational age and fetal hematocrit. *Obstetrics and Gynecology*, **68**, 233–6.

Rizzo, G., Arduini, D., Colosimo, C., and Mancuso, S. (1987). Abnormal fetal cerebral blood flow velocity waveforms as a sign of an aneurysm of the vein of Galen. *Fetal Therapy*, **2**, 75–9.

Rizzo, G., Nicolaides, K. H., Arduini, D., and Campbell, S. (1990). Effects of intravascular fetal blood transfusion on fetal intracardiac Doppler velocity waveforms. *American Journal of Obstetrics and Gynecology*, **163**, 569–71.

Rochelson, B., Schulman, H., Farmakides, G., *et al.* (1987). The significance of absent end-diastolic velocity in umbilical artery velocity waveforms. *American Journal of Obstetrics and Gynecology*, **156**, 1213–18.

Rochelson, B., Coury, A., Schulman, H., Dery, C., Kotz, M., and Shmoys S. (1990). Doppler umbilical artery velocimetry in fetuses with polyhydramnios. *American Journal of Perinatology*, **7**, 340–2.

Soothill, P. W., Nicolaides, K. H., Bilardo, C. M., and Campbell, S. (1986). Relation of fetal hypoxia in growth retardation to mean blood velocity in the fetal aorta. *Lancet*, **ii**, 1118–20.

Soothill, P. W., Nicolaides, K. H., Rodeck, C. H., Clewell, W. H., and Lindridge, J. (1987). Relationship of fetal haemoglobin and oxygen content to lactate concentration in Rh isoimmunized pregnancies. *Obstetrics and Gynecology*, **69**, 268–71.

Soothill, P. W., Nicolaides, K. H., Rodeck, C. H., and Bellingham, A. J. (1988*a*). The effect of replacing fetal with adult hemoglobin on the blood gas and acid-base parameters in human fetuses. *American Journal of Obstetrics and Gynecology*. **158**, 66–9.

Soothill, P. W., Lestas, A. N., Nicolaides, K. H., Rodeck, C. H., and Bellingham, A. J. (1988*b*). 2,3-Diphosphoglycerate in normal, anaemic and transfused human fetuses. *Clinical Science*, **74**, 527–30.

Tonge, H. M., Stewart, P. A., and Wladimiroff, J. W. (1984). Fetal blood flow measurements during fetal cardiac arrythmia. *Early Human Development*, **10**, 23–34.

Trudinger, B. J. and Cook, C. M. (1985). Umbilical and uterine artery flow velocity waveforms in pregnancy associated with major fetal abnormality. *British Journal of Obstetrics and Gynaecology*, **92**, 666–70.

Vaksmann, G., Decouix, E., Mauren, P., Jardin, M., Rey, C., and Dupuis, C. (1989). Evaluation of the vein of Galen arteriovenous malformation in newborns by two dimensional ultrasound, pulsed and colour Doppler method. *European Journal of Pediatrics*, **148**, 510–2.

Van Eyck, J., Wladimirof, J. W., Noordam, M. J., Tonge, H. M., and Prechtl, H. F. R. (1985). The blood velocity waveform in the fetal descending aorta: its relationship to fetal behavioural states in normal pregnancy at 37–38 weeks. *Early Human Development*, **12**, 137–43.

Vyas, S., Nicolaides, K. H., and Campbell, S. (1990). Doppler examination of the middle cerebral artery in anemic fetuses. *American Journal of Obstetrics and Gynecology*, **162**, 1066–8.

Warren, P. S., Gill, R. W., and Fisher, C. C. (1987). Doppler blood flow studies in Rhesus isoimmunization. *Seminars in Perinatology*, **11**, 375–8.

Weiner, C. P. and Anderson, T. L. (1989). The acute effect of cordocentesis with or without fetal cirarization and of intravascular transfusion upon umbilical artery waveform indices. *Obstetrics and Gynecology*, **73**, 219–24.

Weiner, C. P. and Robillard, G. E. (1989). Effect of acute intravascular volume expansion on human fetal prostaglandin concentrations. *American Journal of Obstetrics and Gynecology*, **161**, 1494–7.

Welch, C. R. and Rodeck, C. H. (1990). The effect of intravascular transfusion for Rhesus haemolytic disease on umbilical artery Doppler flow velocity waveforms. *British Journal of Obstetrics and Gynecology*, **97**, 865–6.

Wenstrom, K. D., Weiner, C. P., and Williamson, R. A. (1991). Diverse maternal and fetal pathology associated with absent diastolic flow in the umbilical artery of high risk fetuses. Obstetrics and Gynecology, **77**, 374–8.

Wladimirof, J. W., Tonge, H. M., Stewart, P. A., and Reuss, A. (1986). Severe intrauterine growth retardation; assessment of its origin from fetal arterial flow veolocity waveforms. *European Journal of Obstetrics, Gynecology, and Reproductive Medicine*, **22**, 23–8.

Wootton, R., McFadyen, I. R., and Cooper, J. E. (1977). Measurement of placental blood flow in the pig and its relation to placental and fetal weight. *Biology of the Neonate*, **31**, 333–9.

14. Doppler studies of the cerebral and renal circulations in small-for-gestational age fetuses

Sanjay Vyas and Stuart Campbell

INTRODUCTION

Invasive animal experiments have helped to elucidate the fetal cardio-vascular adjustments in response to hypoxaemia. Thus, Peeters *et al.* (1979) reduced the percentage of oxygen in the gas mixture inhaled by the mother to examine the effect of a reduction in fetal arterial oxygen content (6.1 mmol/l; normal arterial value 5–9.7 mmol/l) on the distribution of blood flow in sheep fetuses at term. Fetal organ perfusion was determined from the amount of radioactivity measured at post mortem after the injection of radioactively labelled microspheres during maternal hypo-oxygenation. The perfusion of fetal organs at different degrees of hypoxaemia was measured, and the responses fell into four groups:

1. Blood flow increased in inverse relation to arterial oxygen content. This response was found in the heart, brain and adrenal glands.

2. Blood flow decreased progressively with a reduction in arterial oxygen content. This response was found only in the lungs.

3. Blood flow was maximal at a certain arterial oxygen content. The gut, carcass, and kidneys had steady blood flow until the arterial oxygen content was reduced to 3 mmol/l, whereafter it fell.

4. Blood flow was unrelated to arterial oxygen content. The thyroid, thymus, and, most importantly, the placenta did not show any altera-tion in blood flow.

These data provide evidence of a redistribution of cardiac output that selectively increases the perfusion of group 1 organs at the expense of those in groups 2 and 3. The effect would be to overcome the reduction in blood oxygen content per unit volume by increasing the amount of blood delivered to selected organs per unit time.

These alterations in fetal organ perfusion might be mediated by neuronal stimulation. Thus, electrical activity has been recorded in the vagus nerves of mature sheep fetuses (Ponte and Purves 1973). Aortic chemoreceptors, which respond to small falls in arterial oxygen levels, are thought to provide the first line of defence to hypoxaemia in fetal lambs (Dawes 1969).

Robillard *et al.* (1986) investigated the role of renal nerves in modulating the renal vasoconstriction during hypoxaemia in chronically catheterized fetal lambs. Changes in renal blood flow were measured by indwelling pulsed Doppler probes, and changes in renal vascular resistance were calculated after taking account of the perfusion pressure (mean aortic pressure − mean inferior vena cava pressure). In each fetus, the left kidney was denervated by severing and stripping the renal nerves around and along the renal artery and vein, followed by the application of 10 per cent phenol in absolute alcohol; the renal pedicle on the right was explored, but only 0.9 per cent saline was applied. Renal vascular resistance increased and renal blood flow fell in both kidneys in response to fetal hypoxaemia. However, the changes in renal blood flow were always smaller in the denervated than in the intact kidney. Robillard *et al.* (1986) concluded that renal vasoconstriction in response to fetal hypoxaemia is modulated by other factors in addition to neuronal stimulation.

The realization that in human pregnancy some small-for-gestational age (SGA) fetuses are hypoxaemic during the antenatal period (Soothill *et al.* 1987; Nicolaides *et al.* 1989) has stimulated workers to investigate similar haemodynamic readjustments in the human fetus. These studies are possible due to the advent of Doppler ultrasonography, which is a non-invasive and safe modality.

DOPPLER STUDIES OF THE FETAL CEREBRAL CIRCULATION

Wladimiroff *et al.* (1986) first described the use of duplex pulsed Doppler ultrasound to obtain flow velocity waveforms (FVWs) from the intracranial vessels. Using real-time imaging they identified the internal carotid artery at its bifurcation into the anterior and middle cerebral arteries on either side of the cerebral peduncles. The pulsed Doppler range gate was then placed on these vessels to obtain FVWs. More recently, van den Wijngaard *et al.* (1989) used similar methodology and investigated the middle cerebral, anterior and posterior communicating, and internal carotid arteries of 14 SGA fetuses. The characteristic finding is an increase in end-diastolic frequencies (EDF), indicating reduced impedance to flow. This morphological abnormality of the FVW is also reflected by a fall in the pulsatility index (PI). Kirkinen *et al.* (1987) also used the same methodology, and reported a fall in resistance index (RI) in 23 of 82 (28 per cent) SGA fetuses.

Table 14.1 Correlation of Doppler measurements with fetal blood gases, pH, and asphyxia index

Measurement	P_{O_2}		P_{CO_2}		pH		Asphyxia index	
	r	RSD	r	RSD	r	RSD	r	RSD
ΔAoV_m	0.51	8.0	−0.59	5.6	0.54	0.044	−0.62	19.7
$\Delta AoPI$	−0.47	8.3	0.57	5.7	−0.57	0.043	0.61	20.0
ΔCCV_m	−0.28	9.0	0.41	6.4	0.38	0.040	−0.43	23.0
$\Delta CCPI$	0.63	7.3	−0.43	6.2	0.51	0.045	−0.60	20.2
Ao–CC index	0.62	7.4	−0.58	5.6	0.58	0.043	−0.67	18.7

Δ, Difference between observed measurement and normal mean for gestational age; r, correlation coefficient; RSD, residual standard deviation; AoV_m, descending thoracic aorta mean blood velocity; AoPI, descending thoracic aorta pulsatility index; CCV_m, common carotid artery mean blood velocity; CCPI, common carotid artery pulsatility index; Ao–CC index, aortic–carotid index (see text).

Bilardo *et al.* (1990) obtained FVWs from the common carotid artery, and correlated the PI and mean blood velocity with umbilical cord blood gases in samples obtained by cordocentesis, in a series of 41 SGA and 10 AGA fetuses. There were significant correlations between the reduction of the PI of FVWs from the common carotid artery and the degree of hypox-

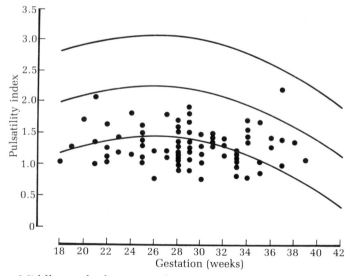

Fig. 14.1 Middle cerebral artery pulsatility index of the 81 SGA fetuses (●) plotted on the reference range for gestation. (From the *British Journal of Obstetrics and Gynaecology*, with permission.)

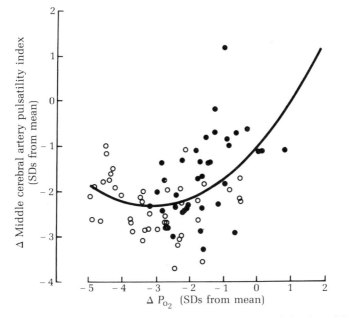

Fig. 14.2 Relationship between fetal hypoxaemia (P_{O_2}) and fetal middle cerebral artery pulsatility index, both expressed as the number of standard deviations by which the observed values differed from the respective normal mean for gestation. The open circles indicate acidaemic fetuses and the closed circles represent non-acidaemic fetuses. (From the *British Journal of Obstetrics and Gynaecology*, with permission.)

aemia, and acidaemia. Furthermore, common carotid artery mean blood velocity was increased in the SGA fetuses, and there was a significant association between the magnitude of this increase and hypoxaemia, and acidaemia. Blood gases and pH were correlated individually and as an asphyxia index, to the Doppler measurements. The asphyxia index was derived by principal component analysis, and defined by the equation:

$$\text{Asphyxia} = -\Delta P_{O_2} + 1.43\,(\Delta P_{CO_2}) - 180.2\,(\Delta pH)$$

where ΔP_{O_2}, ΔP_{CO_2}, and ΔpH are the differences between the observed P_{O_2}, P_{CO_2}, and pH values, respectively, from the normal mean for gestation. Although there were significant correlations between the blood gas results and both the PI and mean blood velocity in the individual vessels, better correlations were found with the ratio of common carotid artery and descending thoracic aorta mean blood velocity and PI. The best predictor of asphyxia (as judged by the lowest residual standard deviation and highest correlation coefficient) was an index comprising the aortic mean blood velocity and the PI of FVWs from the common carotid artery (Table

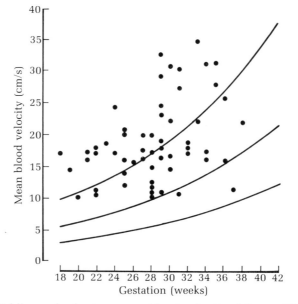

Fig. 14.3 Middle cerebral artery mean blood velocity of the 58 SGA fetuses (●) plotted on the reference range for gestation. (From the British Journal of Obstetrics and Gynaecology, with permission.)

14.1). This index was also derived by principal component analysis, and defined by the equation:

$$\text{Aortic–carotid index} = \Delta\text{Ao}V_m + 4.2\,(\Delta\text{CCPI})$$

where $\Delta\text{Ao}V_m$ and ΔCCPI is the difference between the observed aortic mean blood velocity and common carotid PI, respectively, from the expected mean for gestation.

When the aortic–carotid index was abnormal, all fetuses had an asphyxia index above the mean, 89 per cent of the fetuses had an asphyxia index one standard deviation above the mean; and 60 per cent were more than two standard deviations above the mean. A normal index was always associated with normal blood gases.

Taken as a whole, these results provide indirect evidence of the brain-sparing effect in human SGA fetuses. However, the studies of van den Wijngaard *et al.* (1989) did not include data on fetal blood gases, whilst Bilardo *et al.* (1990) measured fetal blood gases but examined the common carotid artery. This vessel supplies the tissues of the face and neck in addition to the brain. Thus, during fetal hypoxaemia the common carotid artery would reflect the opposing vasoconstrictive effects of the tissues of the head and neck and the vasodilatory effects of the cerebral circulation.

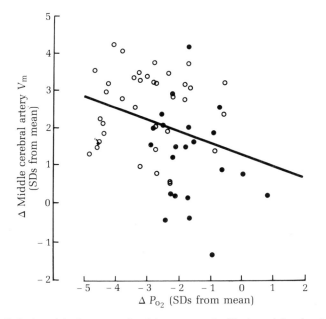

Fig. 14.4 Relationship between fetal hypoxaemia (P_{O_2}) and fetal middle cerebral artery mean blood velocity (V_m), both expressed as the number of standard deviations by which the observed values differed from the respective normal mean for gestation. The open circles indicate acidaemic fetuses and the closed circles represent non-acidaemic fetuses. (From the *British Journal of Obstetrics and Gynaecology*, with permission.)

In an effort to elucidate the fetal cerebral vascular response to hypoxaemia, Vyas *et al.* (1990*a, b*) related umbilical cord blood gases to Doppler indices of velocity and impedance to flow in the fetal middle cerebral artery. In their study of 81 SGA fetuses with an abdominal circumference below the 2.5th centile for gestational age, the middle cerebral artery was examined by colour flow imaging up to 30 min before cordocentesis.

The data were analysed by calculating the delta values of the Doppler or fetal blood gas parameters. The PI of FVWs from the fetal middle cerebral artery was significantly lower than in the reference range (Fig. 14.1). There was a significant quadratic relation between ΔPI and ΔP_{O_2} (Fig. 14.2). Similarly, there was a significant quadratic relation between ΔPI and ΔpH.

The middle cerebral artery mean blood velocity was measured in the last 58 SGA fetuses, and was significantly higher than the reference range (Fig. 14.3). There was a significant correlation between ΔV_m and ΔP_{O_2} (Fig. 14.4). The relation of ΔV_m to ΔpH was best described by a quadratic equation and there was a significant correlation between ΔPI and ΔV_m in the 58 SGA fetuses in which both measurements were performed. There were no significant associations between ΔP_{CO_2} and ΔPI or ΔV_m.

The PI of FVWs represents downstream impedance to flow (Gosling and King 1975), and these data provide evidence of vasodilation in the cerebral vasculature during mild to moderate hypoxaemia. With severe degrees of hypoxaemia (2–4 standard deviations below the mean for gestation), usually with associated acidaemia, the reduction in PI reaches a maximum which probably represents maximum vessel dilatation. In extreme hypoxaemia (> 4 standard deviations below the mean for gestation), the reduction in PI is proportionally less (see Fig. 14.2). Fetal head compression, and therefore increased intracranial pressure, is associated with an increase in the PI of FVWs from the middle cerebral artery (Vyas *et al.* 1990*a*). It could be hypothesized that in severely hypoxaemic SGA fetuses the vasodilatation-mediated decrease in PI is blunted by increased intracranial pressure. This may be due to cerebral oedema and a generalized increase in intracranial pressure, as has been described in hypoxaemic monkey fetuses (Myers *et al.* 1984).

The middle cerebral artery mean blood velocity is higher in the SGA fetuses, and there are significant correlations between the increased mean blood velocity and fetal hypoxaemia and acidaemia. However, the relationship between the increase in mean blood velocity and the decrease in PI is weaker in SGA than in appropriate-growth-for-gestational age (AGA) fetuses ($r = -0.366$ and $r = -0.667$, respectively). These findings suggest that in SGA fetuses blood velocity is not determined by downstream impedance to flow alone and that other factors, such as cardiac contractility, vessel compliance, and blood viscosity, may also play a role.

DOPPLER STUDIES OF THE FETAL RENAL CIRCULATION

The animal model suggests that the increase in cerebral perfusion occurs at the expense of perfusion of the viscera. In order to investigate this hypothesis in the human fetus, Vyas *et al.* (1989) related the degree of fetal hypoxaemia (measured in umbilical cord blood samples) to the PI of FVWs from the fetal renal artery. Although the initial report was based on a small number of fetuses, the current analyses are based on the investigation of 48 SGA fetuses (Vyas *et al.* 1990*a, c*). The fetal abdominal circumference was below the 2.5th centile of the reference range for gestation in all cases, and all fetuses were structurally and karyotypically normal. The renal artery PI of the SGA fetuses was significantly higher than the normal mean for gestation (Fig. 14.5). However, at gestations of 24 weeks or less, six of nine fetuses had renal artery PI values within the 90 per cent confidence intervals of the reference range for gestation. As a group, these nine earlier

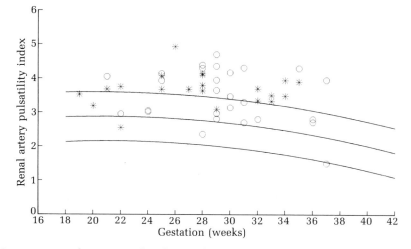

Fig. 14.5 Renal artery pulsatility index of small-for-gestational age fetuses plotted on the reference range for gestation. In 21 cases there was oligohydramnios (*).

gestation fetuses had a higher mean ΔPI than the normal mean for gestation (mean difference = 1.01 SDs, SE = 0.365, $p < 40.05$), but not as high as that of the 39 fetuses at more than 24 weeks' gestation (mean difference = 2.303 SDs, SE = 0.228, $p > 0.0001$).

For the whole group, there was no significant association between ΔPI and ΔP_{O_2}. However, for fetuses at more than 24 weeks' gestation there was a significant association between ΔPI and ΔP_{O_2} (Fig. 14.6; $n = 39$, $p > 0.05$, $r = -0.368$, constant = 1.515, slope = 0.424, residual SD = 1.381). For the subgroup of fetuses at 24 weeks' gestation or less, ΔPI was not significantly related to ΔP_{O_2} ($n = 9$, $r = 0.004$). These findings suggest a gestation-related maturation in renal vascular responsiveness to hypoxaemia.

Oligohydramnios

The ultrasonic diagnosis of olighydramnios was made when the vertical diameter of the largest pool of amniotic fluid was less than 1 cm (Manning *et al.* 1980). There was no significant difference in mean ΔPI from the renal artery between the oligohydramnios and non-oligohydramnios subgroups (mean difference = 0.253, SE = 0.424, $t_{46} = -0.60$, $p = 0.55$). In SGA pregnancies beyond 24 weeks' gestation, the renal artery PI was above the 95th centile of the reference range in 15 of 16 cases (94 per cent) in which an ultrasound diagnosis of oligohydramnios was made. This suggests that increased impedance to flow in the renal vasculature may result in a reduction in fetal urine production and therefore in amniotic fluid volume.

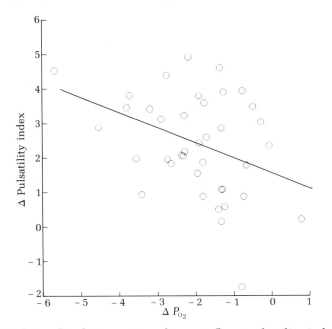

Fig. 14.6 Relationship between impedance to flow (pulsatility index) in the renal artery and hypoxaemia (P_{O_2}), both expressed as the number of standard deviations by which the observed values differed from the respective normal mean for gestation, for fetuses of more than 24 weeks' gestation.

However, in the same group oligohydramnios was present in only 25 of the 28 cases (54 per cent) in which the renal artery PI was above the 95th centile of the reference range. Since the amniotic fluid volume reflects the chronic state, and renal artery PI reflects the acute state, it is possible that oligohydramnios will develop in the remaining 15 cases (48 per cent) in later pregnancy if the renal artery PI remains elevated due to chronic fetal hypoxaemia. This hypothesis needs further evaluation.

Previous studies using pulsed Doppler ultrasound have alluded to alterations in the organ perfusion of SGA human fetuses. Thus, Hackett *et al.* (1987) found that when there was absence of EDF in the fetal descending thoracic aorta, there was an increased incidence of neonatal necrotizing enterocolitis and haemorrhage (Fig. 13.4). The authors speculated that these neonatal complications were the result of hypoperfusion of the fetal gut and liver, respectively. However, exact information was not obtained as the arterial supply of individual organs could not be identified. The use of colour flow imaging has facilitated the investigation of the renal artery, and we presume that the findings are representative of visceral perfusion in SGA fetuses.

Doppler ultrasound examination of the fetal cerebral and renal circulations identifies fetal hypoxaemia. In practice, these changes are usually seen before abnormalities of the cardiotocograph. The exact contribution of this exciting new modality to the care of pregnancies complicated by intra-uterine growth retardation remains to be evaluated.

REFERENCES

Bilardo, C. M., Nicolaides, K. H., and Campbell, S. (1990). Doppler measurement of fetal and uteroplacental circulations: relationship with umbilical venous blood gases measured at cordocentesis. *American Journal of Obstetrics and Gynecology*, **162**, 115–19.

Campbell, S. and Thoms, A. (1975). Ultrasound measurement of the fetal head to abdomen circumference ratio in the assessment of growth retardation. *British Journal of Obstetrics and Gynaecology*, **84**, 165–168.

Dawes, G. S., Duncan, S. L., Lewis, B. V., Merlet, C. L., Owen-Thomas, J. B., and Reeves, J. T. (1969). Cyanide stimulation of the systemic arterial chemoreceptors in foetal lambs. *Journal of Physiology*, **201**, 1171–21.

Gosling, R. G. and King, D. H. (1975). Ultrasonic angiology. In *Arteries and veins* (ed. A. W. Harcus and L. Adamson), p. 61. Churchill Livingstone, Edinburgh.

Hackett, G. A., Campbell, S., Gamsu, H., Cohen-Overbeek, T., and Pearce, J. M. F. (1987). Doppler studies in the growth retarded fetus and prediction of neonatal necrotising enterocolitis, haemorrhage, and neonatal morbidity. *British Medical Journal*, **294**, 13.

Kirkinen, P., Muller, R., Huch, R., and Huch, A. (1987). Blood flow velocity waveforms in human fetal intra-cranial arteries. *Obstetrics and Gynecology*, **70**, 617.

Manninig, F., Platt, L., and Sipos, L. (1980). Antepartum fetal evaluation: Development of a fetal biophysical profile. *American Journal of Obstetrics and Gynecology*, **136**, 787.

Myers, R. E., de Courtney-Myers, G. M., and Wagner, K. R. (1984). Effects of hypoxia on fetal brain. In *Fetal physiology and medicine*, (ed. R. W. Beard and P. W. Nathanielsz), p. 419. Butterworth, London.

Nicolaides, K. N., Economides, D. L., and Soothill, P. W. (1989). Blood gases, pH and lactate in appropriate and small for gestational age fetuses. *American Journal of Obstetrics and Gynecology*, **161**, 996.

Peeters, L. L. H., Sheldon, R. E. Jones, M. D., Makowski, E. L., and Meschia, G. (1979). Blood flow to fetal organs as a functional of arterial oxygen content. *American Journal of Obstetrics and Gynecology*, **135**, 637.

Ponte, J. and Purves, M. J. (1973). Types of different nerve activity which may be measured in the vagus nerve of the sheep fetus. *Journal of Physiology*, **229**, 51.

Robillard, J. E., Nakamura, K. T., and Dibona, G. F. (1986). Effect of renal denervation on renal responses to hypoxaemia in fetal lambs. *American Journal of Physiology*, **19**, F294.

Soothill, P. W., Nicolaides, K. H., and Campbell, S. (1987). Prenatal asphyxia, hyperlacticaemia, hypoglycaemia and erythroblastosis in growth retarded fetuses. *British Medical Journal*, **294**, 1051.

van den Wijngaard, J. A. G. W., Groenenberg, I. A. L., Wladimiroff, J. W., and

Hop, W. C. J. (1989). Cerebral Doppler ultrasound in the human fetus. *British Journal of Obstetrics and Gynaecology,* **96,** 845.

Vyas, S., Nicolaides, K. H., and Campbell, S. (1989). Renal artery flow velocity waveforms in normal and hypoxaemic fetuses. *American Journal of Obstetrics and Gynecology,* **161,** 168.

Vyas, S., Nicolaides, K. H., Bower, S., and Campbell, S. (1990*a*). Middle cerebral artery flow velocity waveforms in fetal hypoxaemia. *British Journal of Obstetrics and Gynaecology,* **97,** 797.

Vyas, S., Campbell, S., Bower, S., and Nicolaides, K. H. (1990*b*). Maternal abdominal pressure alters fetal cerebral blood flow. *British Journal of Obstetrics and Gynaecology,* **97,** 740.

Vyas, S. (1990*c*). Investigation of placental and fetal renal and cerebral circulations by colour Doppler ultrasound. Unpublished MD thesis. University of London.

Wladimiroff, J. W., Tonge, H. M., and Stewart, P. A. (1986). Doppler ultrasound assessment of cerebral blood flow in the human fetus. *British Journal of Obstetrics and Gynaecology,* **93,** 471.

15. Intracardiac Doppler ultrasound studies

Widad Al-Ghazali, Lindsay Allan, Pat Stewart, Darryl Maxwell, and Jurij Wladimiroff

SMALL-FOR-GESTATIONAL AGE FETUSES

Introduction

Pulsed, duplex Doppler systems have allowed the non-invasive investigation of the human fetal circulation. Such equipment has allowed several investigators to study intracardiac haemodynamics in both the normal and abnormal human fetus.

Technique of measurement

Doppler measurements of blood velocities across cardiac valves have been performed by several groups of investigators (Reed *et al.* 1986; Allan *et al.* 1987; de Smedt *et al.* 1987; Kenny *et al.* 1987). In all studies fetal cardiac output from each side of the heart was estimated by placing the sample volume just distal to the arterial valve in the ascending aorta and the main pulmonary artery. Waveforms were accepted only when the angle of insonation was less than 20°.

The internal diameter of the aorta or main pulmonary artery is estimated from a frozen image obtained in diastole. This gives a clear image of the vessel walls with a central echo, representing the closed valve. The measurement is obtained with the ultrasound beam perpendicular to the vessel.

The maximum velocity through each valve is then estimated from the recording of the flow velocity waveform. The mean temporal velocity (see Chapter 1) was calculated by planimetry of the area under the maximum frequency curve for one cardiac cycle. Time-averaged temporal velocity (see Chapter 1) was then obtained by dividing by the length of the cardiac cycle in seconds. The analysis is usually performed automatically by the software in the machine or by a digitizing pad connected to a microcomputer. As the flow velocity profile (see Chapter 1) from the great arteries of the heart is flat, mean flow velocity is obtained by tracing along the maximum velocity envelope of each cycle and along the zero line during diastole. Volume flow (Q) for each arterial valve can then be calculated from:

$$Q = \text{mean temporal velocity} \times \text{vessel area}$$

In post-natal life the two ventricles function in series and have the same cardiac output. In fetal life the ventricles function in parallel and have differing outputs; thus, flows through both great arteries must be added together to provide an estimate of the combined cardiac output (CCO).

The variability of volume flow measurements for CCO is of the order of 10 per cent (Al-Ghazali *et al.* 1989).

Normal pregnancy

In normal pregnancies the right-sided output is dominant, with a right:left ratio of 1.3:1. The maximum velocity through the ascending aorta is greater than that through the pulmonary artery but there appears to be no difference in the mean blood flow velocity between right- and left-sided valves. The CCO is about 500 ml/kg/min and does not change with gestation (Reed *et al.* 1986; Allan *et al.* 1987; de Smedt *et al.* 1987; Kenny *et al.* 1987). The cross-sectional areas of the tricuspid and aortic valves are larger than those of the aortic and mitral valves, thus accounting for the dominance of right-sided cardiac output. Allan *et al.* (1987) reported CCO values of 50 ml/min at 18 weeks' gestation, rising to 1200 ml/min across the great arterial valves, while de Smedt *et al.* (1987) reported higher values of up to 1735 ml/min across the atrioventricular valves. In both studies, however, CCO, expressed in terms of estimated fetal weight, was constant with increasing gestation.

Small-for-gestational age fetuses

Rizzo *et al.* (1988) studied blood velocities across the atrioventricular valves in appropriate-for-gestational age (AGA) and small-for-gestational age (SGA) fetuses. In AGA fetuses, the tricuspid velocities slightly exceed those recorded from the mitral valve, while in SGA fetuses the mitral velocity is greater.

Al-Ghazali *et al.* (1989) compared various haemodynamic parameters in 31 SGA fetuses with those in 92 AGA fetuses. SGA was defined for the purposes of this study as a fetal abdominal circumference of less than two standard deviations from the mean. SGA was subdivided into asymmetrical SGA, in which the head circumference:abdominal circumference ratio was more than two standard deviations above the mean, while in symmetrical SGA the ratio was within normal limits (Campbell and Thoms 1977). Blood flow velocity and volume were recorded in the aorta and pulmonary artery. In the AGA group there was no difference between the mean temporal velocity in the aorta and the pulmonary artery, but the maximum velocity was greater in the aorta (Table 15.1).

Table 15.1 Haemodynamic measurements in normal and growth-retarded fetuses

Group	n	Blood flow velocity			
		Aorta		Pulmonary artery	
		Maximum	Mean	Maximum	Mean
Normal	92	77.0 (14.9)	19.1 (4.4)	68.8 (13.0	18.4 (3.5)
IUGR					
Symmetrical	15	72.6 (12.0)	17.5 (2.5)	68.7 (9.5)	18.3 (2.7)
Asymmetrical	16	75.1 (14.6)	19.0 (4.6)	55.6 (12.6)	13.8 (3.6)

IUGR. Intrauterine growth retardation.
Results are mean values (SD).

The cardiac haemodynamics in the fetuses with symmetrical SGA was not significantly different from that estimated in the AGA fetuses, even though three SGA fetuses had absent end-diastolic frequencies (AEDF) in the umbilical artery. CCO in the symmetrical SGA fetuses was, however, in the low normal range and was abnormal in the three fetuses with AEDF. All three of these fetuses suffered an *in utero* death.

The asymmetrically SGA fetuses all demonstrated a change in intracardiac flow, namely a greater volume flow through the left than the right heart. The mean ratio of right heart volume flow to CCO was 47 per cent in this group, which is statistically significantly less than in the AGA fetuses. The aortic mean and maximum velocities were greater than those observed in the pulmonary artery but did not significantly differ from AGA fetuses. The pulmonary artery maximum and mean velocities were significantly less than those observed in AGA fetuses. The CCO (correcting for gestational age) was reduced or at the lower limits of normal, partly owing to a smaller cross-sectional area of the great vessels and partly owing to the reduced velocities observed in the pulmonary artery (Table 15.1). All 16 fetuses in this group had abnormal umbilical artery waveforms and nine had AEDF. Only four fetuses (all with AEDF) had low cardiac output in terms of ml/kg/min, and all suffered a perinatal death.

These findings confirm the experimental work in animals which demonstrated cardiac redistribution in fetal lambs exposed to both acute and chronic hypoxia (Dawes *et al.* 1968; Ruess *et al.* 1982; Block *et al.* 1984). In sheep, the degree of distribution is related to the degree of hypoxia, and the redistribution appears to mediated through α-adrenergic activity. The work of Al-Ghazali *et al.* (1989) suggests that increased placental resistance (as diagnosed by abnormal umbilical artery waveforms) mainly affects the pulmonary artery flow velocity. This is consistent with experimental work on the fetal lamb where a decrease in the right ventricular output was found in response to increasing the after-load either by inflating a balloon in the fetal aorta (Rudolph 1973) or by peripheral vasoconstriction induced by infusing methoxamine (Gilbert 1982) or phenylephrine (Thornburg and Morton 1983). Less or no effect was observed in the descending aorta in these experiments, perhaps because the aortic isthmus represents the site of functional separation. In the human fetus, cerebral vasodilatation induced by hypoxaemia leads to an increase in the velocities recorded from the ascending aorta.

In summary, the current role of intracardiac Doppler ultrasonography in SGA fetuses is as follows:

1.   Redistribution of cardiac output can be demonstrated in asymmetrical SGA fetuses, and it is believed that the degree of redistribution is proportional to the degree of hypoxemia.

2.   Combined cardiac output (CCO) estimations are time consuming and often difficult to perform. Because reduced CCO has not been observed to occur in the presence of a normal umbilical artery waveform, CCO measurements may only have a role to play in the further evaluation of fetuses with AEDF in the umbilical artery waveforms.

PRENATAL DIAGNOSIS OF CONGENITAL CARDIAC DISEASE

Introduction

Doppler echocardiographic evaluation will display the velocity and direction of blood flow. Blood flow within the fetal heart can be examined with pulsed or colour flow Doppler equipment. Normal flow characteristics can be demonstrated by documenting blood entering and leaving the heart, and by measuring flow through each cardiac valve and across the foramen ovale and the ductus arteriosus (Huhta *et al.* 1982; Allan *et al.* 1987). Abnormal flow such as absence of flow, high velocity flow, or regurgitation can also be recorded in cardiac malformations (Allan 1986; Ludomisky and Huhta 1987; Sharland *et al.* 1989).

Findings in normal fetuses

The course of forward flow from the veins into the atria can be seen on colour flow mapping, from the vena cava to the right atrium and from the pulmonary veins to the left atrium (Fig. 15.1). The blood passes through the atrioventricular valves to the ventricles. Colour flow should look to be equal on both sides of the heart. The velocity of flow across the atrioventricular valves is 40–60 cm/s on both sides of the heart and does not change

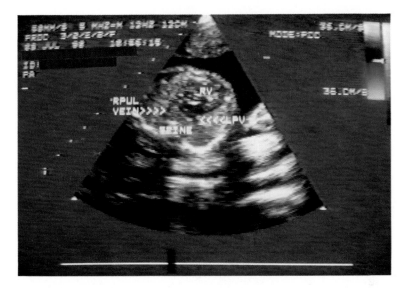

Fig. 15.1 Transverse section of the fetal chest demonstrating the right (RPUL VEIN) and left (LPV) pulmonary veins entering the left atrium. Real-time colour flow mapping clearly demonstrated low velocity flow in these veins. RV, right ventricle.

with gestation. The flow pattern is of a double-peaked waveform with the passive or 'e' wave being smaller than the 'a' or atrial wave in early pregnancy (Fig. 15.2) but becoming more equal as gestation advances. This pattern is the reverse of that seen in post-natal life where the 'e' wave is larger than the atrial complex. This probably indicates that the fetal ventricles are less compliant than they are post-natally.

The velocity of flow in the great arteries ranges from 40 to 100 cm/s between 16 weeks and term respectively. The waveform is a single peak with a fast acceleration and slower decay (Fig. 15.3). The velocity of blood flow in the ductus arteriosus is the highest recorded in the fetal heart, reaching 150 cm/s. There is also a diastolic component to the waveform (Fig. 15.4). Flow can be seen to be passing from the right to left atrium through the foramen ovale on colour flow mapping (Fig. 15.5), and the waveform demonstrates a double peak on pulsed Doppler with a velocity of 10–20 cm/s.

Fetuses with congenital cardiac abnormalities

Valve atresia
No flow is detectable through an atretic valve either on pulsed or colour Doppler examination (Fig. 15.6). Thus, when the chamber or vessel distal

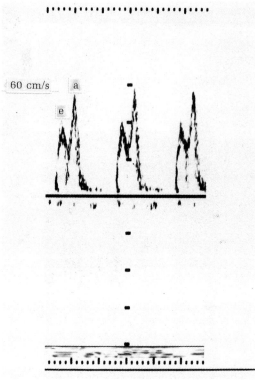

Fig. 15.2 Pulsed Doppler waveforms from the tricuspid valve at 22 weeks' gestation. The 'e' wave (passive filling wave) is smaller than the atrial 'a' component at this gestation. There is no flow through this valve in systole.

to an atretic valve is imaged in real-time, no flow will be detected by placing the pulsed simple volume within the chamber or vessel or after switching to colour Doppler ultrasound. However, lack of flow does not always indicate complete valve atresia, as a stenosed but patent valve associated with poor ventricular function may also demonstrate undetectable flow. In addition, where there is severe incompetence in the upstream valve, such as frequently occurs on the right side of the heart, the pulmonary valve may be anatomically patent but no forward flow will be observed; this is termed functional atresia.

Valve stenosis

In post-natal life, valvular stenosis leads to an increase in the velocity of the blood flowing across the valve. In prenatal life, the velocity across the arterial valves depends upon the interrelationship between ventricular function and the competence of the atrioventricular valves. Thus, in

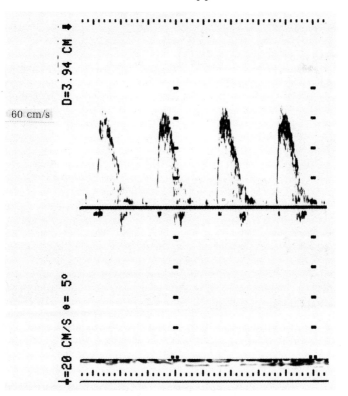

Fig. 15.3 Pulsed Doppler waveforms from the pulmonary valve at 24 weeks' gestation. The maximum velocity is about 60 cm/s. There is no flow through the valve in diastole.

arterial valves, stenosis the velocity of blood flow across the valve may be low, normal, or increased. Figure 15.7 illustrates an example of simple pulmonary stenosis in a fetus with a normal right ventricle and tricuspid valve; in this case the velocity is 2 m/s, twice the upper limit of normal.

A further difficulty in the evaluation of valvular stenosis prenatally is that the degree of obstruction can progress as pregnancy advances. This can result in the artery failing to grow in diameter, probably as the result of the diminished flow through it. The stenosed artery become progressively more hypoplastic, and in some cases stenosis can lead to complete atresia.

Mitral and tricuspid valve stenosis are uncommon in prenatal life but do not result in an increased velocity as the respective atrium is decompressed via the foramen ovale. Other features suggesting a diagnosis such as atrial dilatation and restricted valve excursion have to be used to infer atrioventricular valve stenosis.

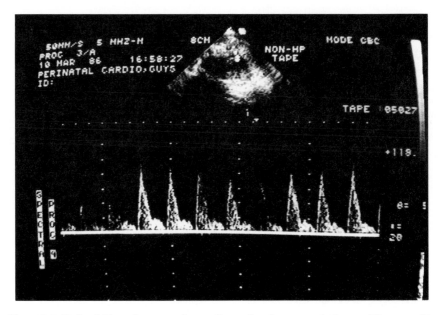

Fig. 15.4 Pulsed Doppler waveforms from the ductus arteriosus. The systolic velocity is more than 80 cm/s and there is always a diastolic component.

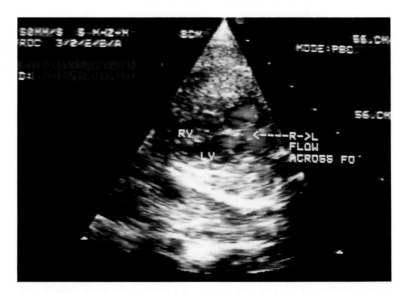

Fig. 15.5 Transverse section of the fetal heart demonstrating the flow (coloured blue) across the foramen ovale (FO) from right to left atrium. RV, right ventricle; LV, left ventricle.

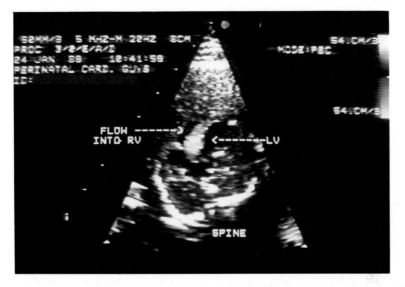

Fig. 15.6 Transverse section through the fetal heart in a case of mitral valve atresia. There is no flow from the left atrium to the left ventricle (LV) during diastole, whereas there is normal flow into the right ventricle (RV).

Valve incompetence

Regurgitation through an abnormal valve can readily be detected on pulsed colour Doppler imaging (Figs 15.8 and 15.9). The extent and breadth of the regurgitant jet will correlate with the severity of the incompetence. Prenatally, valve regurgitation most frequently occurs to a severe degree in the tricuspid valve, but all the cardiac valves can be incompetent in the context of dysplasia. The atrioventricular valves can also be seen to incompetent in fetal tachydysrhythmias, although in this instance the valves themselves are usually anatomically normal and the incompetence resolves once the dysrhythmia is brought under control.

Abnormal ductal and foramenal flow

Reversal of flow in the ductus arteriosus or aortic arch will be found in pulmonary or aortic atresia, respectively, and can be documented on pulsed Doppler or colour flow mapping. Left-to-right shunting through the foramen ovale is seen in conditions in which the left atrial pressure is increased above the right, for example in coarctation of the aorta, aortic or mitral atresia or stenosis (Fig. 15.10). In these conditions, the atrial septum may be closed completely, although this finding is most frequently seen in aortic stenosis or atresia.

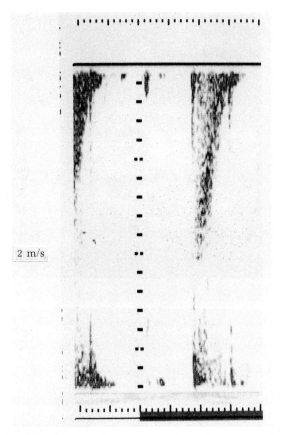

Fig. 15.7 Pulsed Dopler waveforms across the pulmonary valve in a fetus with pulmonary stenosis at 32 weeks' gestation. The maximum velocity is 2 m/s, which is twice the upper limits of normal.

Ventricular septal defects

After the first few weeks of post-natal life, the pressures in the two ventricles are markedly different. The pressure in the left ventricle is of the order of 80–100 mmHg, whereas that in the right ventricle is less than 20 mmHg. Thus, if there is a restrictive defect in the ventricular septum there will be a high velocity jet from the left to right ventricle in systole. This will be readily detectable by colour flow mapping by seeing a turbulent, multi-coloured jet across the defect (Fig. 15.11). Pulsed or continuous wave Doppler ultrasound positioned on the jet can be used to measure the gradient between the two chambers. However, in prenatal life, the ventricular pressure are normally equal. Thus, there will be little or no flow through a small ventricular defect and bidirectional flow through a larger

Sample volume in right atrium

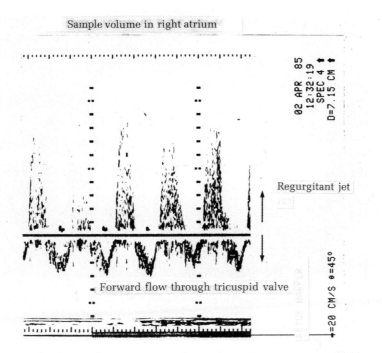

Regurgitant jet

Forward flow through tricuspid valve

Fig. 15.8 Pulsed Doppler waveforms from the right atrium in a fetus with tricuspid regurgitation. With the sample volume positioned in the right atrium, there is normal velocity through the tricuspid valve (the flow below the baseline) but a velocity jet of more than 1 cm/s can be observed passing back into the right atrium during systole.

one. The exception to this would be in cases of obstruction of the outflow of one ventricle where flow through a ventricular septal defect would be in the direction of the unobstructed valve. For example, in tetralogy of Fallot there will be a right-to-left shunt because of the obstruction to the pulmonary outflow tract. Similarly, in co-arctation of the aorta the shunt in a ventricular septal defect will be mainly left to right.

Summary

Pulsed Doppler ultrasonography and colour flow mapping are vital adjuncts to cross-sectional imaging in the accurate evaluation of congenital heart disease prenatally. Their main role is to confirm and clarify a diagnosis suspected by real-time imaging. However, the interpretation of the Doppler results in prenatal life requires a thorough understanding of fetal cardiac function.

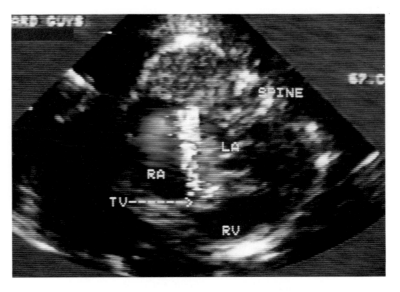

Fig. 15.9 Transverse section of the fetal chest in a case of tricuspid incompetence. The heart can be seen almost to fill the chest, and there is a high velocity jet seen in the right atrium (RA) during systole, indicating severe tricuspid incompetence. LA, left atrium; RV, right ventricle; TV, tricuspid valve.

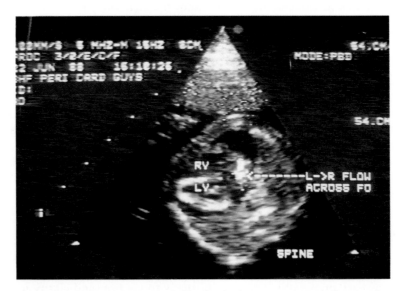

Fig. 15.10 Transverse section of the fetal chest in a case of critical aortic stenosis. The stiff, non-compliant, left ventricle (LV) results in an increased left atrial pressure such that the foramen ovale (FO) flow is from left to right. RV, right ventricle.

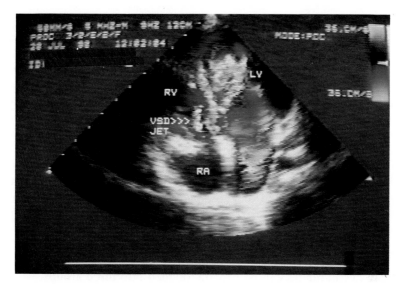

Fig. 15.11 A multi-coloured jet (VSD JET) is seen passing from the left ventricle (LV) to the right ventricle (RV), indicating the site of a small ventricular septal defect in an infant. RA, right atrium.

DIAGNOSIS AND MANAGEMENT OF FETAL DYSRHYTHMIAS

Introduction

Disturbances of fetal heart rate or rhythm are usually discovered incidentally on auscultation or cardiotocographic recordings performed for other reasons. However, increasing attention is now being focused on prenatal cardiac evaluation in high-risk pregnancies (Allan *et al.* 1981, 1983; Devore *et al.* 1983; Kleinman *et al.* 1983; Stewart *et al.* 1987).

The cardiotocograph accurately reflects the rate of rhythm of the fetal heart within the normal range (120–160 b.p.m.), but is often inaccurate in tachydysrhythmias (Kleinman *et al.* 1983; Stewart *et al.* 1983). Fetal electrocardiographic recordings acquired antenatally only reliably record ventricular depolarization; QRS patterns are not clearly seen, and technical difficulties due to vernix caseosa may prevent recordings of any signals during some periods of pregnancy (28–34 weeks).

Real-time directed M-mode echocardiography provides the most useful and accurate method of diagnosing alterations of cardiac rhythm and function, either in isolation or in combination with structural heart disease. Doppler ultrasound techniques may be used to diagnose fetal dysrhythmias but are not as specific as M-mode tracings (Strasburger *et al.* 1986; Steinfeld *et al.* 1986; Reed *et al.* 1987). However, steerable, pulsed Doppler systems allow determination of fetal valvular insufficiency or atrial or venous flow patterns, which may be useful in following the progression (or regression) of cardiac failure. This is of particular importance in assessing the response to therapy in tachydysrhythmias and in following the haemodynamic situation in some conditions such as complete heart block.

Colour flow mapping techniques may be useful in providing immediate information concerning direction of fetal blood flow in intracardiac and extracardiac vessels, but are not useful in determining the type of dysrhythmia. However, adjunctive use of colour flow mapping may shorten the total scanning time as the jet of valvular insufficiency, for example, may be quickly identified to allow placement of the sample gate of the pulsed Doppler system.

Diagnosis of cardiac dysrhythmias

Cardiac dysrhythmias can be broadly divided into three groups:

1. Ectopic beats; defined as persistent irregularities in the fetal heart rate and rhythm.
2. Bradydysrhythmias; defined as a persistent heart rate of less than 100 b.p.m.
3. Tachydysrhythmias; defined as a persistent heart rate of more than 180 b.p.m.

The evaluation of 285 fetuses with a persistent dysrhythmias by the Rotterdam group is illustrated in Table 15.2.

M-mode echocardiography is performed in an attempt to analyse atrial and ventricular mechanical systole. The M-line is directed through the structures to be examined. Atrial systole is identified by movement of the atrial wall towards the atrial septum or aortic root, and ventricular systole

Table 15.2 Evaluation of fetal dysrhythmias (from Stewart *et al.* 1987)

Rhythm abnormality	n	Structural anomaly (%)	Mortality rate (%)
Extrasystoles	216	10 (5)	2 (1)
Bradydysrhythmias	31	16 (52)	10 (32)
Tachydysrhythmias	38	8 (21)	5 (13)
Total	285	34 (12)	17 (6)

is inferred from opening of the atrial valve (Figs 15.12 and 15.13) or from onset of ventricular wall motion towards the septum (Fig. 15.14). Atrial systole may also be inferred from the 'a' wave seen in Figure 15.14 on the tricuspid valve, although the pattern may be difficult to interpret in very high heart rates.

Most workers have adopted the technique of recording the M-mode recording through an atrial wall and an arterial valve. This is readily achieved throughout pregnancy almost regardless of fetal lie.

Ectopic beats

Diagnosis

Supraventricular ectopic beats are frequently encountered (Fig. 15.15). These are not usually accompanied by a ventricular contraction as the atrial contraction occurs during the ventricular refractory period (Fig. 15.16), although this may be observed in fewer than 25 per cent of cases (Fig. 15.17). Premature atrial beats occur in healthy fetuses and neonates (Southall *et al.* 1980*a, b*) and these are associated with a good prognosis. This has been supported by other authors (Devore *et al.* 1983; Kleinman *et al.* 1983) but the Rotterdam group (Table 15.2) reported eight cases (4 per

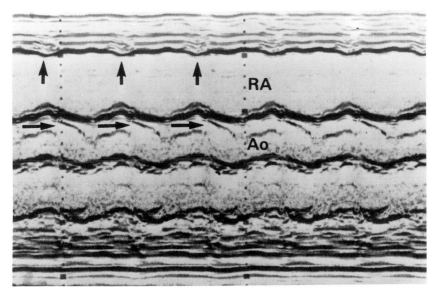

Fig. 15.12 M-mode echocardiogram recorded through the right atrium (RA) and aortic root (Ao). The vertical arrows indicate mechanical atrial systole, and the atrial wall is seen to move towards the aortic wall. The horizontal arrows indicating opening of the aortic valve, inferring mechanical ventricular systole.

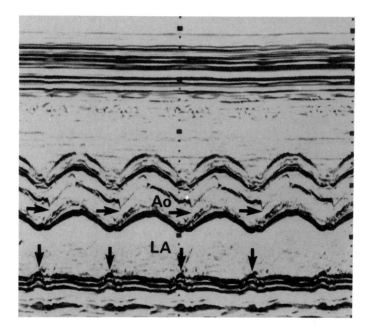

Fig. 15.13 M-mode echocardiogram recorded through the left fetal atrium (LA) and aortic root (Ao). The vertical arrows indicate mechanical atrial systole, and the atrial wall is seen to move towards the aortic wall. The horizontal arrows indicate opening of the aortic valve, inferring mechanical ventricular systole.

cent) of atrial premature beats that were associated with structural anomalies, with fetal death in one case. Thus, all fetuses with atrial premature beats should undergo detailed study of the fetal heart.

Regular screening, probably on a weekly basis, should be carried out on all patients with atrial premature beats, because these may trigger a sustained dysrhythmia in children (Gillette 1976) and this has been observed in a fetus (Stewart *et al.* 1987). In this case, atrial premature beats were observed at 26 weeks' gestation, and these were associated with half-second bursts of atrial flutter. At 32 weeks, the fetus was hydropic with a sustained supraventricular tachydysrhythmia. Following caesarean section, the infant survived and was shown to have the Wolff–Parkinson–White syndrome.

Management

In most fetuses, however, the dysrhythmia is usually benign and either resolves with increasing gestation or within a few days of birth. Rarely, atrial ectopic beats may be associated with aneurysms of the foramen ovale (Stewart and Wladimiroff 1988). Post-natally, these have a totally benign

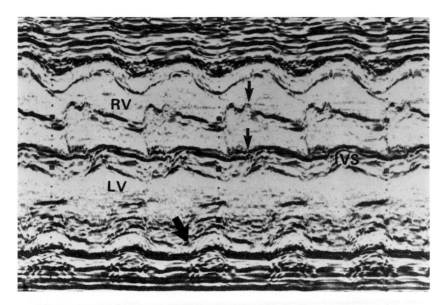

Fig. 15.14 M-mode echocardiogram recorded through the fetal right ventricle (RV) and left ventricle (LV). The heavy arrow indicates the beginning of mechanical systole seen by movement of the ventricular wall towards the intraventricular septum (IVS). The smaller arrows indicate the 'a' wave, indicating mechanical atrial systole.

course, but they should be carefully monitored antenatally because they may obstruct the blood flow through the foramen ovale.

Bradydysrhythmias

Diagnosis

Bradydysrhythmias, especially in the presence of congenital heart disease or hydrops fetalis, have a poor prognosis (Stewart *et al.* 1984; Crawford *et al.* 1985; Wladimiroff *et al.* 1988). Complete heart block in the presence of a structurally normal heart should lead to the search for a maternal connective tissue disorder, particularly systemic lupus erythematosus (Waldimiroff *et al.* 1988).

Congestive cardiac failure will occur in some 20–30 per cent of cases of persistent bradycardia. In the remainder, it appears that, despite the lower heart rate, cardiac output is maintained by an increase in stroke volume (Tonge *et al.* 1986). Cardiac compromise occurs at heart rates of about 45–55 b.p.m., and is presumed to occur as a result of inadequate ventricular

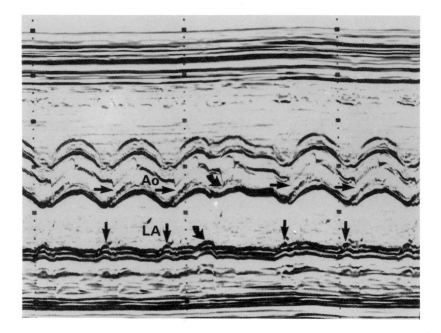

Fig. 15.15 M-mode echocardiogram recorded through the fetal left atrium (LA) and aorta (Ao). The vertical arrows indicate atrial contraction and the horizontal arrows indicate opening of the aortic valve. The curves arrow in the LA shows a premature atrial contraction followed by premature opening of the aortic valve (curved arrow in the Ao).

output due to poor filling rather than from poor ventricular output related to heart rate only.

Bradydysrhythmias are readily diagnosed from M-mode echocardiography (Figs 15.18–15.20). About half will have structural cardiac defects, and karyotyping should be considered (Table 15.2) in these cases. Maternal collagenosis will be present in about one-third of cases.

Management of complete heart block

Structurally normal heart   Maternal connective tissue disorders, predominantly systemic lupus erythematosus (SLE) or Sjögren's syndrome, is present in only 30–50 per cent of women at the time that complete heart block is diagnosed (Scott *et al.* 1988). The majority of asymptomatic women will, however, ultimately develop features of connective tissue disorders (McCune *et al.* 1987). The most commonly detected antibody is Ro(SSA) which is directed against a cytoplasmic RNA binding protein. This is present in almost all mothers whose fetuses have complete heart

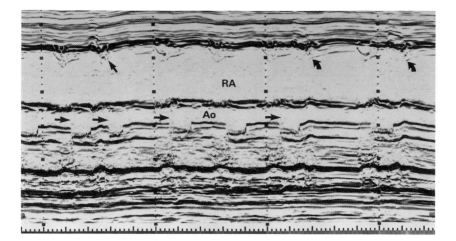

Fig. 15.16 M-mode echocardiogram recorded through the fetal right atrium (RA) and aorta (Ao). The horizontal arrows indicate opening of the aortic valve. The straight arrow in the RA shows a conducted premature atrial contraction. The curved arrows in the RA show a non-conducted premature atrial contraction (note the absence of aortic valve opening).

block and a structurally normal heart, but is present in less than 1 per cent of randomly selected pregnant women (Scott and Bird 1990).

The heart block usually occurs in late pregnancy but has been reported to occur as early as 22 weeks' gestation. Histologically, the major feature is endomyocardial fibrosis with obliteration of the atrioventricular node. The risk of mothers with anti-Ro(SSA) giving birth to infants with complete heart block is unknown, but retrospective data suggest that it is about 6 per cent (Ramsey-Goldman 1986; Scott and Bird 1990). If a previous infant has been affected, the risk increases to about 25 per cent (Ramsey-Goldman 1986). Management of mothers with anti-Ro(SSA) and a previously affected infant is difficult; the use of plasmaphaeresis combined with high-dose dexamethasone has been reported to ameliorate myocarditis, but does not affect the heart block (Buyon *et al.* 1987).

The antenatal management of complete heart block requires referral to a specialist centre that is in close proximity to a paediatric cardiology centre. Regular review looking for chamber enlargement on M-mode echocardiography and decreased cardiac output by pulsed Doppler ultrasonography is necessary, because these precede the development of hydrops fetalis and may be inferred as indicating the development of myocarditis (Buyon *et al.* 1987).

Treatment options are limited, and because of the rarity of the condition

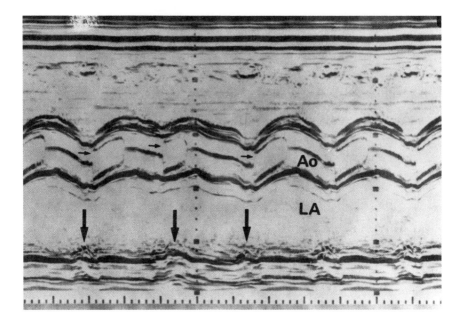

Fig. 15.17 M-mode echocardiogram recorded through the fetal left atrium (LA) and the aorta (Ao). The horizontal arrows indicate opening of the aortic valve. In the second cycle, the aortic valve has opened prematurely and atrial contraction occurs during opening of the aortic valve. This probably represents retrograde conduction to the atria following premature ventricular contractions.

have not been subjected to controlled trials. Dexamethasone or betamethasone cross the placenta and have the added advantage of inducing fetal lung maturity. Transabdominal fetal pacing is technically feasible but often of only short-term benefit. The current advice is that in the presence of fetal lung maturity, the fetus should be delivered.

Delivery in cases of uncomplicated bradydysrhythmias is often carried out by means of caesarean section because conventional heart rate monitoring cannot be used. Atrial rate monitoring may be employed in the assessment of fetal condition but should be combined with repeated fetal scalp pH measurements.

In approximately 15 per cent of cases complete heart block will be fatal and at least a further 20 per cent will require a pacemaker (Scott and Bird 1990). This latter figure is likely to increase as pacemakers are being made smaller and have longer lives. Because there is always a risk of sudden death in individuals with an idioventricular rate of less than 50 b.p.m., the current tendency is to electively pace (D. Ward, personal communication). The heart block is permanent in all individuals and, although there is a

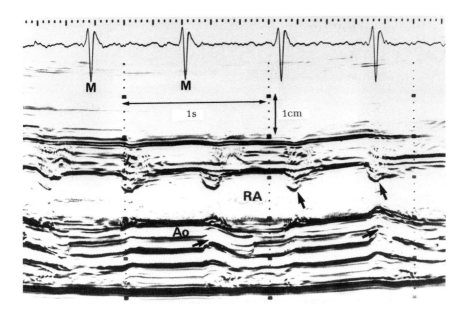

Fig. 15.18 M-mode echocardiogram recorded through the fetal right atrium (RA) and aorta (Ao). The maternal QRS complex is marked with an M. The vertical arrows indicate regular atrial contractions completely dissociated from opening of the aortic valve (horizontal arrows), indicating complete congenital heart block in a fetus with left atrial isomerism and complex heart disease.

close correlation between maternal and neonatal antibody levels at delivery, almost all infants are antibody free by 6 months of age, as anti-Ro(SSA) is immunoglobulin G (Scott and Bird 1990).

Structurally abnormal heart   The outcome for this group is extremely poor (Crawford *et al.* 1985; Allan 1986). Factors to be considered in counselling these patients are the type and severity of the associated structural abnormality, the presence of a chromosomal abnormality, and the gestational age at the time of diagnosis. Antenatal management has to be individualized, bearing in mind the overall poor prognosis.

Tachydysrhythmias

Diagnosis
The estimated incidence of tachydysrhythmias is between 1 in 10 000 and 1 in 25 000 pregnancies, but these figures are likely to be an underestimate

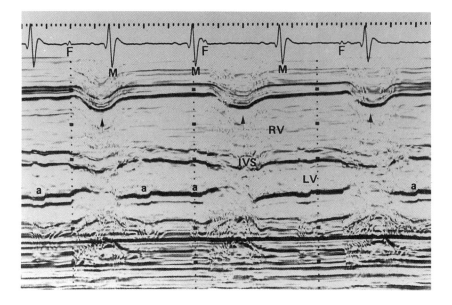

Fig. 15.19 M-mode echocardiogram recorded through the fetal right ventricle (RV) and left ventricle (LV). The vertical arrows indicate ventricular contractions whilst the 'a' reflects atrial contractions on the chordae tendinae of the mitral valve. Fetal cardiac structure was normal in the presence of complete heart block, but the mother was diagnosed as having systemic lupus erythematosus. IVS, intraventricular septum; M, maternal QRS complex; F, fetal QRS complex.

because many cases remain asymptomatic and are therefore undiagnosed (Schreiner *et al.* 1978).

Most tachydysrhythmias are supraventricular in origin. The most common is supraventricular tachycardia (SVT), with heart rates often above 220 b.p.m., which is usually of abrupt onset and termination. Atrial flutter and fibrillation with rates of 300–480 b.p.m. may also occur. Defects of the conducting system have been established in some infants with prenatal tachydysrhythmias (Ho *et al.* 1985) but not in all. Other possible causes may be cardiomyopathy, cardiac tumour, functional instability of the atrial muscle, congenital structural heart disease (5–10 per cent), and congenital infection with cytomegalovirus or Coxsackie B virus. Up to 50 per cent of cases are complicated by hydrops fetalis at presentation (Maxwell *et al.* 1988), and perhaps a further 25 per cent will develop hydrops fetalis (Wladimiroff and Stewart 1985).

The type of tachydysrhythmia is readily diagnosed from the M-mode tracing (Figs 15.21–15.23) and an accurate differentiation should be made before embarking upon treatment (Kleinman *et al.* 1985). It is important to

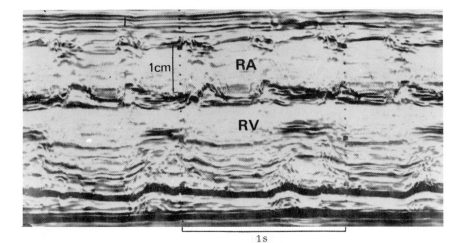

Fig. 15.20 M-mode echocardiogram recorded through the fetal right atrium (RA) and right ventricle (RV). There is complete dissociation between atrial and ventricular contractions, indicating complete heart block.

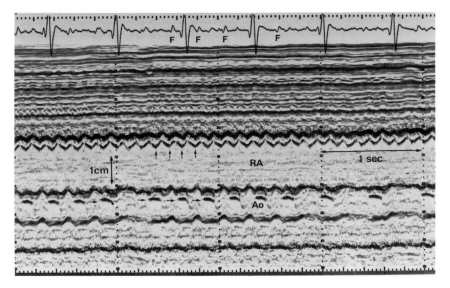

Fig. 15.21 M-mode echocardiogram recorded through the fetal right atrium (RA) and aortic root (Ao) from a fetus with atrial flutter with variable atrioventricular conduction. The small arrows indicate regular atrial contractions, while the horizontal arrows indicate the opening of the aortic valve. F, fetal QRS complex.

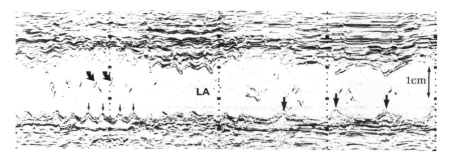

Fig. 15.22 M-mode echocardiogram recorded through the fetal left atrium (LA) from a fetus with paroxysms of atrial flutter (small arrows). The large arrows indicate return to normal rate. This fetus also had frequent episodes of supraventricular extrasystoles. The curved arrows show the movement of the foramen ovale within the LA.

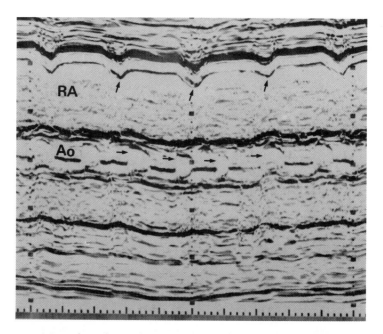

Fig. 15.23 M-mode echocardiogram recorded through the fetal right atrium (RA) and aortic root (Ao), showing complete dissociation. The vertical arrows show atrial contractions, while the horizontal arrows indicate the ventricular rate of about 220 b.p.m. Ventricular tachycardia or A–V junctional tachycardia was suspected. After birth, the diagnosis of tachycardia arising from the bundle of His was diagnosed.

realize that the tachydysrhythmia may be intermittent in both hydropic and non-hydropic fetuses.

Management of tachydysrhythmias

The available options are: (1) expectant management; (2) delivery; and (3) *in utero* treatment. Central to the decision to treat is the knowledge that it is probable that a fetus with a tachycardia has a high chance of developing hydrops fetalis as the pregnancy progresses. It has long been recognized that the prenatal detection of a fetal tachydysrhythmia can be followed by the delivery of a hydropic neonate (Hilrich and Evrard 1955; Herin and Thoren 1973; Newburger and Keane 1979). In the fetal lamb, supraventricular tachycardia produces hydrops fetalis, but this reverses spontaneously when the tachycardiac stimulus is removed (Nimrod *et al.* 1987). In the human fetus, Maxwell *et al.* (1988) have described both the development and worsening of hydrops fetalis *in utero* before control of the tachydysrhythmia has been gained. Currently, there appear to be no specific factors that are predictive of hydrops fetalis.

The common association of polyhydramnios with hydrops fetalis in cases of tachydysrhythmia may lead to pre-term labour and delivery. This suggests that, unless maternal contra-indications are present, prenatal therapy is probably indicated for almost all cases of fetal tachydysrhythmias. Expectant management may be appropriate for a non-hydropic fetus close to term, but careful follow-up is important.

Delivery of an immature fetus with or without hydrops fetalis should be avoided in the absence of compelling obstetric factors as there is little to be gained by adding the complications of prematurity to the management of an uncontrolled tachycardia. The aims of prenatal therapy may be summarized as follows:

(1)   to gain control over the tachydysrhythmia before delivery;

(2)   to prevent hydrops fetalis and polyhydramnios;

(3)   to reverse these complications if present;

(4)   to avoid the complications of pre-term delivery.

The incidence of structural abnormalities with fetal tachydysrhythmias varies from none (Maxwell *et al.* 1988) to 20 per cent (Table 15.2), but all fetuses with a tachydysrhythmia should have detailed real-time study of the cardiac anatomy. Karyotyping in the presence of a structurally normal heart is not indicated. As well as specific treatment for dysrhythmias, the fetus should have regular studies of fetal growth. Cardiotocography (non-stress testing) is unreliable in tachydysrhythmias and Doppler blood flow studies of the fetal circulation are difficult to interpret and are of uncertain value at present.

Non-hydropic fetuses may be managed in the out-patients department once the diagnosis has been established, but all mothers of hydropic fetuses should be admited.

Drug therapy

Maternal administration of anti-dysrhythmic drugs is the mainstay of pre-natal therapy for tachydysrhythmias. The ideal agent would be rapidly effective in controlling the rhythm and would be safe for the mother. Both fetal and maternal drug levels should accurately reflect placental transport, allowing ease of monitoring.

The most commonly used drugs are digoxin, and verapamil. There is limited experienced with other agents, including amiodarone (Arnoux *et al.* 1987), propanolol (Kleinman *et al.* 1985), quinidine (Spinnato *et al.* 1984), flecainide (Wren and Hunter 1988), and adenosine (Clarke *et al.* 1987).

Digoxin   Digoxin is the most frequently reported agent (Lingman *et al.* 1980; Kleinman *et al.* 1985; Wladimiroff and Stewart 1985; Maxwell *et al.* 1988). Maxwell *et al.* (1988) reported that it is most effective in the treatment of atrial fibrillation (AF) and SVT in the non-hydropic fetus. Despite its widespread use, digoxin does not meet the criteria for an ideal agent because the time taken to control the fetal dysrhythmia is highly variable (Maxwell *et al.* 1988) and there is considerable uncertainty as to how much of the drug crosses the placenta (Chan *et al.* 1978; Younis and Granat 1987). Maxwell (personal communication) has demonstrated that fetal levels (obtained by percutaneous umbilical blood sampling) are approximately 40–50 per cent of the maternal level.

The presence of a digoxin-like immunoreactive factor which is detected by digoxin assays has been isolated from both pregnant and non-pregnant women who have never received digoxin (Graves *et al.* 1984; Ebara *et al.* 1986; Gonzales *et al.* 1987). Weiner *et al.* (1987) have demonstrated the presence of a digoxin-like substance in cord blood of fetuses, with and without cardiac abnormalities. These reports mean that fetal levels cannot be inferred from maternal levels. Furthermore, digoxin assays vary widely in their ability to provide true digoxin levels in the mother or fetus (Valdes *et al.* 1984; Soldin 1985; Valdes 1985; Graves *et al.* 1986). These difficulties, together with the fact that digoxin alone is not effective in the presence of hydrops fetalis, has lead to a search for alternative therapies.

Verapamil   Verapamil, given in combination with digoxin, is effective in some cases of tachydysrhythmias in hydropic fetuses (Maxwell *et al.* 1988). Neonatal paediatricians, however, have reservations because of isolated case reports of sudden, unexplained death following verapamil administration.

Flecainide Flecainide is a potent class Ic anti-dysrhythmic drug with applications in the management of atrial, junctional, and ventricular dysrhythmias. It has been used in the paediatric age group with efficacy and apparent safety. However, recent reports of an increase in sudden death in adults following myocardial infarction have led to reservations over its use in patients with myocardial damage (Cardiac arrhythmia suppression trial investigators 1989). Early reports on 16 cases (Allan *et al.* 1991) have suggested that it may be useful in hydropic fetuses with and SVT.

Protocol for treatment A suggested protocol for the treatment of fetal tachydysrhythmias is as follows:

1. *Non-hydropic fetus with an SVT or AF*: Digoxin 0.25 mg twice daily increasing to three times a day if necessary.

2. *Hydrops fetalis with AF*: Digoxin (as above) with verapamil 80 mg three times a day increasing to 160 mg three times a day if necessary.

3. *Hydrops fetalis with SVT*: Flecainide 100 mg three times a day.

Methods of administration The problems of uncertain transfer have led to the suggestion that drugs should be given directly to the fetus. There are case reports of digoxin given directly into the umbilical vein (Gembruch *et al.* 1988*a*) and intramuscularly into the fetus (Weiner and Thompson 1988). Maxwell (personal communication) has also had experience of direct administration of verapamil into the umbilical vein in a fetus that was subsequently shown to be hypoxic and acidotic: asystole occurred.

The new agent adenosine has an extremely short half-life, which makes it inappropriate for maternal administration. Maxwell (personal communication) has used direct intracardiac administration of adenosine, which whilst technically successful failed to cause rhythm conversion. An alternative, recently suggested, route is intraperitoneal injection (Gembruch *et al.* 1988*b*) and depot injections of sustained-release preparations may hold future promise.

Polyhydramnios The maternal discomfort and uterine activity secondary to the associated polyhydramnios is an important aspect of management. There are no randomized, controlled trials to determine the best approach, but the choice of therapy for symptomatic polyhydramnios is continuous drainage or intermittent tapping (Pearce *et al.* 1991). Intermittent tapping with restoration of amniotic pressure to the normal level of a data reference range (Nicolini *et al.* 1989) is gaining popularity. The timing of repeat taps is difficult but can be determined from the size of amniotic columns as measured on real-time ultrasonography; it is usually of the order of 2–3 days in cases of polyhydramnios associated with hydrops fetalis owing to tachydysrhythmias.

Maternal administration of indomethacin has been reported to reduce polyhydramnios by reducing fetal urine production (Cabrol *et al.* 1987). This approach does not seem logical in cases of hydrops fetalis associated with tachydyrhythmias, because the polyhydramnios is the result of a fetal diuresis, an attempt to deal with the heart failure.

Fetal drainage procedures   There are no controlled trials as to the value of drainage of fetal pleural effusions and ascites. Individual cases may benefit from drainage just before delivery, because this allows easier resuscitation after delivery. Determining whether control of paroxysmal tachydysrhythmias has occurred is difficult but may be inferred from resolving pleural effusions. Draining these effusions does not remove the ability to monitor progress as failure of control results in recurrence of the effusions.

Fetal–maternal monitoring

Monitoring of therapy requires frequent attendance at the diagnostic centre. In-patients are scanned every second day to assess rhythm, hydrops, and fetal activity. Out-patients may be assessed on a weekly basis, because all cases of hydrops fetalis should be managed as in-patients.

There are, at present, no easy methods for monitoring fetal heart rate. Conventional heart rate monitors are not suitable because they have logic circuits that halve very fast heart rates. Phonocardiography (Talbert *et al.* 1986) has been reported to be useful, but is not widely available. Most workers use conventional cardiotocographic machines from which the logic circuit have been removed, thus allowing rates of up to 480 b.p.m. to be recorded.

Maternal drug levels should initially be checked at least weekly. All women receiving anti-dysrhythmic drugs should have electrocardiography before therapy, and should probably have a 24-h tape recording a few days after commencing therapy, repeated on a weekly basis.

Conclusion

The treatment of fetal dysrhythmias depends upon accurate diagnosis, which is best performed by M-mode echocardiography. This, however, should be backed up by real-time, pulsed Doppler and colour flow ultrasonography to determine cardiac structure and to estimate cardiac function. It should be remembered that paroxysmal tachydysrhythmias may result in hydrops fetalis, and that this diagnosis may be difficult to make.

Prolonged monitoring by means of a cardiotocography machine with the logic circuit removed appears to be the current best bet.

Prenatal therapy for congenital heart block is limited, mostly to delivery of the fetus who is thought to be mature. Monitoring of ventricular size and function may suggest the development of subendocardial fibrosis, which may indicate the use of steroids.

Tachydysrhythmias always warrant prenatal therapy because pre-term delivery worsens the problems for the perinate. Digoxin alone or with other agents appears to be effective, particularly in non-hydropic fetuses. However, questions still exist over the placental transfer of such drugs and the variable time taken to achieve control. New, invasive methods of therapy are still in the process of being assessed.

REFERENCES

Allan, L. D. (1986). *Manual of fetal echocardiography.* MTP Press.

Allan, L. D., Tynan, M., Campbell, S., and Anderson, R. H. (1981). Normal fetal cardiac anatomy: a basis for echographic detection of abnormalities. *Prenatal Diagnosis,* **1,** 131–5.

Allan, L. D., Anderson, R. H., Sullivan, I. D., Campbell, S., Holt, D. W., and Tynan, M. (1983). Evaluation of fetal arrhythmias by echocardiography. *British Heart Journal,* **50,** 240–5.

Allan, L. D., Chita, S. K., Al-Ghazali, W. H., Crawford, D. C., and Tynan, M. J. (1987). Doppler echocardiographic evaluation of the normal human fetal heart. *British Heart Journal,* **57,** 528–33.

Allan, L. D., Chita, S. K., Sharland, G. K., Maxwell, D., and Priestley, K. (1991). Flecainide in the treatment of feral tachycardias. *British Heart Journal,* (in press).

Al-Ghazali, W. H., Chita, S. K., Chapman, M. G., and Allan, L. D. (1989). Evidence of redistribution of the cardiac output in asymmetrical growth retardation. *British Journal of Obstetrics and Gynaecology,* **96,** 697–704.

Arnoux, P., Seyral, P., Llurens, M., *et al.* (1987). Amiodarone and digoxin for refractory fetal tachycardia. *American Journal of Cardiology,* **59,** 166–7.

Block, B. S. B., Liaos, A. J., and Creasy, R. K. (1984). Responses of the growth retarded fetus to acute hypoxia. *American Journal of Obstetrics and Gynecology,* **148,** 878–92.

Buyon, J. P., Swersky, S. H., Fox, H. E., Bierman, F. Z., and Winchester, R. J. (1987). Intrauterine therapy for presumptive myocarditis with acquired heart block due to systemic lupus erythematosus. *Arthritis and Rheumatism,* **30,** 44–8.

Cabrol, D., Landesman, R., Muller, J., Uzan, M., Sureau, C., and Saxene, B. B. (1987). Treatment of polyhydramnios with prostaglandin synthetase inhibitor (indomethacin). *American Journal of Obstetrics and Gynecology,* **157,** 422–6.

Campbell, S. and Thoms, A. (1977). Ultrasound measurement of the fetal head to abdominal circumference ratio in the assessment of growth retardation. *British Journal of Obstetrics and Gynaecology,* **84,** 165–74.

Cardiac arrythmia suppression trial investigators (1989). *New England Journal of Medicine,* **321,** 406–12.

Chan, V., Tse, T. F., and Wong, V. (1978). Transfer of digoxin across the placenta and into the breast milk. *British Journal of Obstetrics and Gynaecology*, **85**, 605–9.

Clarke, B., Rowland, E., Barnes, P. J., Till, J., Ward, D. E., and Shinebourne, E. A. (1987). Rapid and safe termination of supraventricular tachycardia in children with adenosine. *Lancet*, **i**, 299–300.

Crawford, D. L., Chapman, M., and Allan, L. D. (1985). The assessment of persistent bradycardia in prenatal life. *British Journal of Obstetrics and Gynaecology*, **92**, 941–4.

Dawes, G. S., Lewis, B. V., Milligar, J. E., Roach, M. R., and Talner, N. S. (1968). Vasomotor responses in the hind limbs of fetal and new-born lambs to asphyxia and aortic chemoreceptor stimulation. *Journal of Physiology*, **195**, 55–81.

de Smedt, G. H., Visser, G. H., and Meijboom, E. J. (1987). Fetal cardiac output estimated by Doppler echocardiography during mild and late gestation. *American Journal of Cardiology*, **60**, 338–42.

Devore, G. R., Siassi, B., and Platt, L. D. (1983). Fetal echocardiography. The diagnosis of cardiac arrhythmias using real-time-directed M-mode ultrasound. *American Journal of Obstetrics and Gynecology*, **146**, 792–9.

Ebara, H., Suzuki, S., Hagashima, K., *et al.* (1986). Digoxin and digitoxin-like immunoreactive substances in amniotic fluid, cord blood and serum neonates. *Pediatric Research*, **20**, 28–31.

Gembruch, U., Hansmann, M., and Bald, R. (1988*a*). Direct intrauterine treatment of fetal tachyarrhythmias and severe hydrops fetalis by antiarrhythmic drugs. *Fetal Therapy*, **3**, 210–15.

Gembruch, U., Hansmann, M., Redel, D. A., and Bald, R. (1988*b*). Intrauterine therapy of fetal tachyarrhythmic drugs to intraperitoneal tachyarrhythmias with severe hydrops fetalis. *Journal of Perinatal Medicine*, **16**, 39–44.

Gilbert, E. D. (1982). Effects of afterload and baroreceptors on cardiac function in fetal sheep. *Journal of Developmental Physiology*, **4**, 299–36.

Gillette, P. C. (1976). The mechanism of supraventricular tachycardia in children. *Circulation*, **54**, 133–40.

Gonzalez, A. R., Phelps, S. J., Cochran, E. B., and Sibai, B. M. (1987). Digoxin-like immunoreactive substance in pregnancy. *American Journal of Obstetrics and Gynecology*, **157**, 660–4.

Graves, S. W., Valdes, R., Brown, B. A., Knight, A. B., and Craig, H. R. (1984). Endogenous digoxin-immunoreactive substance in human pregnancies. *Journal of Clinical Endocrinology and Metabolism*, **58**, 748–51.

Graves, S. W., Sharma, K., and Chandler, A. B. (1986). Methods for eliminating interferences in digoxin immunoassays caused by digoxin-like factors. *Clinical Chemistry*, **32**, 1506–9.

Herin, P. and Thoren, C. (1973). Congenital arrhythymias with supraventricular tachycardia in the perinatal period. *Acta Obstetricia et Gynaecologica Scandinavica*, **52**, 381–6.

Hilrich, N. M. and Evrard, J. R. (1955). Supraventricular tachycardia in the newborn with onset in utero. *American Journal of Obstetrics and Gynecology*, **70**, 1139–42.

Ho, S. Y., Mortimer, G., and Anderson, R. H. (1985). Conduction system defects in three perinatal patients with arrhythmia. *British Heart Journal*, **53**, 158–63.

Huhta, J. C., Strasburger, J. F., and Carpenter, R. J. (1982). Pulsed Doppler feral echocardiography. *Journal of Clinical Ultrasound*, **13**, 247–54.

Kenny, J. P., Plappert, T., Doubilet, P., Saltzman, D. H., Cartier, M., Zollars, L., Leatherman, G. F., and St. John Sutton, M. G. (1986). Changes in the cardiac blood flow velocities and right and left ventricular stroke volumes with gestrional age in the normal human fetus: a prospective Doppler echo cardiographic study. *Circulation*, **74**, 1208–16.

Kleinman, C. S., Donnerstein, R. L., Jaffe, C. C., Dekore, G. R., Weinstein, E. M., Lynch, D. C., Talner, N. S., Burkowitz, R. L., and Hobbins, J. C. (1983). Fetal echocardiography. A tool for evaluation of in utero cardiac dysrhythmias and monitoring of in utero therapy. *American Journal of Cardiology*, **51**, 237–43.

Maxwell, D. J., Crawford, D. C., Curry, P. V. M., Tynan, M. J., and Allan, L. D. (1988). Obstetric importance of the diagnosis and management of feral tachycardias. *British Medical Journal*, **297**, 107–10.

Newburger, J. W. and Keane, J. F. (1979). Intrauterine supraventricular tachycardia. *Journal of Pediatrics*, **95**, 780–6.

Nicolini, U., Fisk, N. M., Talbert, D. G., *et al.* (1989). Intrauterine manometry: technique and application to fetal pathology. *Prenatal Diagnosis*, **9**, 243–54.

Nimrod, C., Davies, D., Harder, J., Iwanicki, S., Kondo, C., Takahaski, Y., Maloney, J., Persaud, D., and Nicholson, S. (1987). Ultrasound evaluation of tachycardia-induced hydrops in the fetal lamb. *American Journal of Obstetrics and Gynecology*, **157**, 655–9.

Pearce, J. M., Fisk, N., and Rodeck, C. (1991). The operative management of abnormalities of amniotic fluid volume. In *An atlas of ultrasound* (ed. F. Chervanek). Little, Brown & Co., New York (in press).

Ramsey-Goldman, R. (1986). Anti-SSA antibodies and fetal outcomes in maternal systemic lupus erythematosus. *Arthritis and Rheumatism*, **39**, 1269–73.

Reed, K. L., Meijboom, E. J., Sahn, D. J., Scagnelli, S. A., Valdes-Cruz, L. M., and Shenker, A. L. (1986). Cardiac Doppler flow velocities in human fetuses. *Circulation*, **73**, 41–6.

Reed, K. L., Sahn, D. J., Marx, G. R., Anderson, C. F., and Shenker, L. (1987). Cardiac Doppler flows during fetal arrhythmias: physiologic consequences. *Obstetrics and Gynecology*, **70**, 1–6.

Rizzo, G., Arduini, D., Romanini, C., and Mancuso, S. (1988). Doppler echocardiographic assessment of atrioventricular velocity waveforms in normal and small for gestation age fetuses. *British Journal of Obstetrics and Gynaecology*, **95**, 65–9.

Rudolph, A. M. (1973). Control of the fetal circulation. In *Proceedings of the Sir Barcroft centenary symposium on fetal physiology*, pp. 88–111. Cambridge University Press, Cambridge.

Ruess, M. L., Parer, J. I., Harris, J. L., and Kreuger, T. R. (1982). Haemodynamic effects of alpha-adrenergic blockade during hypoxia in fetal sheep. *American Journal of Obstetrics and Gynecology*, **18**, 199–205.

Schreiner, R. L., Hurwitz, R. A., Rosenfeld, C. R., and Miller, W. (1978). Atrial tachyarrhythmias associated with massive edema in the newborn. *Journal of Perinatal Medicine*, **6**, 274–9.

Scott, J. S. and Bird, H. A. (1990). *Pregnancy, autoimmunity and connective tissue disorders*. Oxford University Press, Oxford.

Scott, J. S., Maddison, P. J., Taylor, P. V., Esscher, E., Scott, O., and Skinner, R. P. (1983). Connective tissue disease, antibodies to ribonucleoprotein, and congenital heart block. *New England Journal of Medicine*, **309**, 209–12.

Sharland, G. K., Chita, S. K., and Allan, L. D. (1989). The use of colour Doppler in fetal echocardiography. *International Journal of Cardiology*, **28**, 229–36.

Soldin, S. J. (1985). Digoxin: issues and controversies. *Clinical Chemistry*, **32**, 5–12.

Southall, D. P., Johnston, A. M., and Shinebourne, E. A. (1980*a*). Study of the nature and natural history of disorders of cardiac rhythm and conduction in the apparently healthy infant. In *Paediatric cardiology. Proceedings of the first world congress in paediatric cardiology* (ed. P. Goodman), pp. 67–73. Churchill Livingstone, London.

Steinfeld, L., Rappaport, H. L., Rossbach, H. C., and Martinez, E. (1986). Diagnosis of fetal arrhythmias using echocardiographic and Doppler techniques. *Journal of the American College of Cardiology*, —, 1425–33.

Spinnato, J. A., Shaver, D. C., Flinn, G. S., Sibai, B. M., Watson, D. L., and Marin-Garcia, J. (1984). Fetal supraventricular tachycardia; *in utero* therapy with digoxin and quinidine. *American Journal of Obstetrics and Gynecology*, **64**, 730–5.

Steinfeld, L., Rappaport, H. L., Rossbach, H. C., and Martinez, E. (1986). Diagnosis of fetal arrhythmias using echocardiographic and Doppler techniques. *Journal of the American College of Cardiology*, **8**, 1425–33.

Stewart, P. A., Tonge, H. M., and Wladimiroff, J. W. (1983). Arrhythmia and structural abnormalities of the fetal heart. *British Heart Journal*, **50**, 550–4.

Stewart, P. A., Becker, A. E., and Wladimiroff, J. W. (1984). Left atrial isomerism associated with asplenia: prenatal echocardiographic detection of complex congenital cardiac malformation. *Journal of the American College of Cardiology*, **4**, 1015–20.

16. Neonatal cerebral blood flow

Alan Fenton and Malcolm Levene

INTRODUCTION

Little (1843) called attention to the fact that certain complications of the birth process resulted in mental retardation and bilateral spasticity. This was seen particularly in pre-term and asphyxiated infants. The role of impaired cerebral perfusion in the aetiology of such brain injury in the newborn has been recognized since Parrot (1873) attributed pathological changes in the periventricular white matter to cerebrovascular insufficiency. Many studies since that time have implicated disordered cerebrovascular regulation in both term and pre-term cerebral injury, although much of the pathophysiology remains incompletely understood.

FACTORS INFLUENCING CEREBRAL BLOOD FLOW

The control of cerebral blood flow is extremely complex and is influenced by many interrelated physiological variables. Those factors that have been examined in detail include arterial blood pressure (ABP), arterial carbon dioxide and oxygen tensions (P_{A,CO_2} and P_{a,O_2} respectively), and autonomic innervation.

It was widely believed for many years that cerebral blood flow varied directly with ABP. This concept, known as the Monro–Kellie doctrine, persisted until 1938 when Fog demonstrated the ability of the cerebral circulation to respond independently to oppose changes in ABP. From this and subsequent studies it was concluded that over a range of blood pressures, changes in vessel diameter maintained cerebral blood flow relatively constant by altering cerebrovascular resistance.

These observations gave rise to the concept of autoregulation, which may be defined as the intrinsic tendency of an organ to maintain constant blood flow despite changes in perfusion pressure. Within certain limits the ability to maintain adequate cerebral blood flow over a considerable range of blood pressures has been demonstrated both in animal studies (Rapela and Green 1964; Harper 1966; Yoshida *et al.* 1966; Strandgaard *et al.* 1974) and in humans (Agnoli *et al.* 1968; Olesen 1973). In pre-term animals, however, the blood pressure range over which autoregulation occurs has been found to be narrower than in the adult, and in addition the mean blood pressure was close to the lower limit of autoregulation (Papile *et al.* 1985). This may be one factor that predisposes the pre-term brain to ischaemic injury.

It is important to note that whilst global hemispheric blood flow is maintained at a fairly constant level, there may be great variation in regional blood flow which corresponds to neuronal activity. For example, during voluntary muscle contraction in the hand, blood flow is seen to increase in the sensorimotor cortical hand area (Olesen *et al.* 1971). The increase in neuronal activity is analogous to an increase in physical work performed by voluntary muscles, and thus requires an increase in energy supply and hence blood flow. This suggests the linking of cerebral blood flow to metabolic demands, although the exact mechanisms involved are uncertain. Clearly autoregulation is not simply a function of the responses to changes in perfusion pressure. It may also be defined as the capability of an organ to regulate its blood supply in accordance with its needs. This involves the interraction of several other factors in addition to perfusion pressure on cerebrovascular resistance to maintain cerebral blood flow at an adequate level to support cerebral function.

Changes in the calibre of blood vessels on the surface of the brain resulting from experimental asphyxia were first observed more than 100 years ago in animal studies (Donders 1851) but it was not until the studies of Wolff and Lennox (1930) that this effect was shown to be largely due to changes in P_{A,CO_2}, and to a lesser extent to changes in P_{A,O_2}. The cerebrovascular response to P_{A,CO_2} is mainly a local and intrinsic phenomenon mediated by changes in extracellular fluid pH, hypercapnia leading to a fall in cerebrovascular resistance and consequently to a rise in cerebral blood flow. Wolff and Lennox (1930) studied the effects of hypoxia separately from hypercapnia and demonstrated that the cerebral vessels were more sensitive to changes in P_{A,CO_2} than changes in P_{A,O_2}. Hypoxia was shown to cause vasodilatation, and hyperoxia to cause vasoconstriction, the response to hyperoxia decreasing after the neonatal period (Kennedy *et al.* 1971).

The role of the autonomic nervous system in the regulation of cerebral blood flow has been the subject of much controversy, and a full review is given by Edvinsson and MacKenzie (1976). In summary, however, although various studies have demonstrated that cerebral blood vessels have the capacity to respond to autonomic stimulation, they do not prove that such a capacity subserves an important physiological function under normal conditions. It may, however, be of use in situations where normal regulatory limits have been reached (Berntman *et al.* 1979) or, in the extreme preterm situation, if normal regulatory mechanisms have not been fully established.

Measurement of cerebral blood flow

In choosing a method for measurement of cerebral blood flow, there is a need to consider safety, clinical applicability, quantitative performance, and the actual physiological or clinical questions being asked. Additionally, in view of the considerable differences in regional blood flow that may occur, any method of assessing cerebral blood flow will give only a crude overall estimation.

Measurement of cerebral blood flow in the newborn has been attempted by a variety of techniques including: (a) the Kety–Schmidt method; (b) radio-labelled isotope clearance (e.g. ^{133}Xe); (c) venous occlusion plethysmography; (d) electrical impedance plethysmography; (e) positron emission tomography; and (f) near infra-red spectroscopy. The major drawbacks of these methods include the need for repeated blood sampling (a), the use of ionizing radiation (b and e), variability of skull compliance and the inclusion of extracerebral blood flow in measurements (c) lack of validation against volumetric flow (d), non-portability of equipment (e), and the assumption of constant cerebral blood volume and oxygen extraction during measurements (f).

Following a report by Bada *et al.* (1979, Doppler ultrasonography has also been used to examine cerebral haemodynamics in infants. Early studies utilized continuous wave equipment, and results were therefore given in terms of angle-independent indices such as the Pourcelot resistance index (RI). Subsequently, duplex systems allowed accurate, reproducible placement of the Doppler sample volume for measurement of cerebral blood flow velocity in cm/s. This is unlike the techniques above, which express cerebral blood flow in volumetric terms per unit brain weight per minute (apart from electrical impedance plethysmography). The major limitation of this method in terms of assessing absolute volumetric changes in cerebral blood flow is that it assumes a constant blood vessel cross-sectional area, and measurement of cerebral arterial diameter in neonates is beyond the resolution powers of current imaging equipment. However, changes in cerebral blood flow velocity have been shown to be closely related to changes in cerebral blood flow (Batton *et al.* 1983; Hansen *et al.* 1983), and within certain limitations this technique provides a non-invasive bedside method of assessing changes within the cerebral circulation, even in extremely sick infants.

SIGNAL ACQUISITION AND ANALYSIS

The anterior fontanelle is most commonly used in neonates to insonate one anterior cerebral artery (ACA), although in practice it is not possible to distinguish the side being insonated, since the arteries run almost adjacent to each other. The ACA is visualized in the sagittal plane, and insonation at a point mid-way between the inferior-most border of the corpus callosum and the vessel's origin from the circle of Willis enables the angle of insonation to be kept below 10° (Fig. 16.1). Alternatively, the middle cerebral artery (MCA) may be visualized through the ipsilateral temporal bone in the fold of the temporal lobe. Using this approach, both the course

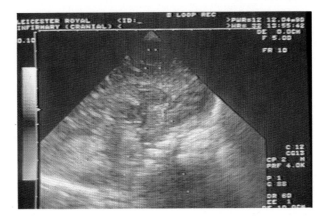

Fig. 16.1 Anterior cerebral artery visualized in the parasagittal plane, using colour Doppler ultrasonography for clarity. The vessel's course allows the angle of insonation via the anterior fontanelle to be kept to less than 20°

of the vessel and blood flow in its straight mid-portion will be directly towards the transducer, again minimizing the angle of insonation (Fig. 16.2). Sick pre-term infants tolerate repeated handling poorly, but intermittent sampling over a period of hours from the MCA is possible, using a miniature probe recently described, which is simply fixed to the infant's skin (Fenton *et al.* 1990*a*).

In addition to the arterial side, the venous component of the cerebral circulation has been studied using both conventional (Cowan and Thoresen 1985; Pfannschmidt and Jorch 1989) and colour flow (Fenton *et al.* 1990*b*) Doppler techniques. The latter simplifies identification of the relatively low flow, non-pulsatile veins and allows the optimal angle of insonation to be obtained (Fig. 16.3).

It is good practice to record Doppler signals on to digital audiotape and to perform analysis at a later time. The advantages of digital over analogue tape have recently been reviewed (Evans *et al.* 1989*b*). A maximum frequency follower is used to determine cerebral blood flow velocity from the

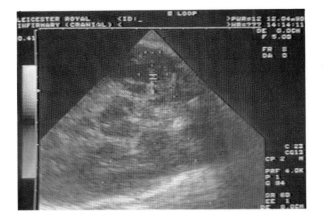

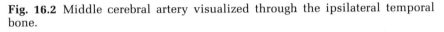

Fig. 16.2 Middle cerebral artery visualized through the ipsilateral temporal bone.

sonogram, since the haemodynamic conditions that prevail in the neonatal brain, that is, predominantly unidirectional, established laminar flow, are particularly suited to the application of this method. The major advantages of this method are that it is resistant to noise and to measures designed to reduce noise such as high-pass filters (Evans *et al.* 1989*a*). In addition, its output is independent of the way in which the ultrasound beam samples the blood vessel. The maximum frequency outline is superimposed on the sonogram display to ensure that the desired part of the spectrum is being followed. Using this method and assuming a parabolic flow velocity

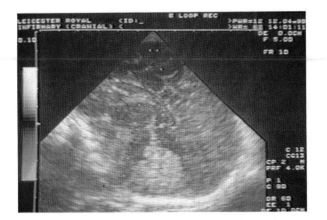

Fig. 16.3 Vein of Galen. Colour Doppler ultrasonography allows easy identification of such relatively low-flow vessels.

profile, the time-averaged maximum velocity obtained will be twice the time-averaged mean (Evans 1985).

Use of waveforms and reference ranges

Doppler waveforms in the newborn have been used mostly for research purposes. The transition from intra-uterine to independent life requires many major physiological changes, most notably in the cardiovascular and respiratory systems. The elimination of the umbilico-placental circulation and the closure of vascular shunts at birth dramatically alter the haemodynamics of the circulation. In particular, the umbilico-placental circulation tends to dampen the reactivity of the fetal circulation to the effects of vaso-active agents, and after birth the circulatory response to both physiological and pathological stress is enhanced. The ability of the brain and other organs to regulate their blood flow depending on their metabolic requirements during this change-over period is essential to the maintenance of normal function.

Wigglesworth and Pape's model for cerebral injury in the pre-term neonate (1978) has prompted many studies directed at elucidating the sequence of events that results in neurodevelopmental injury. The majority of this work has been directed at examining circulatory parameters, in particular blood pressure and cerebral blood flow, and relating these to subsequent outcome.

Many clinical events in the sick neonate such as apnoea, bradycardia, endotracheal tube suction, pneumothorax, and seizures result in profound changes in the cerebral circulation as assessed by Doppler ultrasonography. Many of the changes detected in this way result primarily from disturbances in blood pressure and are therefore to be expected; they do not contribute further to the management of such conditions. In addition, relatively minor events such as rotation of the infant's head during normal nursing care may produce cessation of blood flow in the cerebral veins without apparent ill-effect (Cowan and Thoresen 1985). Clearly, the information obtained using these techniques requires further evaluation before its use is extended beyond the research setting. However, these and similar studies may provide information on the mechanisms responsible for the regulation of cerebral blood flow in the neonate.

Normal ranges for cerebral blood flow velocity and RI in both the ACA and MCA during the first days of life have been established for pre-term (Evans *et al.* 1988) and term infants (Fenton *et al.* 1990c). These are shown in Table 16.1. The main feature of note is the increase in velocity and fall in RI in the first 2–3 days of life, which may represent post-natal cerebrovascular dilatation. As discussed previously, vessel diameter cannot be accurately measured and thus cerebrovascular resistance (mean blood pressure

Table 16.1 Normal range (±1SD) for cerebral blood flow velocity in the anterior cerebral artery (ACA) and middle cerebral artery (MCA) in term and pre-term infants during the first week of life. (From Evans *et al.* 1988 and Fenton et al. *1990c*, with permission)

Age (h)	ACA (cm/s)		mCA (cm/s)	
Term	Pre-term	Term	Pre-term	Term
6		6.20 (2.10)		6.90 (2.00)
12	3.35 (1.60)		4.75 (2.45)	
18		8.40 (2.00)		10.00 (2.30)
36	4.65 (1.75)	8.70 (2.40)	6.50 (2.10)	11.50 (2.30)
60	6.30 (2.60)	9.70 (3.10)	8.15 (2.95)	11.80 (2.70)
84	6.05 (2.10)		8.10 (3.10)	
96		11.50 (3.60)		15.00 (3.90)
108	6.90 (2.50)		9.25 (4.20)	
132	5.70 (1.75)		8.90 (2.20)	
156	6.35 (2.05)	10.90 (2.70)	8.95 (2.70)	13.90 (3.10)

divided by mean blood flow) cannot be obtained directly. Evans *et al.* (1988) suggested the use of an index of resistance which is calculated by dividing mean blood pressure by mean velocity. This index is therefore the product of the peripheral resistance and the cross-sectional area of the vessel at the site of insonation, and is termed the resistance area product.

CLINICAL APPLICATIONS

The main area of clinical use of these ranges is in the management of post-asphyxial encephalopathy (PAE), which remains a major cause of morbidity in term infants. There has been no significant advance in the treatment of this condition, and invasive techniques such as intracranial pressure monitoring have been shown to be of no benefit. Previous work has demonstrated disordered cerebral blood flow patterns in this condition, and Archer *et al.* (1986) found that the positive predictive value of an abnormal RI for death or severe impairment was 83 per cent. In addition, abnormal cerebral blood flow velocity (less than two standard deviations below the mean and/or more than three standard deviations above the mean) had a positive predictive value for a similar outcome of 94 per cent (Levene *et al.* 1989). The abnormal cerebral blood flow velocity, which is argued to represent extreme variations in cerebral blood flow (see above), was felt to arise as a result of vasoparalysis, but whether it contributes to the pathophysiology of PAE or is merely symptomatic of it remains uncertain.

Two other clinical situations in which changes in RI have been suggested to be of value are, first, in the diagnosis of neonatal brain death, in which McMenamin and Volpe (1983) described a gradual diminution in and disappearance of Doppler signals. Hill and Volpe (1982) observed an abnormally high RI in hydrocephalus, which returned to more normal values after drainage. Neither of these suggested applications has found widespread use. The study of venous flow may provide information on the postulated role of venous infarction in certain types of parenchymal injury (Gould *et al.* 1987).

In summary, Doppler ultrasonography provides a useful non-invasive research tool for the study of neonatal cerebral blood flow. Its clinical use is currently lmited to a prognostic indicator in PAE. It may, however, provide information in the future on factors that regulate cerebral blood flow.

REFERENCES

Agnoli, A., Fieschi, C., Bozzao, L., Battistini, N., and Prencipe, M. (1968). Autoregulation of cerebral blood flow. *Circulation,* **38,** 800–12.

Archer, L. N. J., Levene, M. I., and Evans, D. H. (1986). Cerebral artery Doppler ultrasonography for prediction of outcome after perinatal asphyxia. *Lancet,* **ii,** 1116–18.

Bada, H. S., Hajjar, W., Chua, C., and Sumner, D. S. (1979). Noninvasive diagnosis of neonatal asphyxia and intraventricular haemorrhage by Doppler ultrasound. *Journal of Pediatrics,* **95,** 775–9.

Batton, D. G., Hellmann, J., Hernandez, M. J., and Maisels, M. J. (1983). Regional cerebral blood flow, cerebral blood velocity and pulsatility index in newborn dogs. *Pediatric Research,* **17,** 908–12.

Berntman, L., Dahlgren, N., and Siesjo, B. K. (1979). Cerebral blood flow and oxygen consumption in the rat brain during extreme hypercapnia. *Anaesthesiology,* **50,** 299–305.

Cowan, F. and Thoresen, M. (1985). Changes in superior sagittal sinus blood velocity due to postural alterations and pressure on the head of the newborn infant. *Pediatrics,* **75,** 1038–47.

Donders, F. C. (1851). Die Bewegungen des Gehirns und die Veranderungen der Gefäßfullung der Pia mater. *Schmid's Fahrbucher,* **69,** 16–20.

Edvinsson, L. and MacKenzie, E. T. (1976). Amine mechanisms in the cerebral circulation. *Pharmacological Reviews,* **28,** 275–348.

Evans, D. H. (1985). On the measurement of the mean velocity of blood flow over the cardiac cycle using Doppler ultrasound. *Ultrasound in Medicine and Biology,* **11,** 735–41.

Evans, D. H., Levene, M. I., Shortland, D. B., and Archer, L. N. J. (1988). Resistance index, blood flow velocity, and resistance area product in the cerebral arteries of very low birth weight infants during the first week of life. *Ultrasound in Medicine and Biology,* **14,** 103–10.

Evans, D. H., Schlindwein, F. S., and Levene, M. I. (1989*a*). The relationship between time averaged intensity weighted mean velocity and time averaged maximum velocity in neonatal cerebral arteries. *Ultrasound in Medicine and Biology,* **15**, 429–35.

Evans, D. H., McDicken, W. N., Skidmore, R., and Woodcock, J. P. (1989*b*). *Doppler ultrasound: physics, instrumentation and clinical application.* Wiley, Chichester.

Fenton, A. C., Evans, D. H., and Levene, M. I. (1990*a*). On-line cerebral blood flow velocity and blood pressure measurement in neonates: a new method. *Archives of Disease in Childhood,* **65**, 11–14.

Fenton, A. C., Papathoma, E., Evans, D. H., and Levene, M. I. (1990*b*). Neonatal cerebral venous flow velocity measurement using a colour flow Doppler system. *Journal of Clinical Ultrasound* (in press).

Fenton, A. C., Shortland, D. B., Papathoma, E., Evans, D. H., and Levene, M. I. (1990*c*). Normal range for blood flow velocity in cerebral arteries of newly born term infants. *Early Human Development* (in press).

Fog, M. (1938). The relationship between the blood pressure and the tonic regulation of the pial arteries. *Journal of Neurology and Psychiatry,* **1**, 187–97.

Gould, S. J., Howard, S., Hope, P. L., and Reynolds, E. O. R. (1987). Periventricular ischaemia/parenchymal cerebral haemorrhage in preterm infants: the role of venous infarction. *Journal of Pathology,* **151**, 197–202.

Hansen, N. B., Stonestreet, B. S., Rosenkrantz, T. S., and Oh, W. (1983). Validity of Doppler measurements of anterior cerebral artery blood flow velocity: correlation with brain blood flow in piglets. *Pediatrics,* **72**, 526–31.

Harper, A. M. (1966). Autoregulation of cerebral blood flow: influence of the arterial blood pressure on the blood flow through the cerebral cortex. *Journal of Neurology, Neurosurgery and Psychiatry,* **29**, 398–403.

Hill, A. and Volpe, J. J. (1982). Decrease in pulsatile flow in the anterior cerebral arteries in infantile hydrocephalus. *Pediatrics,* **69**, 4–7.

Kennedy, C., Grave, G. D., and Jehle, J. W. (1971). Effect of hyperoxia on the cerebral circulation of the newborn puppy. *Pediatric Research,* **5**, 659–67.

Levene, M. I., Fenton, A. C., Evans, D. H., Archer, L. N. J., Shortland, D. B., and Gibson, N. A. (1989). Severe birth asphyxia and abnormal cerebral blood flow velocity. *Developmental Medicine and Child Neurology,* **31**, 427–43.

Little, W. J. (1843). Course of lectures on the deformities of the human frame. Lecture viii. *Lancet,* **i**, 318–22.

McMenamin, J. B. and Volpe, J. J. (1983). Doppler ultrasonography in the determination of neonatal brain death. *Annals of Neurology,* **14**, 302–7.

Olesen, J. (1973). Quantitative evaluation of normal and pathologic cerebral blood flow regulation to perfusion pressure. *Archives of Neurology,* **28**, 143–50.

Olesen, J., Paulson, O. B., and Lassen, N. A. (1971). Regional CBF in man determined by the initial slope of the intrarterially injected ^{133}Xenon. *Stroke,* **2**, 519–40.

Papile, L.-A., Rudolph, A. M., and Heymann, M. A. (1985). Autoregulation of cerebral blood flow in the preterm fetal lamb. *Pediatric Research,* **19**, 159–61.

Parrot, M. J. (1873). Etude sur le ramollissement de l'encephale chez le nouveau-ne. *Archives de Physiologie Normale et Pathologique (Paris),* **5**, 283–303.

Pfannschmidt, J. and Jorch, G. (1989). Transfontanelle pulsed Doppler measurement of blood flow velocity in the internal jugular vein, straight sinus, and internal cerebral vein in preterm and term neonates. *Ultrasound in Medicine and Biology,* **15**, 9–12.

Rapela, C. E. and Green, H. D. (1964). Autoregulation of canine cerebral blood flow. *Circulation Research,* **15** (Supplement), 205–12.

Strandgaard, S., MacKenzie, E. T., Sengupta, D., Rowan, J. O., Lassen, N. A., and Harper, A. M. (1974). Upper limit of autoregulation of cerebral blood flow in the baboon. *Circulation Research,* **34,** 435–40.

Wigglesworth, J. S. and Pape, K. E. (1978). An integrated model for haemorrhagic and ischaemic lesions in the newborn brain. *Early Human Development,* **2,** 179–99.

Wolff, H. G. and Lennox, W. G. (1930). The cerebral circulation: xii. The effect on pial vessels of variations in the O_2 and CO_2 content of the blood. *Archives of Neurology and Psychiatry,* **23,** 1097–120.

Yoshida, K., Meyer, J. S., Sakamoto, K., and Handa, J. (1966). Autoregulation of cerebral blood flow. *Circulation Research,* **19,** 726–38.

17. Doppler measurements of maternal cardiac output

Stephen Robson and William Dunlop

INTRODUCTION

The maternal cardiovascular system undergoes major adaptations during normal pregnancy. Understanding of the physiological changes in the heart and peripheral circulation are important if women with pre-existing and pregnancy-induced cardiovascular disease are to be managed appropriately during pregnancy and delivery.

Cardiac output is the ultimate measure of cardiac pump performance. It is influenced by four distinct, although interrelated, mechanisms: pre-load, after-load, the inotropic or contractile state of the myocardium, and heart rate. While studies during pregnancy have consistently shown an increase in cardiac output, the pattern of change and the mechanisms underlying this increase remain unclear. These differences probably reflect variations in investigative method and study design. Early measurements of cardiac output were made using the direct Fick and dye dilution techniques. Because of the inherent risks of cardiac catheterization, most studies were cross-sectional in design and were of limited value in view of the wide variations in cardiac output between individuals. With the development of non-invasive methodology, serial measurements of cardiac output can now be performed without risk or discomfort, and women can act as their own non-pregnant controls. M-mode echocardiography and impedance cardiography were the first two non-invasive techniques applied to pregnancy. Although both have been validated and widely used in non-pregnant subjects, they have a number of limitations when applied to pregnant subjects (Robson *et al*. 1987*c*). More recently, cardiac output has been measured by cross-sectional and Doppler echocardiography. This chapter reviews the principles of volumetric flow measurement using this combined technique and describes studies of cardiac output in normal and hypertensive pregnancy.

FLOW MEASUREMENT USING CROSS-SECTIONAL AND DOPPLER ECHOCARDIOGRAPHY

Principles

Flow through a blood vessel or across a valve orifice may be calculated as:

$$Q_{(t)} = V_{(t)} \times \text{CSA}_{(t)}$$

where Q is the blood flow, V is the spatial mean velocity, CSA is the cross-sectional area, and (t) indicates that the variables are functions of time.

Measurement of blood velocity by Doppler varies with the cosine of the angle (θ) between the ultrasound beam and flow. If cosine θ is close to unity ($\theta = 0$–$20°$) and if one assumes a constant CSA of flow during the cardiac cycle, stroke volume (SV) can be calculated as:

$$\text{SV} = \text{CSA} \times \int v_{(t)} dt$$

where $\int v_{(t)} dt$ is the time velocity integral, the integral of the instantaneous velocities over the period within the cardiac cycle during which flow occurs. This velocity integral (VI) is equal to the distance that the column of blood moves during the ejection period. Cardiac output (CO) may then be calculated as:

$$\text{CO (ml/min)} = \text{SV (ml)} \times \text{heart rate (beats/min)}$$

where SV (ml) = VI (cm) × CSA (cm^2).

Flow velocities can be measured by either pulsed or continuous wave Doppler ultrasound. One theoretical advantage of using pulsed Doppler is that simultaneous imaging allows the cross-sectional area to be determined at the site of velocity sampling. In addition, the beam-flow intercept angle (θ) can be estimated. In practice, the sample volume is positioned within the annulus of the valve or in one of the great vessels, utilizing an appropriate window that places the ultrasound beam in an orientation nearly parallel with blood flow. Measurement of systolic or diastolic velocity integral can be done on-line, using a computer within the Doppler instrument, or off-line, usually by planimetry of the area under the velocity recoding using a computer-assisted digitizer.

Absolute measurement of cross-sectional area requires imaging the vessel or valve annulus in a transverse plane. While this is possible for some sites (i.e. mitral valve, aorta), it is not feasible for all. Thus, area is often derived from a diameter measurement utilizing a geometric model.

Techniques

Flow can be measured at any of the four intracardiac valves or in the great vessels. For most studies, flow was measured across the pulmonary, mitral, and aortic valves, allowing three estimates of cardiac output. The techniques employed (Robson *et al.* 1987*c*) may be summarized as:

Pulmonary valve   Pulmonary velocities (Fig. 17.2) are recorded from the parasternal short-axis view using pulsed Doppler ultrasound. Pulmonary artery area is calculated from the maximal systolic annular diameter recorded from the same view (Fig. 17.1).

Mitral valve   Mitral velocities (see Fig. 17.2) are recorded from the apical four-chamber view using pulsed Doppler ultrasound. Maximal mitral annular area is measured during diastole from parasternal short-axis echocardiographs using a tracker-ball technique (Fig. 17.1).

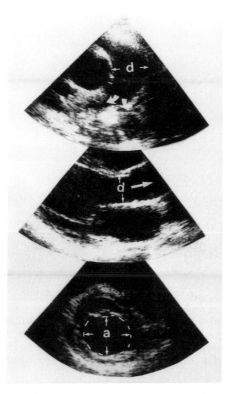

Fig. 17.1 Cross-sectional echocardiographs. Top: parasternal short-axis view at the level of the great arteries, illustrating site of measurement of pulmonary artery diameter (d). Middle: parasternal long-axis view, illustrating site of measurement of aortic diameter (d). Bottom: parasternal short-axis view at the level of the mitral valve, illustrating the site of measurement of mitral annular cross-sectional area (a).

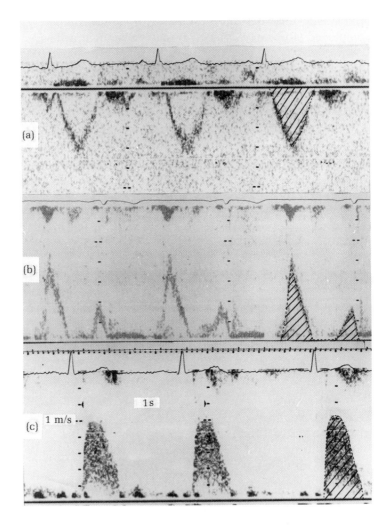

Fig. 17.2 Typical Doppler velocity traces from (a) pulmonary artery and (b) mitral valve, using pulsed Doppler, and from (c) ascending aorta using continuous wave Doppler ultrasound. Cross-hatched area indicates the velocity integral. (From the *British Journal of Obstetrics and Gynaecology*, with permission.)

Aortic valve Ascending aortic velocities (see Fig. 17.2) are recorded from the suprasternal notch using continuous wave Doppler ultrasound. Although attempts have been made to measure velocities using the pulsed mode it is difficult to obtain good quality velocities owing to the size and configuration of the pulsed Doppler transducer. Aortic area is calculated from the maximal systolic annular diameter recorded from the parasternal long-axis view (Fig. 17.1). Using these methods, good quality recordings are obtainable in more than 90 per cent of pregnant subjects.

Most workers who have used this technique in pregnancy have concentrated on aortic flow measurements. Caton and Banner (1987) and Easterling *et al.* (1987, 1990*a*) employed an identical technique to measure aortic velocities but measured aortic diameter using A-mode echocardiography. Lee *et al.* (1988) recorded left ventricular outflow velocities using pulsed Doppler ultrasound from the apical four-chamber view. Aortic diameter was measured using cross-sectional echocardiography from the parasternal short-axis plane, as described above.

Assumptions and sources of error

Velocity measurement   The velocity profile recorded is assumed to represent the velocity across the entire vessel or valve orifice (spatial average velocity). Flow acceleration and convergence of flow, as occurs in the ventricular outflow tracts and in the immediate proximity of the semi-lunar valves, flattens the velocity profile, and there is some evidence in humans to suggest that a flat velocity profile at these sites is a reasonable assumption (Schultz *et al.* 1969; Taylor and Whammond 1976; Bogren *et al.* 1988). The effect of pregnancy-induced changes in blood viscosity is complex and poorly understood. Failure to correct for such changes may theoretically lead to a small but probably haemodynamically insignificant overestimation of cardiac output (Robson *et al.* 1987*c*). Calculation of velocity ideally requires knowledge of the beam-flow intercept angle (θ). This angle cannot be measured accurately from a two-dimensional image because of the problem of estimating the angle in the third (elevational) place. Consequently most workers have attempted to align the ultrasound beam parallel with flow and then assumed cosine θ to be equal to one. Provided that the intercept angle is less than 20° to the flow axis, such an assumption will underestimate velocity by less than 6 per cent. One further assumption, when using continuous wave Doppler ultrasound, is that the maximum velocity recorded corresponds to the velocity at the level where cross-sectional area has been measured.

Cross-sectional area measurement   Areas derived from vessel diameters assume that the area through which blood flows is circular and of constant size throughout the period of flow. The assumption of circular geometry is reasonable but the cross-sectional area does change during ejection. The variation of area during systole is smaller for the proximal aorta (11 per cent) than for the pulmonary artery (23 per cent) (Greenfield and Griggs 1962, 1963). Such large changes do not occur at the level of the fibro-muscular valve orifice, and Ihlen *et al.* (1984) reported no change in aortic orifice area during systole. Studies comparing different echocardiographic methods of measuring aortic diameter have shown that Doppler flows calculated from cross-sectional echocardiographic measurements at the level of the valve annulus correlate the closest with invasive measurements (Ihlen *et al.* 1984; Gardin *et al.* 1985; Christie *et al.* 1987).

The method of determining mitral area also assumes a constant size during diastole. Ormiston *et al.* (1981) showed that there are changes in the orifice area during diastole, although this change is much less marked at the mitral inlet (at the level of the valve annulus), where the change is about 10 per cent, than at the outlet (at the free cusp margin).

Validation and reproducibility

Despite the assumptions of flow estimation by the Doppler method, studies that have compared cardiac output measured by invasive techniques with Doppler-derived flows across the pulmonary (Gillam *et al.* 1985; Kolev *et al.* 1986), mitral (Goldberg *et al.* 1985; Hoit *et al.* 1988), and aortic valves (Huntsman *et al.* 1983; Nishimura *et al.* 1984) in non-pregnant subjects have close agreement. Robson *et al.* (1987*c*) obtained comparable results when pulmonary, mitral, and aortic Doppler flows were compared with cardiac output measured by the direct Fick technique in non-pregnant subjects. Although there was no systematic difference between the two methods, there were significant individual differences in a number of paired measurements. However, in all but one comparison the difference between Cardiac output measured by the two methods was less than 25 per cent. Even larger individual differences have been reported when the Fick method has been compared with the dye dilution method, 25 per cent of paired measurements differing by more than 25 per cent, and individual differences ranging from + 58 to − 57 per cent (Taylor and Shillingford 1959; Reddy *et al.* 1976). Two groups have compared Doppler aortic flow measurements with thermodilution in pregnant women (Easterling *et al.* 1987, 1990*a* Lee *et al.* 1988); Table 17.1). Their results show that Doppler cardiac outputs correlate closely with those measured by thermodilution.

A large number of studies have investigated the reproducibility of Doppler flow measurements. Irrespective of the site of measurement, inter-observer and intra-observer variability, expressed as a mean percentage error, has generally been between 5 and 10 per cent (Lewis *et al.* 1984; Ihlen *et al* 1987; Nicolosi *et al.* 1988). With particular reference to serial studies in pregnant subjects, Robson *et al.* (1988*a*) reported the temporal variability of Doppler flow measurements. Under ideal circumstances of good echocardiographic subjects and an experienced echocardiographer, the 95 per cent confidence interval for Doppler flow measurements ranged from 0.49 l/min at the mitral valve to 0.56 l/min at the aortic valve. When multiple echocardiographers perform measurements on unselected sub-

Table 17.1 Results of validatory studies in which cardiac output measured by Doppler ultrasound at the aortic valve was compared with cardiac output measured by thermodilution in pregnant subjects

Reference	n	r	SD (1/min)	Slope	Intercept
Easterling *et al.* (1987)	12	0.91		1.11	−0.98
Lee *et al.* (1988)	16	0.94	0.64	0.74	+1.91
Easterling *et al.* (1990*b*)	11	0.95		1.05	−0.35

n, Number of subjects; r, correlation coefficient; SD, residual standard deviation.

jects, the 95 per cent confidence interval is approximately twice this value (Robson *et al.* 1988*b*).

In conclusion, good quality velocity and cross-sectional echocardiographic recordings can be obtained in more than 90 per cent of pregnant subjects. In this group, the technique allows accurate and reproducible measurements of cardiac output. Over the past few years several workers have systematically used this method to study the haemodynamic changes during normal and hypertensive pregnancy. The results of these studies are reviewed below.

HAEMODYNAMIC CHANGES DURING NORMAL PREGNANCY

Singleton pregnancy

Newman (1982) first used the Doppler technique to study mean aortic velocity during Caesarean section. Haites *et al.* (1985) and McLennan *et al.* (1987) subsequently reported increases in aortic velocity integral during pregnancy of 43 and 20 per cent, respectively. None of these workers measured vessel cross-sectional area and therefore calculation of stroke volume was not possible. Caton and Banner (1987) reported the first serial study of Doppler cardiac output during pregnancy. Ascending aortic flow was measured in 20 women and, although results were grouped in 2–3-week intervals, each subject was not studied during every interval. Cardiac output increased during pregnancy but mean values were not reported. Easterling *et al.* (1988) performed serial measurements of aortic flow in 71 nulliparous women from 16 weeks' gestation. Forty-seven of this group remained normotensive and were studied at 1–4-weekly intervals during pregnancy and at 6 weeks' post-partum. Cardiac output was increased at 16 weeks' gestation (6.0 l/min) but this was not compared statistically with post-natal control values (4.9 l/min). Maximum values of cardiac output were recorded at 34 weeks' gestation (7.4 l/min), representing an increase of 51 per cent over post-natal values. Thereafter, there was a statistically significant decrease in cardiac output, such that by 40 weeks' gestation mean cardiac output was 6.4 l/min.

The main drawback of these and most previous serial studies of cardiac output during pregnancy was that non-pregnant measurements were performed after delivery and little information existed concerning changes in cardiac output during the first trimester. To overcome this, Robson *et al.* (1989*b*) performed serial measurements of cardiac output at three intracardiac sites in 13 women recruited before conception. Studies were performed in the luteal phase of two consecutive menstrual cycles and then immediately after pregnancy was confirmed (mean 35 days). Subsequent studies were performed at monthly intervals from 8 weeks till 36 weeks, with a final investigation at 38 weeks' gestation. All subjects were again studied at 6 months after delivery. To avoid caval compression by the gravid uterus, all measurements were performed in the left semi-lateral position. Flows from the three sites correlated closely ($r = 0.91$–0.93). The mean Doppler cardiac output and stroke volume (calculated as the average of the three measurement sites) together with mean heart rate are shown in Figure 17.3.

The most noticeable and previously unreported finding was the very early increase in cardiac output, this being statistically significant by 5 weeks' gestation. Heart rate was increased at 5 weeks' gestation, confirming the findings of Clapp (1985), while the increase in stroke volume was not significant until 8 weeks. This early increase in cardiac output was subsequently confirmed by Capeless and Clapp (1989) who demonstrated an increase in stroke volume and cardiac output, measured by M-mode echocardiography, at 8 weeks' gestation, the time of their first post-conception measurement.

Maximal values of cardiac output were attained by the end of the second trimester, when cardiac output was 46 per cent above pre-pregnancy values (Robson *et al.* 1989*b*). The results of 10 previous studies in which cardiac output was measured serially in the left lateral position are shown in Table 17.2 (Pyorala 1966; Ueland *et al.* 1969; Katz *et al.* 1978; Atkins *et al.* 1981; Myhrman *et al.* 1982; Castillon *et al.* 1984; Hirata *et al.* 1984; Kagiya *et al.* 1984; Matsunga 1984; Mashini *et al.* 1987). The timing and size of this maximum increase varied considerably, although average increases were similar to those found in recent work (Robson *et al.* 1989*b*). Recently, Clark *et al.* (1989) reported thermodilution measurements in 10 women at 36–38 weeks of pregnancy and at 11–13 weeks post-partum. Cardiac output decreased from 6.2 l/min during pregnancy to 4.3 l/min after delivery. Although these figures are slightly lower than those reported from Doppler studies, the percentage increase in cardiac output (43 per cent) is comparable.

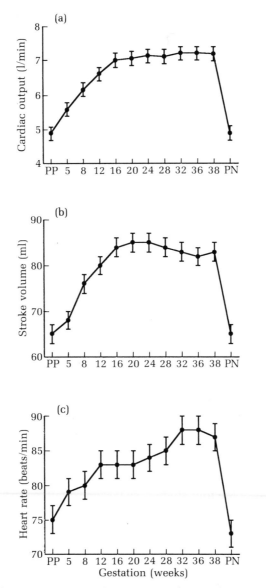

Fig. 17.3 Serial measurements of mean Doppler cardiac output (a), stroke volume (b), and heart rate (c) during 13 singleton pregnancies. Figures represent mean and within-subject 95 per cent confidence intervals. (From Robson *et al.* 1989*b*.)

Table 17.2 Maximum increase in cardiac output, stroke volume, and heart rate during pregnancy: comparison of cross-sectional and Doppler echocardiographic results obtained by Robson et al. (1981b) with those from 10 previous serial studies in which measurements were performed in the left lateral position

	Previous studies		Robson et al. (1989b)	
	Absolute	Percentage	Absolute	Percentage
Cardiac output (l/min)	1.9	40	2.3	46
	(0.7–3.2)	(13–65)		
Stroke volume (ml)	13	19 17	27	
	(−3–30)	(−3–38)		
Heart rate (beats/min)	12	19	12	17
	(3–19)	(4–33)		

Values are mean (range) and percentage differences from non-pregnant values.

Unlike Easterling *et al.* (1988), Robson *et al.* (1989*b*) did not find a decrease in cardiac output during the third trimester. This may be because Robson's last serial measurements were performed at 38 weeks' gestation, but results from other studies between 37–41 weeks' gestation have consistently shown mean values of cardiac output above 7 l/min (Robson *et al.* 1987*b, d*, 1989*a*, 1989*d*), suggesting that there is no fall in cardiac output during the last weeks of pregnancy. Previous studies have also shown conflicting results, with some workers reporting a fall in cardiac output during the third trimester, secondary to a reduction in stroke volume (Ueland *et al.* 1969; Atkins *et al.* 1981; Myhrman *et al.* 1982; Kagiya *et al.* 1984), while others have found no change (Pyorala 1966; Matsunga 1984; Mashini *et al.* 1987). Cardiac output was measured by impedance cardiography in three of the four studies, suggesting a fall in cardiac output. This method correlates poorly with invasively determined cardiac output during the third trimester (Secher *et al.* 1979; Easterling *et al.* 1989).

In addition to the functional changes, a number of structural adaptations appear to occur in the heart during pregnancy. As well as an increase in ventricular wall thickness, valve cross-sectional areas increase progressively throughout gestation. In serial study aortic, pulmonary, and mitral annular areas increased by 12–14 per cent (Robson *et al.* 1989*b*). A comparable increase in tricuspid area was reported by Limacher *et al.* (1985). This is an important finding in view of the recent interest in Doppler aortic minute distance (velocity integral × heart rate), which has been reported to reflect changes in cardiac output in the non-pregnant state (Haites *et al.* 1985). Use of this parameter in pregnancy (McLennan *et al.* 1987) is likely to underestimate changes in cardiac output, because no account is made of the changes in valve area.

Twin pregnancy

Much less information is available regarding the changes in cardiac output during twin pregnancy. Robson *et al.* (1989c) recently reported the first serial study of haemodynamics during twin pregnancy. Cardiac output was measured, using the Doppler methods described, at monthly intervals from 20 to 36 weeks' gestation and then at 6 months after delivery. The results of mean Doppler cardiac output in 10 women with twin pregnancies, compared with the 13 with singleton pregnancies, are shown in Figure 17.4.

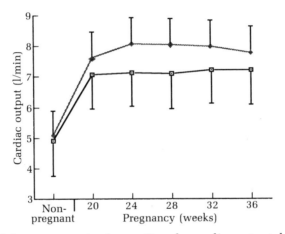

Fig. 17.4 Serial measurements of mean Doppler cardiac output during 10 twin (◆) and 13 singleton (□) pregnancies. Figures represent mean and 95 per cent confidence intervals. (From Robson *et al.* 1989c.)

Maximum values of cardiac output, stroke volume, and heart rate were 58, 24 and 31 per cent above post-natal values, respectively. Comparison of the twin and singleton groups showed a significantly higher cardiac output and heart rate during twin pregnancy.

Factors responsible for the increase in cardiac output during pregnancy

The increase in cardiac output during pregnancy appears to be the result of changes in all four of normal regulatory mechanisms.

Preload

Venous return is likely to be increased during pregnancy in view of the marked increase (40 per cent) in blood volume (Hytten 1985). Indirect evidence for this comes from M-mode echocardiographic studies in which left atrial and left ventricular end-diastolic dimensions have been shown to increase during pregnancy (Katz *et al.* 1978; Hirata *et al.* 1984; Robson *et al.* 1989*b*). This increase is evident from the beginning of the second trimester, corresponding to the time when plasma volume increases (Hytten and Paintin 1963).

Afterload   Serial studies of blood pressure during pregnancy have consistently shown a fall in blood pressure during the first half of pregnancy and then a progressive increase to term (Schwarz 1964; MacGillivray *et al.* 1969; Robson *et al.* 1989*b*). Total peripheral resistance must therefore fall dramatically during pregnancy. In serial studies (Robson *et al.* 1989*b*), peripheral resistance, calculated from mean Doppler cardiac output and mean arterial pressure, had decreased by 34 per cent at 20 weeks' gestation. Thereafter, there was small increase towards term but values remained lower than in non-pregnant controls. In addition to the fall in peripheral resistance, aortic compliance is increased during pregnancy (Hart *et al.* 1986). These factors, together with the reduction in blood viscosity, suggest that cardiac after-load is likely to be reduced during pregnancy, especially during the first 20 weeks.

Myocardial contractility   *In vivo* assessment of contractility is extremely difficult. A number of non-invasive studies using M-mode echocardiography and systolic time intervals have suggested an increased inotropic state during the first and second trimesters of pregnancy (Laird-Meeter *et al.* 1979; Cellina *et al.* 1983; Castillon *et al.* 1984; Kagiya *et al.* 1984; Robson *et al.* 1989*b*). However, interpretation of M-mode indices of left ventricular function during pregnancy is difficult because measurements are affected by changes in heart rate, pre-load, and particularly after-load. Clerk *et al.* (1989) are the only group to have studied intrinsic left ventricular contractility, as assessed by left ventricular work index, in normal pregnant subjects. They found a statistically insignificant increase at 36–38 weeks' gestation when compared with post-natal control values. Thus, any increase in myocardial contractility during pregnancy appears to be confined to the first two trimesters.

Heart rate   Heart rate has been consistently shown to increase during pregnancy. This appears to be the earliest haemodynamic change and the increase continues until the third trimester.

HAEMODYNAMIC CHANGES DURING LABOUR AND THE PUERPERIUM

Labour

Most previous studies of cardiac output during labour have been performed on supine subjects in whom caval compression may have reduced cardiac output. Robson *et al*. (1987*b*) studied 15 non-epiduralized women in the left semi-lateral position during the first stage of labour. Cardiac output was measured at the pulmonary valve before and at the peak of uterine contractions. The results are shown in Figure 17.5.

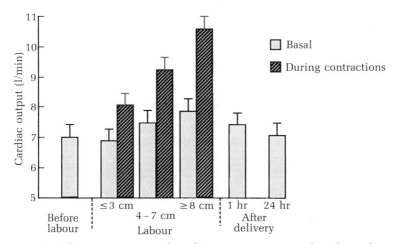

Fig. 17.5 Serial measurements of cardiac output, measured at the pulmonary valve, in 15 non-epiduralized women before labour, during the first stage of labour (at ≤3, 4–7, and ≥8 cm cervical dilatation), and at 1 and 24 h after delivery. Figures represent mean and within-subject 95 per cent confidence intervals. (From Robson *et al*. 1987*b*.)

Basal cardiac output (between uterine contractions) increased by 12 per cent due to an increase in stroke volume. Relative to basal values, cardiac output increased during uterine contractions. The increment became progressively greater as labour advanced such that at 8 cm or more of cervical dilatation, cardiac output had increased by 34 per cent. At 3 cm or less of dilatation, the increase in cardiac output during contractions was due to an increase in stroke volume, whereas later both stroke volume and heart rate increased. In a more recent Doppler study, Lee *et al*. (1989) measured aortic flow before and during uterine contractions at a mean cervical dilatation of 5.4 cm. They reported a 16 per cent increase in stroke volume and an 11 per cent increase in cardiac output during contractions. Heart rate remained unchanged, possibly due to the pain relief afforded by epidural analgesia in their subjects. These results are consistent with previous dye dilution studies in which cardiac output has been measured in the supine position (Adams and Alexander 1958; Ueland and Hansen 1969; Kjeldsen 1979).

In contrast to the first stage of labour, little is known about the haemodynamic changes during the second stage. Ueland and Hansen (1969) suggested that cardiac output, measured by dye dilution, increased from 7.7 l/min between contractions to 8.5 l/min during contractions. This change is considerably smaller than might be expected from the results of Doppler studies. One likely explanation for this is that determination of cardiac output by dye dilution assumes stable flow during the period of recording. Such an assumption may not be valid during uterine contractions, especially immediately before deliver. To date, no data exist regarding the haemodynamic changes associated with active pushing.

Puerperium

Aortic Doppler studies during Caesarean section have shown that there is an increase in stroke volume of approximately 15 per cent immediately after delivery of the placenta (Robson *et al.* 1989*d*). This presumably reflects an increase in venous return as blood is returned to the central circulation from the choriodecidual space when the uterus contracts down after delivery. This conclusion is supported by the marked increase in M-mode left atrial end-diastolic dimension shortly after delivery (Robson *et al.* 1987*a*).

Based on isolated puerperal measurements, previous studies had suggested that cardiac output returns to non-pregnant values by about 6 weeks after delivery (Ueland *et al.* 1969; Katz *et al.* 1978; Atkins *et al.* 1981). In order to determine the timing of this fall, Robson *et al.* (1987*d*) serially measured cardiac output in 15 women between 2 weeks and 6 months after delivery. The results suggested that cardiac output and heart rate had returned to non-pregnant values by 2 weeks. Stroke volume had also decreased by 2 weeks, although there was a further small reduction between 2 weeks and 6 months after delivery. The results of a more detailed study of 30 women during the first 2 weeks of the puerperium (Robson *et al.* 1989*a*) are shown in Figure 17.6. Stroke volume remained at pregnancy levels during the first 2 days after normal delivery and then fell to values 10 per cent lower than those recorded at the end of pregnancy by 14 days. Heart rate and cardiac output remained elevated during the first 24 h after delivery. Thereafter, both fell until the 10th day when values were 16 and 25 per cent, respectively, below those obtained at the end of pregnancy. A

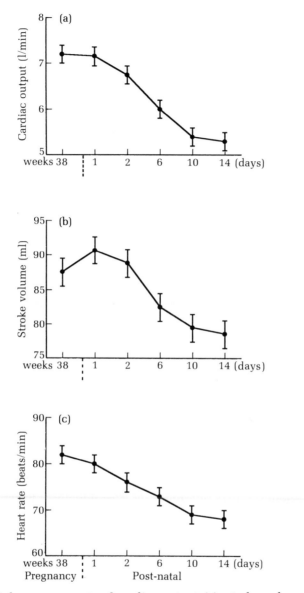

Fig. 17.6 Serial measurements of cardiac output (a), stroke volume (b), and heart rate (c), measured at the aortic valve in 30 women after a normal vaginal delivery. Figures represent mean and within-subject 95 per cent confidence intervals. (From Robson *et al.* 1989a.)

similar reduction in cardiac output has been reported in women 2 weeks after caesarean section (Robson *et al.* 1989*d*). Interestingly, ventricular wall thickness and valve cross-sectional areas take considerably longer to return to non-pregnant values (Robson *et al.* 1987*d*).

HAEMODYNAMIC CHANGES DURING HYPERTENSIVE PREGNANCY

In contrast to the changes during normal pregnancy, the central haemo-dynamic alterations in pregnancy-induced hypertension are poorly under-stood. Cardiac output has been reported to be normal, increased, and decreased. These differences are probably related to: (1) small numbers of subjects in each series; (2) variable methodology used to measure cardiac output; (3) differences in disease severity and duration; and (4) therapeutic interventions before haemodynamic measurements (Mabie *et al.* 1989). Reliable thermodilution measurements have been peformed in some un-treated hypertensive women but, because of the need for cardiac catheter-ization, these have been limited to women with severe disease (Wallenburg 1988; Mabie *et al.* 1989).

Easterling *et al.* (1987) first reported cardiac output measurements in 36 pre-eclamptic women using Doppler and A-mode echocardiography. Twelve of the subjects had received magnesium sulphate, although none had been given antihypertensive treatment. The mean cardiac output was 7.4 (range 3.9–13.2) l/min, which was not significantly different from the mean cardiac output in 18 normal women. In an attempt to explain the haemodynamic heterogeneity of their results, the authors hypothesized that early pre-eclampsia might be characterized by a high output, low resistance state, and that as the disease became more severe a low cardiac output, high resistance state might supervene. To test the hypothesis that pregnancy-induced hypertension is, at least initially, a hyperdynamic high cardiac output state, the same group serially studied 71 nulliparous women from 16 weeks of pregnancy (Easterling *et al.* 1988). Twenty (28 per cent) developed hypertension and four (6 per cent) developed proteinuric pre-eclampsia. Interestingly, cardiac output was consistently higher in the hypertensive compared with the normotensive group. This increase was evident at 16 weeks' gestation and persisted at 6 weeks after delivery. The data for the four women who developed proteinuria were not presented separately and therefore it was not possible to determine whether the development of proteinuria coincided with a decline in cardiac output. More recently, Easterling *et al.* (1990*b*) reported serial haemodynamic measurements in 76 women who developed hypertension at weeks' or less gestation. They divided women into three groups depending on the calculated total peripheral vascular resistance; low resistance group (n = 36, mean cardiac output 9.6 l/min), high resistance group (n = 32, mean cardiac output 6.4 l/min), and a cross-over group (n = 8) in whom resistance changed from low to high. The incidence of proteinuria in each group was not reported. Mean arterial pressure was higher, birth-weight was lower, and fetal death was more common in the high resistance group. These findings suggest that the development of a high resistance state may signify a form of cardiovascular decompensation associated with a worsening of hypertension and an increased risk of fetal complication.

Robson *et al.* (1990) have measured cardiac output using Doppler and cross-sectional echocardiography at the aortic valve in 44 primigravid women with proteinuric pregnancy-induced hypertension. Results were compared with a group of normotensive women matched for age and gestation. Cardiac output was significantly lower in the hypertensive group (6.06 versus 6.83 l/min), although there was considerable overlap between the two groups. Within the proteinuric group, subjects with more severe hypertension (diastolic blood pressure > 100 mmHg) had a significantly lower mean cardiac output than those with mild hypertension (5.50 versus 6.60 l/min). These results confirm those of Wallenburg (1988) who showed low cardiac indices in 44 untreated women with severe proteinuric hypertension (median diastolic pressure 110 mmHg).

Thus, many women with severe proteinuric hypertension have a low cardiac output and a high systemic vascular resistance, but this haemodynamic profile is by no means universal (Mabie *et al.* 1989). Further Doppler studies are needed to confirm whether hypertension is preceded by a high output phase and to determine the relationship between disease progression and the development of a low output/high resistance state.

REFERENCES

Adams, J. Q. and Alexander, A. M. (1958). Alterations in cardiovascular physiology during labour. *Obstetrics and Gynecology*, **12**, 542–9.

Atkins, A. J. F., Watt, J. M., Milan, P., Davies, P., and Selwyn Crawford, J. (1981). A longitudinal study of cardiovascular dynamic. *European Journal of Obstetrics, Gynecology, and Reproductive Biology*, **12**, 215–24.

Bogren, H., Klipstein, R. H., Mohiadden, R., *et al.* (1988). *British Heart Journal*, **59**, 141–2.

Capeless, E. L. and Clapp, J. F. (1989). Cardiovascular changes in early phase of pregnancy. *American Journal of Obstetrics and Gynecology*, **161**, 1449–53.

Castillon, G., Weissenburger, J., Rouffett, M., Castillon, V., and Barrat, J. (1984). Etude echocardiographique des modifications hemodynamiques de la grossesse *Journal of Obstetrics, Gynecology, and the Biology of Reproduction*, **13**, 499–505.

Caton, D. and Banner T. E. (1978). Doppler estimates of cardiac output during pregnancy. *Bulletin of the New York Academy of Medicine*, **63**, 727–31.

Cellina, G., Binaghi, P., Limonta, A., Locicero, G., Montanari, C., and Brina, A. (1983). Modificazione dei tempi sistolica durante la gravidanza e il puerperio. *G Italiano Cardiologica*, **11**, 63–7.

Christie, J., Sheldahl, L. M., Tristani, F. E., Saga, K. B., Ptacin, M. J., and Wann, S. (1987). Determination of stroke volume and cardiac output during exercise: comparison of two-dimensional and Doppler echocardiography, Fick oximetry and thermodilution. *Circulation*, **76**, 539–47.

Clapp, J. F. (1985). Maternal heart rate in pregnancy. *American Journal of Obstetrics and Gynecology*, **152**, 859–60.

Clark, S. L., Cotton, D. B., and Lee, W. (1989). Central hemodynamic assessment of normal term pregnancy. *American Journal of Obstetrics and Gynecology*, **161**, 1439–42.

Easterling, T. R., Watts, D. H., Schmucker, B. C., and Benedetti, T. J. (1987). Measurement of cardiac output during pregnancy; validation of Doppler technique and clinical observations during pre-eclampsia. *Obstetrics and Gynecology*, **69**, 845–50.

Easterling, T. R., Benedetti, T. J., and Shmucker, B. C. (1988). Maternal cardiac output in pregnancy induced hypertension: a longitudinal study. *Sixth international congress of the Internation Society for the Study of Hypertension in pregnancy*, Montreal, Canada. Abstract 276.

Easterling, T. R., Benedetti, T. J., Carlson, K. L., and Watts, D. H. (1989). Measurement of cardiac output in pregnancy by thermodilution and impedance techniques. *British Journal of Obstetrics and Gynecology*, **96**, 67–9.

Easterling, T. R., Carlson, K. L., Shmucker, B. C., Brateng, D. A., and Benedetti, T. J. (1990*a*). Measurement of cardiac output in pregnancy by Doppler technique. *American Journal of Perinatology*. **7**, 220–2.

Easterling, T. R., Benedetti, T. J., Shmucker, B. C., Carlson, K. L., Brateng, D. A., and Wilson, J. (1990*b*). Maternal hemodynamics and fetal outcome in pregnancies complicated by hypertension. *Seventh international congress of the International Society for the Study of Hypertension in Pregnancy*. Perugia, Italy. Abstract 317.

Gardin, J. M., Tobis, J. M., Dabestani, A., *et al.* (1985). Superiority of two dimensional measurement of aortic vessel diameter in Doppler estimates of left ventricular stroke volume. *Journal of American College of Cardiology*, **6**, 66–74.

Gillam, L. D., Kritzner, G. L., Ascah, K. J., Wilkins, G. T., and Marshall, G. T. (1985). Which cardiac valve provides the best Doppler estimate of cardiac output in humans? *Circulation*, **72**, 99 (Abstract).

Goldberg, S. J., Dickinson, D. F., and Wilson, N. (1985). Evaluation of an elliptical area technique for calculating mitral blood flow by Doppler echocardiography. *British Heart Journal*, **54**, 68–75.

Greenfield, J. C. and Griggs, D. M. (1963). Relationship between pressure and diameter in the pulmonary artery of man. *Journal of Applied Physiology*, **18**, 557–9.

Greenfield, J. C. and Patel, D. J. (1962). Relationship between pressure and diameter in the descending aorta of man. *Circulation Research*, **10**, 778–81.

Haites, N. E., McLennon, F., Mowat, D. H. R., and Rawles, J. M. (1985). Assessment of cardiac output by Doppler ultrasound technique alone. *British Heart Journal*, **53**, 123–9.

Heart, M. V., Morton, M. J., Hosenpud, J. D., and Metcalfe, J. (1986). Aortic function during normal pregnancy. *American Journal of Obstetrics and Gynecology*, **154**, 887–91.

Hirata. F., Nishida, N., and Kanamura, S. (1984). Non-invasive estimates of hemodynamics in normal pregnancy. *Journal of Cardiography*, **14**, 775–84.

Hoit, B. D., Rashwan, M., Watt, C., Sahn, D. J., and Bhargava, V. (1988). Calculating cardiac output from transmitral volume flow using Doppler and M-mode echocardiography. *American Journal of Cardiology*, **62**, 131–5.

Huntsman, L. L., Stewart, D. K., Barnes, S. R., Franklin, S. B., Colocousis, M. D., and Hessel, E. A. (1983). Non-invasive Doppler determination of cardiac output in man: clinical validation. *Circulation*, **67**, 593–602.

Hytten, F. E. (1985). Blood volume changes in normal pregnancy. *Clinics in Haematology*, **14**, 601–12.

Hytten, F. E. and Paintin, D. B. (1963). Increase in plasma volume during normal pregnancy. *Journal of Obstetrics and Gynaecology of the British Commonwealth*, **70**, 402–7.

Ihlen, H., Amlie, J. P., Forfang, K., *et al.* (1987). Determination of cardiac output by Doppler echocardiography. *British Heart Journal*, **51**, 54–60.

Kagiya, A., Shiratori, H., Shinagawa, S., and Seki, K. (1984). Systolic time intervals and impedance cardiogram in pregnant and toxaemic women. *Nippon Sanka Fujinka Gakkai Zasshi*, **36**, 1087–94.

Katz, R., Karliner, J. S., and Resnik, R. (1978). Effects of natural volume overload state (pregnancy) on left ventricular performance in normal human subjects. *Circulation*, **58**, 434–41.

Kjeldsen, J. (1979). Haemodynamic investigations during labour and delivery. *Acta Obstetricia et Gynecologica Scandinavica*, **89**, (Supplement) 77–195.

Kolev, N., Lazarova, M., and Lengyel, M. (1986). Doppler two-dimensional echocardiographic determinations of right ventricular output and diastlic filling. *Journal of Cardiography*, **16**, 659–67.

Laird-Meeter, K., van de Ley, G., Bom, T. H., and Wladimiroff, J. W. (1979). Cardiocirculatory adjustments during pregnancy—an echocardiographic study. *Clinical Cardiology*, **2**, 328–32

Lee, W., Rokey, R., and Cotton, D. B. (1988). Noninvasive maternal stroke volume and cardiac output determinations by pulsed Doppler echocardiography. *American Journal of Obstetrics and Gynecology*, **158**, 505–10.

Lee, W., Rokey, R., Miller, J., and Cotton, D. B. (1989). Maternal hemodynamic effects of uterine contractions by M-mode and pulsed Doppler echocardiography. *American Journal of Obstetrics and Gynecology*, **161**, 974–7.

Lewis, J., Lawrence, C. K., Nelson, J. G., Limacher, M. C., and Quinones, M. A. (1984). Pulsed Doppler echocardiographic determination of stroke volume and cardiac output: clinical validation of two new methods using an apical window. *Circulation*, **79**, 425–31.

Limacher, M. C., Ware, A., O'Meara, M. E., Fernandez, G. C., and Young, J. B. (1985). Two-dimensional and pulsed Doppler echocardiographic observations. *American Journal of Cardiology*, **55**, 1059–62.

Mabie, W. C., Ratts, T. E., and Sibi, B. M. (1989). The central hemodynamics in severe pre-eclampsia. *American Journal of Obstetrics and Gynecology*, **161**, 1443–8.

MacGillivray, I., Rose, G. A., and Rowe, B. (1969). Blood pressure survey in pregnancy. *Clinical Science*. **37**, 395–407.

McLennan, F. M., Haites, N. E., and Rawles, J. M. (1987). Stroke and minute distance in pregnancy: a longitudinal study using Doppler ultrasound. *British Journal of Obstetrics and Gynaecology*, **94**, 499–506.

Mashini, I. S., Albazzaz, S. J., Fadel, H. E., *et al.* (1987). Serial non-invasive elevation of cardiovascular hemodynamics during pregnancy. *American Journal of Obstetrics and Gynecology*, **156**, 1208–13.

Matsunga, T. (1984). Studies on maternal hemodynamics during normal pregnancy: correlation between maternal hemodynamics and fetal growth. *Nippon Sanka Fujinka Gakkai Zasshi*, **36**, 795–804.

Myhrman, P., Granerus, G., Karlsson, K., and Lundgren, Y. (1982). Cardiac output in normal pregnancy measured by impedance cardiography. *Scandinavian Journal of Clinical and Laboratory Investigation*, **42**, 513–20.

Newman, B. (1982). Cardiac output changes during Caesarean section. Measurements by transcutaneous aortovelography. *Anaesthesia*, **37**, 270–3.

Nicolosi, G. L., Pungercic, E., Cervesato, E., *et al.* (1988). Feasibility and variability of six methods for the echocardiographic and Doppler determination of cardiac output. *British Heart Journal*, **59**, 299–303.

Nishimura, R. A., Callahan, M. J., Schaff, H. V., Ilstrup, D. M., Miller, F. A., and Tajik, A. J. (1984). Non-invasive measurements of cardiac output by continuous wave Doppler echocardiography: initial experience and review of the literature. *Mayo Clinic Proceedings*, **59**, 484–9.

Ormiston, J. A., Shah, P. M., Tei, C., and Wong, M. (1981). Size and motion of the mitral valve annulus in man. 1. A two dimensional echocardiographic method and findings in normal subjects. *Circulation*, **64**, 113–20

Pyorala, T. (1966). Cardiovascular response to the upright position in pregnancy. *Acta Obstetricia et Gynecologica Scandinavica*, **45**, (Supplement 5), 44–74.

Reddy, P. S., Curtiss, E. I., Bell, B., *et al.* (1976). Determinations of variations between the Fick and indicator dilution estimates of cardiac output during diagnostic catheterization. *Journal of Clinical and Laboratory Medicine*, **87**, 568–76.

Robson, S. C., Hunter, S., and Dunlop, W. (1987*a*). Left atrial dimension during early puerperium. *Lancet*, **ii**, 111–12.

Robson, S. C., Dunlop, W., Boys, R. J., and Hunter, S. (1987*b*). Cardiac output during labour. *British Medical Journal*, **295**, 1162–72.

Robson, S. C., Dunlop, W., Moore, M., and Hunter, S. (1987*c*). Combined Doppler and echocardiographic measurement of cardiac output: theory and application in pregnancy. *British Journal of Obstetrics and Gynaecology*, **94**, 1014–27.

Robson, S. C., Hunter, S., Moore, M., and Dunlop, W. (1987*d*). Haemodynamic changes in the puerperium: a Doppler and M-mode echocardiographic study. *British Journal of Obstetrics and Gynaecology*, **94**, 1028–39.

Robson, S. C., Boys, R. J., and Hunter, S. (1988*a*). Doppler echocardiographic estimation of cardiac output: analysis of temporal variability. *European Heart Journal*, **9**, 313–18.

Robson, S. C., Murray, A., Peart, I., Heads, A., and Hunter, S. (1988*b*). Reproducibility of cardiac output measurements by cross sectional and Doppler echocardiography. *British Heart Journal*, **59**, 680–4.

Robson, S. C., Boys, R. J., Hunter, S., and Dunlop, W. (1989*a*). Maternal hemodynamics after normal delivery and delivery complicated by postpartum haemorrhage. *Obstetrics and Gynecology*, **74**, 234–9.

Robson, S. C., Hunter, S., Boys, R. J., and Dunlop, W. (1989*b*). Serial study of factors influencing changes in cardiac output during human pregnancy. *American Journal of Physiology*, **256**, H1060–5.

Robson, S. C., Hunter, S., Boys, R. J., and Dunlop, W. (1989c). Hemodynamic changes in twin pregnancy: a Doppler and M-mode echocardiographic study. *American Journal of Obstetrics and Gynecology*, **161**, 1273–8.

Robson, S. C., Dunlop, W., Hunter, S., Boys, R. J., and Bryson, M. (1989d). Haemodynamic changes associated with Caesarean section under epidural anaesthesia. *British Journal of Obstetrics and Gynaecology*, **96**, 642–7.

Robson, S. C., McPhail, S, Rodeck, C., and Dunlop, W. (1990). Haemodynamics in pregnancy-induced hypertension: a Doppler and cross-sectional echocardiographic study. *Seventh international congress of the International Society for the Study of Hypertension in Pregnancy*, Perugia, Italy. Abstract 156.

Schultz, D. L., Tunstal-Pedoe, D. S., Lee, D. de J., Gunning, A. J., and Bellhouse, B. J. (1969). Circulation and respiratory mass transport. *Ciba Foundation Symposium*, pp. 172–99.

Schwarz, R. (1964). Das Verhalten des Kreislaufs in der normalen Schwangerschaft. *Archives fur Gynakologie*, **199**, 549–70.

Secher, N. J., Arnsbo, P., Heslet Anderson, L., and Thompson, A. (1979). Measurement of cardiac stroke volumes in various body positions in pregnancy and during Caesarean section: a comparison between thermodilution and impedance cardiography. *Scandinavian Journal of Laboratory Investigation*, **39**, 569–76.

Taylor, S. H. and Shillingford, J. P. (1959). Clinical applications of coomassie blue. *British Heart Journal*, **21**, 497–505.

Taylor, D. E. M. and Whammond, J. S. (1976). Velocity profile and impedance of the healthy mitral valve. In *The mitral valve: a pluridisciplinary approach* (ed, D. Kalmanson), pp. 127–36. Edward Arnold, London.

Ueland, K. and Hansen, J. M. (1969b). Maternal cardiovascular dynamics. III. Labor and delivery under local and caudal analgesia. *American Journal of Obstetrics and Gynecology*, **103**, 8–18.

Ueland, K., Novy, M. J., Peterson, E. N., and Metcalfe, J. (1969). Maternal cardiovascular dynamics. IV. The influence of gestational age on the maternal cardiovascular response to posture and exercise. *American Journal of Obstetrics and Gynecology*, **104**, 856–64.

Wallenburg, H. C. S. (1988). Hemodynamics in hypertensive pregnancy. In *Hypertension in pregnancy* (ed. P. C. Rubin), pp. 66–101. Elsevier Holland.

Subject index